和英対訳

医療機器の製造販売承認申請等に必要な生物学的安全性評価の基本的考え方について
第2版

Bilingual in Japanese and English

Basic Principles of Biological Safety Evaluation Required for Application for Approval to Market Medical Devices
2nd Edition

ISO/TC 194 国内委員会 訳
Translated by The Japanese domestic committee of ISO/TC 194

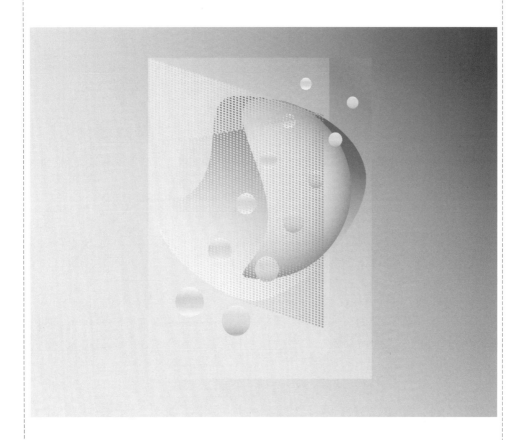

薬事日報社　YAKUJI NIPPO,LTD.

目次／CONTENTS

序

　医療機器の製造販売承認申請に際して添付すべき資料の一つである「生物学的安全性評価の基本的考え方」及び「医療機器の生物学的安全性試験法ガイダンス」がそれぞれ改正され，令和2年1月6日付け薬生機審発0106第1号：厚生労働省医薬・生活衛生局医療機器審査管理課長通知「医療機器の製造販売承認申請等に必要な生物学的安全性評価の基本的考え方についての改正について」の別紙及び別添として発出されました．

　当該通知の英訳は，海外規制当局及び海外医療機器メーカと国内審査部門との相互理解を深め，審査の迅速化を図る上で有益なツールとなりますので，本冊子の発行に至りました．

　英文翻訳は，ISO/TC 194国内委員会に設立した国内ガイダンス改定準備特別作業班に参画した専門家の皆様にご担当頂きました．ここに感謝の意を表します．

　令和3年4月吉日

編集責任者　酒島由二
（ISO/TC 194国内委員会委員長）

Preface

MHLW Notification by Director, Pharmaceutical Safety and Environmental Health Bureau, Medical Device Evaluation Division, Yakuseikishin-hatsu 0106 No. 1 "Basic Principles of Biological Safety Evaluation Required for Application for Approval to Market Medical Devices" was issued on January 6, 2020. The notification consists of an annex "Basic Principles for Biological Safety Evaluation of Medical Devices" and an attachment "Guidance on test methods for biological safety evaluation of medical devices".

We thought that the English translation of the notification would be useful to deepen mutual understanding with overseas regulatory bodies and medical devices manufacturers, resulting in a rapid approval review of medical devices. That led us to the publication of this booklet.

The English translation was done by experts of "working group on the revision of domestic guidance" established in the Japanese domestic committee of ISO/TC 194. I would like to express thanks to them.

Editor-in-chief Yuji Haishima, April, 2021
(Chairman, the Japanese domestic committee of ISO/TC 194)

翻訳担当者

蓜島由二　　　　　国立医薬品食品衛生研究所　医療機器部　部長

坂口圭介　　　　　テルモ株式会社　研究開発センター　研究開発推進部　評価センター　センター長

山影康次　　　　　一般財団法人食品薬品安全センター　秦野研究所　研究顧問

金澤由基子　　　　独立行政法人　医薬品医療機器総合機構　医療機器ユニット　医療機器調査・基準部　医療機器基準課　テクニカルエキスパート

松岡厚子　　　　　国立医薬品食品衛生研究所　医療機器部　客員研究員

橋本裕介　　　　　アボットメディカルジャパン合同会社　薬事部　マネージャー

中村鉄平　　　　　一般財団法人　日本食品分析センター　千歳研究所　安全性試験部　生物科学課　課長補佐

加藤玲子　　　　　国立医薬品食品衛生研究所　医療機器部　第二室　主任研究官

谷川隆洋　　　　　テルモ株式会社　研究開発センター　研究開発推進部　評価センター　研究員

中岡竜介　　　　　国立医薬品食品衛生研究所　医療機器部　埋植医療機器評価室　室長

Translators

Dr. Yuji Haishima	Director, Division of Medical Devices, National Institute of Health Sciences
Mr. Keisuke Sakaguchi	General Manager, Evaluation Center, TERUMO Corporation
Dr. Kohji Yamakage	Advisor for Research, Hatano Research Institute, Food and Drug Safety Center
Ms. Yukiko Kanazawa	Technical Expert, Office of Standards and Compliance for Medical Devices, Pharmaceuticals and Medical Devices Agency
Dr. Atsuko Matsuoka	Visiting Researcher, Division of Medical Devices, National Institute of Health Sciences
Dr. Yusuke Hashimoto	Manager, Regulatory Affairs, Abbott Medical Japan LLC
Dr. Teppei Nakamura	Deputy Section Head, Section of Biological Science, Chitose Laboratory, Japan Food Research Laboratories
Dr. Reiko Kato	Senior Researcher, Division of Medical Devices, National Institute of Health Sciences
Mr. Takahiro Tanigawa	Research Leader, Evaluation Center, TERUMO Corporation
Dr. Ryusuke Nakaoka	Section Chief, Division of Medical Devices, National Institute of Health Sciences

厚生労働省　医薬・生活衛生局　医療機器審査管理課長通知
令和2年1月6日　薬生機審発 0106 第1号

医療機器の製造販売承認申請等に必要な
生物学的安全性評価の基本的考え方について

別紙：医療機器の生物学的安全性評価の基本的考え方

別添：医療機器の生物学的安全性試験法ガイダンス

MHLW Notification by Director, Pharmaceutical Safety and Environmental Health Bureau, Medical Device Evaluation Division, Yakuseikishin-hatsu 0106 No. 1

January 6, 2020

Basic Principles of Biological Safety Evaluation Required for Application for Approval to Market Medical Devices

Annex: Basic Principles for Biological Safety Evaluation of Medical Devices

Attachment: Guidance on Test Methods for Biological Safety Evaluation of Medical Devices

医療機器の生物学的安全性評価の基本的考え方

1．目的

　医療機器の生物学的安全性評価は，医療機器の使用によって生じる潜在的な生物学的リスクからヒトを保護するために実施するものであり，JIS T 14971「医療機器―リスクマネジメントの医療機器への適用」（以下，JIS T 14971）又は国際規格である ISO 14971, Medical devices-Application of risk management to medical devices （以下，ISO 14971）に規定されるリスクマネジメントプロセスの検証作業の一つとして位置づけられる（10項の1)項参照）．本文書は，医療機器の安全性評価の一環として，生物学的有害作用（毒性ハザード）のリスク評価を行うための生物学的安全性評価に関する基本的考え方を示すものである．

2．定義

　本文書において用いられる用語の定義は以下によるものとする．

1)　原材料

　医療機器を構成する材料又は医療機器の製造工程中で用いられる材料であり，合成又は天然高分子化合物，金属，合金，セラミックス，その他の化学物質などをいう．

2)　最終製品

　包装を含む全ての製造工程を終えた医療機器又は医療機器の構成部材をいう．該当する場合は滅菌処理も含む．ただし，出荷後，用時加工・調製され使用されるものにあっては，実際に使用される状態の製品をいう．

3)　ハザード

　ヒトの健康に不利益な影響を及ぼす原因となり得る遺伝毒性，感作性，慢性全身毒性などの要素をいう．

4)　リスク

　ハザードにより引き起こされる，ヒトの健康に及ぼす不利益な影響の発生確率及びその重大さとの組合せをいう．

5)　エンドポイント

　医療機器の生物学的安全性を評価するために必要な項目をいう．

3．公的規格の活用

　医療機器の生物学的安全性評価は，原則として，JIS T 0993-1「医療機器の生物学的評価―第1部：リスクマネジメントプロセスにおける評価及び試験」（以下，JIS T 0993-1）あるいは国際規格である最新の ISO 10993 シリーズ（医療機器の生物学的評価関連の規格群）に準拠して行うこととする．すなわち，JIS T 0993-1 及び ISO 10993-1, Biological evaluation of medical devices-Part 1: Evaluation and testing within a risk management process（以下 ISO 10993-1）に準拠して，個々の医療機器の接触部位と接触期間に応じて必要な評価項目を選定する．各評価項目は ISO 10993 シリーズの各試験法ガイダンスを参考として適切な試験法を選定し安全性評価を行うこととする．各試験法については，医療機器の安全性評価を適切に実施できるのであれば，他の公的規格に準拠した試験法

Basic Principles for Biological Safety Evaluation of Medical Devices

1. Purpose

    The purpose of biological safety evaluation of medical devices is the protection of humans from potential biological risks arising from the use of medical devices, and is one of verification works in the risk management process specified in JIS T 14971 "Medical Devices-Application of Risk Management to Medical Devices" (hereinafter referred to as JIS T 14971) or ISO 14971 "Medical devices-Application of risk management to medical devices" (hereinafter referred to as ISO 14971), which is an international standard (see 10.1)). This document provides basic principles for biological safety evaluation to evaluate the risk of adverse biological effects (toxic hazards), as a part of safety evaluation of medical devices.

2. Terms and definitions

    Definitions of terminology utilized in this document shall be as follows:

    1) Raw material

        Refers to a material constituting medical devices or a material used in the manufacturing processes for medical devices such as synthetic or natural polymer compounds, metals, alloys, ceramics and other chemical substances.

    2) Final products

        Refers to medical devices or components of medical devices after the whole manufacturing processes including packaging and, where applicable, refers to sterilization treatment. However, in the event that the shipped product is to be processed and prepared for use, "final product" is a product in a state where it is actually used.

    3) Hazard

        Refers to a factor that may cause adverse effects on human health, such as genotoxicity, sensitization or chronic systemic toxicity.

    4) Risk

        Refers to a combination of a probability of occurrence and severity of an adverse effect on human health caused by such a hazard.

    5) Endpoint

        Refers to an index required to evaluate biological safety of a medical device.

3. Adoption of official standards

    As a rule, biological safety evaluation of medical devices shall be performed in compliance with JIS T 0993-1 "Biological evaluation of medical devices-Part 1: Evaluation and testing within a risk management process" (hereinafter referred to as JIS T 0993-1), or the latest version of international standards ISO 10993 series (a group of standards related to biological evaluation of medical devices). Specifically, based on the framework and principles of JIS T 0993-1 and ISO10993-1, "Biological evaluation of medical devices-Part 1: Evaluation and testing within a risk management process" (hereinafter referred to as ISO 10993-1), the necessary endpoints shall be selected corresponding to the nature and duration of contact of individual medical devices with the body. Safety evaluation is conducted through the selection of appropriate test methods for each endpoint by referring to the guidance on test

による評価で代替することができる．また ISO 10993 シリーズの各試験法ガイダンスとして，多くの場合，評価項目ごとに複数の試験法が提示されているが，個々の医療機器についてどの試験法をいかに適用するか，また試験結果に基づいてそれぞれの医療機器をどのように評価すべきかについては明確に規定されていない．このため，試験実施に当たっては，4 項以下を踏まえて適切な試験法を選択することが必要である．本文書及び別添の「医療機器の生物学的安全性試験法ガイダンス」では，生物学的安全性評価で留意すべき点を追記している．

　なお，公的規格及び基準は科学技術の進展に伴って逐次改訂されるものであるため，試験を実施する時点における最新の規格及び基準を参照し，適切な試験法を選択する必要がある．

表　本文書で引用する ISO 10993 シリーズ及び関連国際規格

ISO 規格番号	表題
ISO 10993-1	Biological evaluation of medical devices-Part 1: Evaluation and testing within a risk management process
ISO 10993-2	Biological evaluation of medical devices-Part 2: Animal welfare requirements
ISO 10993-3	Biological evaluation of medical devices-Part 3: Tests for genotoxicity, carcinogenicity and reproductive toxicity
ISO 10993-5	Biological evaluation of medical devices-Part 5: Tests for *in vitro* cytotoxicity
ISO 10993-9	Biological evaluation of medical devices-Part 9: Framework for identification and quantification of potential degradation products
ISO 10993-10	Biological evaluation of medical devices-Part 10: Tests for irritation and skin sensitization
ISO 10993-11	Biological evaluation of medical devices-Part 11: Tests for systemic toxicity
ISO 10993-12	Biological evaluation of medical devices-Part 12: Sample preparation and reference materials
ISO 10993-13	Biological evaluation of medical devices-Part 13: Identification and quantification of degradation products from polymeric medical devices
ISO 10993-14	Biological evaluation of medical devices-Part 14: Identification and quantification of degradation products from ceramics
ISO 10993-15	Biological evaluation of medical devices-Part 15: Identification and quantification of degradation products from metals and alloys
ISO 10993-17	Biological evaluation of medical devices-Part 17: Establishment of allowable limits for leachable substances
ISO 10993-18	Biological evaluation of medical devices-Part 18: Chemical characterization of materials
ISO/TS 10993-19	Biological evaluation of medical devices-Part 19: 2 Physico-chemical, morphological and topographical characterization of materials
ISO/TR 10993-22	Biological evaluation of medical devices-Part 22: Guidance on nanomaterials
ISO/TS 21726	Biological evaluation of medical devices-Application of the threshold of toxicological concern (TTC) for assessing biocompatibility of medical device constituents
ISO 18562-1	Biocompatibility evaluation of breathing gas pathways in healthcare applications-Part 1: Evaluation and testing within a risk management process

methods described in the ISO 10993 series. Any test methods in accordance with the other appropriate official standards can be substitutable, if biological safety evaluation of medical devices can be adequately performed with them.

The test method guidance in the ISO 10993 series generally provides multiple test methods for each endpoint. For those test methods indicated, it is not clearly specified how to apply a given test method to each medical device or how to evaluate each medical device based on the test results. Before conducting the tests, therefore, it is important to select an appropriate test method based on the following clauses 4 and after. Points to consider in the biological safety evaluation are added in this document and the attachment "Guidance on test methods for biological safety evaluation of medical devices."

The official standards have been continuously revised according to the development of science and technology. Accordingly, an appropriate test method must be selected, considering the most current standards at the time when testing is conducted.

Table   ISO 10993 series and related international standards quoted in this document

ISO Standard No.	Title
ISO 10993-1	Biological evaluation of medical devices-Part 1: Evaluation and testing within a risk management process
ISO 10993-2	Biological evaluation of medical devices-Part 2: Animal welfare requirements
ISO 10993-3	Biological evaluation of medical devices-Part 3: Tests for genotoxicity, carcinogenicity and reproductive toxicity
ISO 10993-5	Biological evaluation of medical devices-Part 5: Tests for *in vitro* cytotoxicity
ISO 10993-9	Biological evaluation of medical devices-Part 9: Framework for identification and quantification of potential degradation products
ISO 10993-10	Biological evaluation of medical devices-Part 10: Tests for irritation and skin sensitization
ISO 10993-11	Biological evaluation of medical devices-Part 11: Tests for systemic toxicity
ISO 10993-12	Biological evaluation of medical devices-Part 12: Sample preparation and reference materials
ISO 10993-13	Biological evaluation of medical devices-Part 13: Identification and quantification of degradation products from polymeric medical devices
ISO 10993-14	Biological evaluation of medical devices-Part 14: Identification and quantification of degradation products from ceramics
ISO 10993-15	Biological evaluation of medical devices-Part 15: Identification and quantification of degradation products from metals and alloys
ISO 10993-17	Biological evaluation of medical devices-Part 17: Establishment of allowable limits for leachable substances
ISO 10993-18	Biological evaluation of medical devices-Part 18: Chemical characterization of materials
ISO/TS 10993-19	Biological evaluation of medical devices-Part 19: 2 Physico-chemical, morphological and topographical characterization of materials
ISO/TR 10993-22	Biological evaluation of medical devices-Part 22: Guidance on nanomaterials
ISO/TS 21726	Biological evaluation of medical devices-Application of the threshold of toxicological concern (TTC) for assessing biocompatibility of medical device constituents
ISO 18562-1	Biocompatibility evaluation of breathing gas pathways in healthcare applications-Part 1: Evaluation and testing within a risk management process

4．生物学的安全性評価の原則

1) 医療機器及び原材料の生物学的安全性評価は，JIS T 14971 又は ISO 14971 に示されたリスク分析手法により実施されなければならない．すなわち，意図する使用又は意図する目的及び医療機器の安全性に関する特質を明確化し，既知又は予見できるハザードを特定し，各ハザードによる不利益のリスクを推定する必要がある．このようなリスク分析手法のアプローチにおいては，「陽性」の結果は，ハザードが検出・特定できたことを意味するものであって，それが直ちに医療機器としての不適格性を意味するものではなく，当該医療機器の安全性は，引き続き行われるリスク評価により判断される．上市後の医療機器も JIS T 14971 又は ISO 14971 により管理されるべきであり，本ガイダンス及び ISO 10993 シリーズの改訂ごとに，生物学的安全性の再評価を必ずしも求めるものではない．

2) 生物学的安全性評価は，次のア～クに示す情報及び本文書に準拠して実施された安全性試験結果，当該医療機器に特有の安全性評価項目の試験結果，関連の最新科学文献，非臨床試験，臨床使用経験（市販後調査を含む）などを踏まえて，リスク・ベネフィットを考慮しつつ，総合的に行う必要がある．

　　ア）　構成材料（直接的又は間接的に人体組織と接触する全ての材料）

　　イ）　添加物，製造工程での混入物及び残存物（残留エチレンオキサイドについては JIS T 0993-7「医療機器の生物学的評価―第 7 部：エチレンオキサイド滅菌残留物」を参照）

　　ウ）　包装材料（直接的又は間接的に医療機器と接触することにより化学物質が医療機器に移行し，結果的に患者や医療従事者に移行する可能性）

　　エ）　溶出物（ISO 10993-17 及び ISO 10993-18 参照）

　　オ）　分解生成物（一般原則は ISO 10993-9，高分子・セラミックス・金属の分解生成物はそれぞれ ISO 10993-13，ISO 10993-14，及び ISO 10993-15 を参照）

　　カ）　最終製品中のア）～オ）以外の成分及びそれらの相互作用

　　キ）　最終製品の性質，特徴

　　ク）　最終製品の物理学的特性（多孔率，粒径，形状，表面形態を含む）

3) 生物学的安全性評価は，教育・訓練が十分になされ，経験豊富な専門家によって行われなければならない．

4) 原材料及び医療機器において，以下の項目のいずれかに該当する変更や事象が確認された場合には，再度，生物学的リスクの評価を行わなければならない．

　　ア）　製品の製造に使用される材料の供給元又は仕様の変更

　　イ）　製品の成分・配合，加工，一次包装又は滅菌方法の変更

　　ウ）　保管中，最終製品（用時加工・調整される前の製品を含む）に化学変化が認められた場合，有効期限，保管条件及び輸送条件の変更

　　エ）　最終製品の使用目的に変更があった場合

　　オ）　製品が人体に使用された際，何らかの有害な作用を生じる可能性を示す知見が得られた場合

4. Principles of biological safety evaluation
1) Biological safety evaluation of raw materials or medical devices must be carried out using risk analysis techniques specified in JIS T 14971 or ISO 14971. The intended use or intended purpose and the safety properties of a medical device must be clarified, known or foreseeable hazards must be identified, and the risk of disadvantage caused by each hazard must be anticipated. If such a risk analysis technique is employed, its "positive results represent detection and identification of some hazards and do not necessarily mean non-conformity of the medical device. The safety of such medical device must be determined through continued risk analyses. Medical devices on the market must be also controlled in accordance with JIS T 14971 or ISO 14971 and are not necessarily required reevaluation of biological safety for each revision of this guidance and ISO 10993 series.

2) Biological safety evaluation must be comprehensively carried out based on the results of safety evaluation conducted in accordance with the information provided in a) to h) below and this document, test results for safety evaluation items specific to the medical device, the latest relevant scientific literature and other non-clinical tests and clinical experiences (including post-marketing surveillance), taking the risk-benefit profile into consideration.

a) The material (s) of construction (i.e. all direct and indirect tissue contacting materials)

b) Intended additives, process contaminants and residues (see JIS T 0993-7 "Biological evaluation of medical devices-Part 7: Ethylene oxide sterilization residuals" for ethylene oxide sterilization residuals)

c) Packaging materials that directly or indirectly contact the medical device can transfer chemicals to the medical device and then indirectly to the patient or clinician

d) Leachable substances (see ISO 10993-17 and ISO 10993-18)

e) Degradation products (see ISO 10993-9, for general principles and 10993-13, 10993-14 and 10993-15 for degradation products from polymers, ceramics and metals, respectively)

f) Components other than Items (a) to (e) of the final product and their interactions

g) The performance and characteristics of the final product

h) Physical characteristics of the final product, including but not limited to, porosity, particle size, shape and surface morphology

3) Biological safety evaluation must be conducted by experienced specialists with sufficient education and training.

4) In the case where any changes and events that falls under any of the following conditions on the raw materials and medical devices are found, biological risk must be evaluated again.

a) Change of suppliers or any changes in the specifications of the materials used for the manufacturing the product.

b) Any change in the components and their formulation, processing, primary packaging or sterilization of the product.

c) Any chemical change observed in the final products (including the products before processing or preparing for use) during the storage period, and change in the expiration date, storage and shipment conditions.

d) Any change in the intended use of the final products.

e) Any evidence in that the product may cause adverse events when the product is used for the human body.

　　上記条件に該当しても，例えば最終製品からの溶出化学物質とその溶出量を分析し，毒性学的情報に基づいた摂取許容値との対比により生物学的安全性が確保できる場合には，必ずしも生物学的安全性試験を再実施する必要はない．

5)　再使用可能な医療機器では，再使用に係る洗浄・滅菌などにおける原材料の材質に対する影響など，検証済みの再使用可能な最大サイクルを考慮した評価を実施する．

6)　医療機器の生物学的安全性について評価すべき項目の選択については，ISO 10993-1に示されているとおり，医療機器あるいは構成部材ごとの接触部位及び接触期間によるカテゴリ分類に応じて，原則として，表1に示すエンドポイントを評価することが望ましい．カテゴリのいずれにも該当しない医療機器を評価する場合には，最も近いと考えられるカテゴリを選択すること（10項の3)参照）．医療機器が複数の接触期間のカテゴリに該当する場合は，より長期間のカテゴリに適用される項目について評価すること．また複数の接触部位のカテゴリに該当する場合は，それぞれのカテゴリに適用される項目について評価すること．

①　医療機器の接触部位によるカテゴリ分類

　ア）　非接触機器：直接/間接を問わず，患者の身体に接触しない医療機器

　イ）　表面接触機器

　　　　○皮膚：健常な皮膚の表面のみに接触する医療機器

　　　　○粘膜：健常な口腔，食道，尿道などの粘膜組織に接触する医療機器

　　　　○損傷表面：創傷皮膚あるいは粘膜組織に接触する医療機器

　ウ）　体内と体外とを連結する機器

　　　　○血液流路間接的：血管と一点で接触し，血管に薬液などを注入する医療機器

　　　　○組織/骨/歯質：軟組織，骨，歯髄又は歯質と接触する医療機器

　　　　○循環血液：循環血液と接触する医療機器

　エ）　体内植込み機器（インプラント）

　　　　○組織/骨：主として軟組織又は骨と接触する医療機器

　　　　○血液：主として血液と接触する医療機器

②　接触期間によるカテゴリ分類

　　　　○一時的接触：単回又は複数回使用され，その累積接触期間が24時間以内の医療機器

　　　　○短・中期的接触：単回又は複数回使用され，その累積接触期間が24時間を超えるが30日以内の医療機器

　　　　○長期的接触：単回又は複数回使用され，その累積接触期間が30日を超える医療機器

5．評価の進め方

　　生物学的安全性評価は，図1のフローチャートに従って行う．

1)　生物学的安全性評価を実施する上で，対象となる医療機器及びその構成成分の物理学的及び化学的情報を収集することが重要である．これらの情報は図1のフローチャートの材料，製造方法，滅菌方法，形状，物理学的特性，身体接触及び臨床使用

Even in the case that falls under the above conditions, for example, if analyses of chemicals leached from final products and their amounts ensure biological safety by contrast with the intake limit based on toxicological information, it is not necessarily required to conduct the retests.

5) Biological safety of reusable medical devices shall be evaluated for the maximum number of validated processing cycles such as how cleaning, sterilization, etc. before reuse may affect the quality of a material.

6) Items to be evaluated for the biological safety of medical devices shall be selected by following the requirements specified in ISO 10993-1. As a general rule, evaluation must be made for the endpoints shown in Table 1, depending on the categorization in accordance with the nature of body contact and the duration of contact with medical devices and each component. When a medical device does not directly fall into any of the categories, the closest category should be selected (see 10.3)). If multiple categories for the duration of contact apply to the medical devices, the item that corresponds to the category with the longer duration should be evaluated. If multiple categories for the nature of body contact apply to the medical devices, the item that corresponds to each category should be evaluated.

(i)   Categorization by nature of body contact

a)   Non-contacting medical devices: Medical devices that have neither direct nor indirect contact with the body

b)   Surface-contacting medical devices

○Skin: Medical devices that contact intact skin surfaces only

○Mucosal membranes: Medical devices that contact intact mucosal membranes such as oral cavity, esophagus and urethra

○Breached or compromised surfaces: Medical devices that contact breached or otherwise compromised body surfaces or mucosal membranes

c)   Externally communicating medical devices

○Blood path, indirect: Medical devices that contact blood path at one point and serve as a conduit for drug entry into the vascular system

○Tissue/bone/dentin: Medical devices that contact soft tissue, bone or pulp and dentin systems

○Circulating blood: Medical devices that contact circulating blood

d)   Implant medical devices

○Tissue/bone: Medical devices that principally contacting soft tissue and/or bone

○Blood: Medical devices principally contacting circulating blood

(ii)   Categorization by duration of contact

○Limited exposure: Medical devices whose cumulative sum of single, multiple or repeated duration of contact is up to 24 hours

○Prolonged exposure: Medical devices whose cumulative sum of single, multiple or repeated contact time is likely to exceed 24 hours but not exceed 30 days

○Long-term exposure: Medical devices whose cumulative sum of single, multiple or repeated contact time exceeds 30 days

5. Evaluation procedures

Biological safety evaluation should be conducted in accordance with the flow chart shown in Figure 1.

1) In biological safety evaluation, it is important to gather physical and chemical information on the target medical device and its components. These information should satisfy the question regarding the materials, manufacturing method, sterilization, shape, physi-

に関する質問を充足できる内容であることが望まれる．また毒性学的リスク評価のために，少なくとも最終製品の化学的成分及び製造時に使用した残留する可能性のある加工助剤又は添加物を可能な限り明らかにしなければならない．

　材料の化学的特性評価を実施する場合には，ISO 10993-18 を参照する．医療機器から溶出し得る化学物質の種類と量を化学的特性評価によって把握することにより，毒性学的閾値，並びに摂取許容値に基づく安全性評価（ISO 10993-17 参照）が可能となり，新たな生物学的安全性試験の実施の要否を判断することができる．インプラント又は血液と接触する医療機器の評価においては，物理学的特性評価に関する情報（ISO/TS 10993-19 参照）が必要となるものがある．ナノマテリアル（nanomaterial）の特性評価には，ISO/TR 10993-22 を参照する．

2)　対象の医療機器と既承認／認証医療機器との生物学的安全性における同等性を判断する．ISO 10993-1 では，①原材料（配合組成など），②製造工程・滅菌の種類／工程，③幾何学的形状及び物理学的特性，④接触部位及び臨床適用における同等性の確認を要求している．

3)　2)において既承認／認証医療機器との同等性が確認できなかった場合，以下の 3 点を充足する情報又はデータにより，当該医療機器の臨床適用における生物学的安全性の担保が可能か否かを判断する．これらは，生物学的安全性におけるリスク評価の実施を正当化できる根拠及び当該医療機器の臨床適用に関連性のある化学的及び生物学的なデータとなる．
　　①　原材料の化学物質毒性データ
　　②　①は他の化学物質混合時にも適用可能なデータであること
　　③　①は当該医療機器の安全性評価可能な用量及びばく露経路を踏まえたデータであること

4)　2)及び 3)を充足しない場合には，表 1 の評価すべき生物学的安全性評価項目及び参考情報（10 項の 3)~6)参照）を検討して，試験を行う．

5)　1)~4)で得られた情報及びデータから毒性学的リスク評価を実施する（10 項の 7)参照）．JIS T 0993-1 の B.2.1（ISO 10993-1 Annex B の B.2.1）に記載されているとおり，生物学的ハザードを特定するために，当該医療機器を構成する原材料情報から，ハザードとなり得る化学物質を特定するとともに，臨床ばく露量の推定などにより評価を行う．これらの情報と表 1 に示す項目の評価を対比させて過不足を判断する．表 1 は，印を付したエンドポイントとなる全試験の実施を必ずしも要求するものではない．ただし，公表文献による評価を行う場合には，JIS T0993-1 の附属書 C（ISO 10993-1 Annex C）を参考とし，客観性及び第三者による検証に耐え得るよう，その妥当性を明らかにする必要がある．

6)　表 1 に示されたエンドポイントのみでは，当該医療機器の生物学的安全性評価が不十分と考えられる場合，その特質を十分考慮して評価項目を検討する必要がある．例えば，歯科裏装用セメントに関する歯髄・象牙質使用模擬試験やコンタクトレンズに係る家兎眼装用試験のように医療機器固有の試験が必要となる場合の他，毒性試験結果などから免疫系への影響が疑われた場合に免疫毒性に関する評価が必要となる場合，あるいは細胞／組織を使用した医療機器の評価など，表 1 に示された試験を単純に適用するのが困難な場合もある．また生体内で経時的に吸収され性状が変化する医療機器では，その変化を考慮した試験条件などを設定することも必要である．

cal properties, body contact and clinical use in the flowchart of Figure 1. In addition, for toxicological risk evaluation, at least chemical constituents of final products, and processing aids and additives which have possibility of remaining as residues after manufacturing should be identified as much as possible.

Chemical properties evaluation of materials shall be carried out, referring to ISO 10993–18. Determining the types and amounts of chemicals which may leach from medical devices by chemical property evaluation enables the safety evaluation based on the toxicological threshold and uptake tolerance (see ISO 10993–17) and judgement on necessity of a new biological safety test. Some evaluations for implant and external communicating devices require information associated with physical property evaluation (see ISO/TS 10993–19). See ISO/TR 10993–22 for property evaluation of nanomaterials.

2) Equivalence of the said medical device to already approved or accredited medical devices in biological safety should be considered. ISO 10993–1 requires confirmation of equivalence in i) raw materials including formulation, ii) manufacturing process and type and process of sterilization, iii) geometric form and physical properties, iv) confirmation of equivalence in nature of body contact and clinical use.

3) If the equivalence to already approved or accredited medical devices cannot be confirmed in 2), whether biological safety in the clinical use of the medical device can be secured should be judged by the information or data satisfying the following three items. These can be the grounds which enable to justify the risk evaluation in the biological safety evaluation and chemical and physical data related to the clinical use the medical devices.
    i)   chemical toxicity data of raw materials
    ii)   The data of i) should be applicable at the time of mixing other chemicals
    iii)   The data of i) should be based on a dose and an exposure path which are evaluable in safety of the medical device

4) If it does not satisfy 2) and 3), the test should be conducted considering Table 1 "Endpoint to be addressed in a biological risk assessment" and reference information (see 10.3) to 6)).

5) Toxicological risk evaluation should be conducted from information and data obtained in 1) to 4) (see 10.7)). As described in JIS T 0993–1 B.2.1 (ISO 10993–1 Annex B B.2.1), in order to identify a biological hazard, evaluation is conducted by estimating clinical exposure along with identifying chemicals which can be hazards using information on the raw materials constituting the medical devices. It should be judged whether it is adequate by comparing these information with the endpoints shown in Table 1. It is not necessarily required to conduct all of the tests with marked endpoints in Table 1. In this case, however, it is necessary to refer to JIS T 0993–1 Annex C (ISO 10993–1 Annex C) and to clearly determine such appropriateness to show concreteness and withstand inspection by a third party.

6) In the case where the biological safety evaluation of the medical device with only those endpoints shown in Table 1 is insufficient, the endpoints must be investigated, taking the properties of the medical devices into account adequately. For example, device specific tests, such as pulp/dentine simulated use testing for dental liner cement or ocular simulation testing with rabbit eyes for contact lenses may be needed. Or in other cases, it is necessary to conduct the evaluation on immunotoxicity, if any effect on the immune system is suspected from the results of toxicity tests and other data. Also, it may be difficult to simply apply the tests shown in Table 1 to evaluations of cell/tissue engineered medical devices. In the case of medical devices whose property changes during use by being absorbed in human body, it is necessary to set test conditions considering the change.

6．試験法

1) ISO 10993 シリーズの各試験法ガイダンスには，それぞれの評価項目ごとに多様な試験法が並列的に記述されており，その中のどの試験法を選択すべきかについては，明確に規定されていない．ある評価項目に関して複数の試験法の中からどれを選択すべきかについては，目的とする医療機器の生物学的安全性評価の意義との関連において，試験の原理，感度，選択性，定量性，再現性，試験試料の適用方法とその制限などを勘案して決めるべきである．

　　ア) 細胞毒性試験に関しては，ISO 10993-5 に，抽出液による試験法，直接接触法，及び間接接触法（寒天重層法，フィルター拡散法）が示されている．これらの試験法は，感度，定量性などが異なるため，リスク評価のためのハザード検出に当たっては，感度が高く定量性のある方法を用いる必要がある．一般的に，抽出液による試験法は感度が高いため，この方法で試験するのが望ましいが，当該試験法以外を選択した場合にはその妥当性を説明する必要がある．

　　イ) 感作性試験及び遺伝毒性試験のハザード検出に当たっては ISO 10993-12 の抽出溶媒に関する規定や ISO 10993-3 及び ISO 10993-10 に記載されている抽出法を参照し，各材料に適したものであって，かつ抽出率の高い溶媒を選択して医療機器の安全性を評価することが必要である．その際，抽出溶媒の種類や抽出条件によって試料溶液中の溶出物の濃度や種類が異なることから，結果が偽陰性を示す可能性があることに留意する．

　　ウ) 亜急性全身毒性，亜慢性全身毒性，及び慢性全身毒性試験に関しては，埋植試験あるいは使用模擬試験が各毒性試験で必要とされる観察項目及び生化学データなどを含んでいる場合，これらの毒性試験に代えることができる．

　　エ) インプラントのリスク評価では，全身的影響及び局所的影響を考慮しなければならない．

2) 全ての医療機器について一律の試験法を定めることは合理性に欠ける．また特定の試験法を固守するよう求めるものでもないが，選定した試験法から得られた結果が臨床適用上の安全性を評価するに足るものであると判断した根拠と妥当性を明らかにする必要がある．

7．試験試料

1) 医療機器の生物学的安全性試験を実施する場合の試験試料としては，最終製品，最終製品の一部及び原材料などが考えられる．試験試料の選択においては，最終製品の安全性を十分に評価できるか否かを検討し，その選択の妥当性を明らかにする必要がある．

2) 医療機器は複数の材料を組合せて製造されることが多く，滅菌を含む製造工程において材料が化学的に変化する可能性がある．またそれら複数の材料は人体へ複合的に直接又は間接ばく露され得る．このため生物学的安全性試験を実施する際には，最終製品，最終製品が人体と接触する部分を切り出した試験試料，最終仕様の試作品あるいは同じ条件で製造した模擬試験試料を用いて実施することを基本とする．一方，製造工程において材料が化学的に変化しないことが確認できる場合には，原材料を試験試料として試験を実施しても差し支えない．

3) 原材料の一部の成分を新規の化学物質に変更し，かつ，それが材料中で化学的に変

6. Test methods
  1) In the guidance for test methods specified in the ISO 10993 series, various test methods
      for each endpoint are listed in parallel, but which test method should be selected among
      them is not indicated. When there are multiple test methods for a given endpoint, selec-
      tion must be done taking into account the principles, sensitivity, selectivity, quantitative
      capability, and reproducibility of the test methods as well as application method and limi-
      tation of test samples, with respect to the significance of the biological safety evaluation
      for the medical device in question.
    a) In the case of cytotoxicity, ISO 10993-5 includes the extraction test method, the di-
        rect contact method and the indirect contact method (the agar overlay method, the
        filter disffusion method). Since the sensitivity, quantitative capability, etc. of these
        test methods are varied, in order to detect potential hazards for risk evaluation, it is
        necessary to use a quantitative test method with high detection sensitivity. As the
        extraction method, in general, has a high sensitivity, it is desirable to be used. The
        use of other test methods shall be justified.
    b) In the tests for sensitization and genotoxicity, biological safety evaluation of medical
        devices shall be carried out using an appropriate solvent with a high percentage of
        extractables in order to detect potential hazards for risk evaluation, referring to the
        provisions relating to extraction solvents in ISO 10993-12 and extraction methods
        desctibed in ISO 10993-3 and -10. In that case, concentration and nature of leached
        substances in the extract varies depending on extraction solvents and conditions,
        which may lead to false negative results.
    c) As for subacute systemic toxicity, subchronic toxicity and chronic toxicity, if the im-
        plant testing or simulated use testing includes observation items and biochemical
        data that are needed for those toxicity tests, it is possible to use the testing results
        in lieu of those of such toxicity tests.
    d) Both systemic and local effects shall be considered in risk evaluation of implant de-
        vices.
  2) It is not logical to establish a uniform test method nor is it necessary to adhere to specif-
      ic test method. However, it is essential to clarify the basis and justification for the judge-
      ment that the results obtained using the selected test methods meet the requirements
      for evaluating safety in clinical use.

7. Test samples
  1) Test samples used in testing for biological safety evaluation of medical devices include
      final products, parts of a final product and raw materials, etc. Among them, a suitable
      test sample must be selected by assessing its ability to appropriately evaluate the safety
      of a final product and by demonstrating scientific justification for the selection.
  2) Many medical devices are manufactured by combining multiple materials, and the manu-
      facturing processes including the sterilization process can chemically alter the materials.
      In addition, human bodies can be complexly exposed to those materials directly or indi-
      rectly. Therefore, biological safety testing basically must be conducted using the final
      product, test samples taken from the area where the final product contacts the human
      body, the trial product in the final specification or simulated test samples manufactured
      under the same conditions. If it can be confirmed that the manufacturing processes do
      not alter the materials chemically, testing may be conducted using the raw materials as
      the test sample.
  3) When the chemical substances, as part of the raw materials, are changed to new chemi-

化しない場合，原材料又は最終製品を用いて試験を実施するよりも当該化学物質について試験を行った方が合理的なこともある．このような場合は，当該化学物質の試験をもって，原材料又は最終製品の試験に代えることができる．

8．Good Laboratory Practice の適用

　5項の4)に規定する生物学的安全性試験は，「医薬品，医療機器及び再生医療等製品の製造販売承認申請等の際に添付すべき医薬品，医療機器及び再生医療等製品の安全性に関する非臨床試験に係る資料の取扱い等について（平成26年薬食審査発1121第9号・薬食機参発1121第13号）」に基づき，「医療機器の安全性に関する非臨床試験の実施の基準に関する省令（平成17年厚生労働省令第37号）」で定める基準（Good Laboratory Practice，「GLP」という）に従って実施すること．ただし当該製品に求められる機能性/有効性を評価する試験で安全性評価の目的が副次的である場合には，「医薬品，医療機器等の品質，有効性及び安全性の確保等に関する法律施行規則（昭和36年厚生省令第1号）」第114条の22を順守すること．

　生物学的安全性評価を目的とした試験はGLPに準拠した実施が求められる．性能確認試験など，その他の目的で実施する場合は，必ずしもGLP準拠が求められるものではないことに留意する必要がある．

9．動物福祉

　試験に動物を用いる際の動物の取扱いについては，「動物の愛護及び管理に関する法律（昭和48年法律第105号）」，「厚生労働省の所管する実施機関における動物実験等の実施に関する基本指針（平成27年科発0220第1号）」，「実験動物の飼養及び保管並びに苦痛の軽減に関する基準（平成18年環境省告示第88号）」及びISO 10993-2などに従い，動物実験の代替法の3Rの原則［1．Replacement（実験動物の置き換え），2．Reduction（実験動物数の削減），3．Refinement（実験方法の改善による動物の苦痛の軽減）］に則り動物の福祉[1)]に努めつつ，適正な動物実験を実施すること．

10．参考情報

1) リスクマネジメントプロセスにおける生物学的評価

　医療機器のリスクマネジメントに係る規格であるJIS T 14971又はISO 14971には，医療機器のライフサイクル全体の安全性確保に不可欠な要求事項が示されている．生物学的安全性評価は，その要求事項に従い実施するリスクマネジメントプロセスの一環であり，検証上の重要なプロセスに位置している．リスクマネジメントプロセスの概要，及び評価全般の注意事項は，JIS T 0993-1の附属書B（ISO 10993-1 Annex B）を参照するとよい．

2) Transitory-contacting medical device

　ISO 10993-1: 2018 5.3.2項及び対応するJIS T 0993-1の5.3.2項では，使用時間が1分未満のランセットや皮下注射針など，人体との接触が非常に短時間又は一時的である医療機器として定義され，通常，生物学的安全性試験の実施を要求しないことが記載されている．しかし，これらの医療機器に使用されているコーティング材や潤滑材が組織に接触し残留する可能性もあるため，詳細な評価が必要となる場合のあること

cal substances but are not chemically altered, it may be more reasonable to conduct tests on such chemical substances rather than performing tests using the raw materials or a final product. In this case, the former tests can replace the latter.

8. Application of Good Laboratory Practice

The biological safety tests prescribed in 5.4) shall be conducted in accordance with "Good Laboratory Practice (GLP)" stipulated in "the Ministerial Order on Standards for Non-Clinical Studies Concerning Safety of Medical Devices" (Order of the Ministry of Health, Labour and Welfare No. 37 in 2005) based on "Handling of materials pertaining to non-clinical studies concerning safety of pharmaceuticals, medical devices and regenerative medicine products to be attached for application for the manufacture and sales approval of pharmaceuticals, medical devices and regenerative medicine products (Yakushokusinsa-hatsu 1121 No. 9, Yakushokukisan-hatsu 1121 No. 13, 2014). However, the objective of the safety evaluation is secondary in the test required for the product to evaluate the functionality or effectiveness, "Regulation for Enforcement of the Act on Securing Quality, Efficacy and Safety of Products Including Pharmaceuticals and Medical Devices" (Order of the Ministry of Health, Labour and Welfare No. 1 Article 114 -22 of February 1, 1961) shall be complied. Tests aimed for biological safety evaluation must be conformed to GLP. It should be noted that other tests such as performance verification tests are not necessarily required to conform to GLP.

9. Animal welfare

The use of animals for testing must follow the laws and regulations such as "Act on welfare and Management of Animals (Act No. 105 of October 1, 1973)", "Guidelines for Conduct of Animal Experiments in Institutions under the Ministry of Health, Labor and Welfare" (Kahatsu 0220 No. 1, 2015), "Standards relating to the Care and Keeping and Reducing Pain of Laboratory Animals" (Notice of the Ministry of the Environment No. 88 of 2006) and ISO 10993-2. The proper conduct of animal experiments shall be considered for animal welfare and alternatives to animal experiments; 3R's tenet comprised with 1) replacement (to replace animals to other methods), 2) reduction (to use fewer animals) and 3) refinement (to prevent, alleviate or minimize pain suffering, distress or lasting harm).

10.   Reference information

1) Biological evaluation within a risk management process

JIS T 14971 or ISO 14971, standards pertaining to the risk management of medical devices, provides the requirements which are essential to ensure the safety over the whole life cycle of the medical devices. Biological safety evaluation is part of the risk management process implemented in accordance with the requirements and play an important role in the verification process. The outline of the risk management process and the general notes for the whole evaluation can be found in JIS T 0993-1 Annex B (ISO 10993-1 Annex B).

2) Transitory-contacting medical device

ISO 10993-1: 2018 5.3.2 and corresponding JIS T 0993-1 5.3.2 define some medical device with limited exposure have very brief/transitory contact with the body such as lancets, hypodermic needles that are used for less than one minute. These generally would not require testing to address biocompatibility. However, for products made with materials such as coatings and lubricants that could be left in contact with body tissues after the medical device is removed. Therefore, it is possible that a more detailed assessment

も考えておかねばならない．また累積的使用時のリスクも考慮する必要がある．

3）　考慮すべき評価項目（表1）の改訂について

　　本文書は，ISO 10993-1: 2018 及び対応する JIS T 0993-1 と整合させる目的で，考慮すべき評価項目（表1）を改訂した．今回の ISO 改訂により米国 FDA 発出の生物学的安全性評価指針[2]とも差異がほとんどなくなり，国際調和が図られたことになる．物理学的・化学的情報に関する項目は，医療機器及び構成成分の基本的情報を収集することを指す（5項の1)参照）．このプロセスは生物学的評価の最初のステップとして ISO 10993-1: 2009 及び JIS T 0993-1: 2012 においても規定されていたものであって，新たな要求事項ではない．

　　また JIS T 14971 又は ISO 14971 に基づくリスクマネジメントプロセスの下，より詳細に毒性学的影響を評価して，医療機器の生物学的安全性を確保することが目的であり，表1に記されたエンドポイント別に独立した試験を実施することを求めるものではない．例えば「埋植」がエンドポイントと記されたカテゴリで，当該医療機器の臨床適用部位での全身毒性試験又は刺激性試験が行われ，適用部位の病理組織学的検査が適切に実施されている場合には，その試験結果を評価することも可能と考えられる．

4）　生分解性評価

　　生分解性の材料が使用された医療機器など，臨床適用時に原材料が体内で分解することが予測される場合には，その過程で発生する化学物質及びその量を検討することが望ましい．ISO 10993-9，ISO 10993-13，ISO 10993-14 及び ISO 10993-15 を参考とし，それらの化学物質の安全性情報の収集に努め，生物学的安全性評価に利用すべきである．また実施された試験において試験系にそれらの化学物質がばく露されていることを検証することも重要になる．分解の過程でナノ粒子が発生するおそれがある場合には ISO/TR 10993-22 を考慮した評価を行うこと．

5）　生殖発生毒性の評価

　　ISO 10993-1: 2018 及び対応する JIS T 0993-1 の発行に伴い，表1の評価項目に生殖発生毒性を追加した．この評価の推奨される医療機器のカテゴリは存在しないが，例えば評価対象となる医療機器の原材料に生殖発生毒性や内分泌かく乱作用を有すると考えられる化学物質が含まれる場合には，評価が必要となる．

6）　がん原性の評価

　　ISO 10993-1: 2018 及び対応する JIS T 0993-1 の発行に伴い，表1の評価項目にがん原性を追加した．人体に長期的に使用される医療機器においては，がん原性のリスク評価が必要となる．ISO 10993-3 では，医療機器及びその原材料の発がん性の評価方法に関する情報が記述されている．原材料の不純物及び医療機器からの溶出物の化学的同定と，これらの化学物質のばく露量などから，発がんリスクを評価することが基本となる．発がん性の情報[3]から，当該医療機器の接触部位（経路）及び接触期間に対して適切なものを選択する．重大な発がんリスクが存在しない医療機器に対し，発がん性試験を実施する必要性は低いと考えられる．最終製品の発がん性試験が必要であると判断される場合には，遺伝子組み換えモデルや OECD 試験ガイドライン 453[4]に記述されている慢性全身毒性と腫瘍形成性を評価する試験法が参考になる．

7）　毒性学的リスク評価について

　　毒性学的リスク評価には ISO 10993-17 が参照可能である．当該規格では，医療機

will be necessary. In addition, the risk by cumulative uses should also be considered.

3) Revisions to "Endpoint to be addressed in a biological risk assessment" (Table 1)

Endpoint to be addressed in a biological risk assessment (Table 1) was revised in this document to make consistent with ISO 10993-1: 2018 and corresponding JIS T 0993-1. This revision almost eliminate the difference from the guidance for biological safety evaluation[2] issued by U.S. Food and Drug Administration (FDA), which means the realization of international harmonization. Items pertaining to the physical and chemical information mean collecting the basic information on the medical devices and components (see 5.1)). This process is stipulated in ISO 10993-1: 2009 and JIS T 0993-1: 2012 as a first step of biological evaluation and not a new requirement.

The purpose is to secure the biological safety of medical devices by evaluating toxicological effect in detail under the risk management process based on JIS T 14971 or ISO 14971 and not to require a specific test for every endpoint shown in Table 1. For example, in the category with the endpoint of "implantation", when a systemic toxicity test or an irritation test is conducted in the clinical use site and the histopathologic examination in the site is appropriately performed, it may be possible to evaluate the results.

4) Biodegradation evaluation

When biodegradable materials are used in medical devices, and are estimated to degrade within the human body during clinical use, the types and amount of the chemicals generated in the process should be determined. The safety information on those chemicals should be collected and utilized for the biological safety evaluation, referring to ISO 10993-9, 13, 14 and 15. It is also important to verify that the chemicals are exposed in the test system. When nanoparticles are likely to be generated in the degradation process, the evaluation must be conducted taking ISO/TR 10993-22 into consideration.

5) Reproductive and developmental toxicity evaluation

With the issuance of ISO 10993-1: 2018 and corresponding JIS T 0993-1, reproductive and development toxicity was added to the endpoint in Table 1. There is no medical device category that should undergo this evaluation. However, this evaluation becomes necessary if medical devices contain any chemicals that may cause reproductive and developmental toxicity or endocrine disruption effect.

6) Carcinogenicity evaluation

With the issuance of ISO 10993-1: 2018 and corresponding JIS T 0993-1, carcinogenicity was added to the endpoint in Table 1. Medical devices with long term use for human body shall evaluate the risk of carcinogenicity. The information on the evaluation methods for carcinogenicity of medical devices and their raw materials are described in ISO 10993-3. It is fundamental to evaluate the carcinogenicity risks from chemical identification of impurities in raw materials and their leachable substances and those chemicals exposure levels. Appropriate tests should be selected considering the nature of body contact (the route) and the contact duration of the medical device by referring to the carcinogenicity information[3]. The medical devices that have no major carcinogenicity risk do not seem to require carcinogenicity tests. In the case where the carcinogenicity test of a final product is judged to be necessary, test methods to evaluate chronic toxicity and tumorigenicity provided in OECD Guidelines for the Testing of Chemicals No. 453[4], and transgenic models are helpful.

7) Toxicological risk assessment

For toxicological risk may be evaluated referring to ISO 10993-17, which describes the method in which risk assessment is performed using the information on the toxicological threshold and others of the chemicals confirmed leaching from a medical device. As of November 2018, the title was changed from "Establishment of allowable limits for

器からの溶出が確認された化学物質の毒性学的閾値などの情報を用いてリスク評価する方法が説明されている．2018 年 11 月現在，表題を「Establishment of allowable limitsforleachable substances」から「Toxicological risk assessment of medical device constituents」へ変更して，ISO/TC 194/WG 11 において改訂作業が進められている．

　これに関連して，TTC（Threshold of Toxicological Concern：毒性学的懸念の閾値）の概念が提唱された．TTC とは，製品の主体以外の化学物質で，意図する / しないに関わらず製品に存在する全ての化学物質を対象として，その閾値未満であればヒトへの健康に明らかなリスクを示さないとされるばく露閾値のことである．医薬品不純物の評価及び管理ガイドライン[5]，食品における香料及び間接添加物の許容ばく露閾値[6,7]の根拠に TTC が用いられている．一方で，医療機器分野では ISO/TS 21726 が発行された．

11. 薬食機発 0301 第 20 号からの変更点

ISO 10993-1: 2018 及び対応する JIS T 0993-1」との調和を考慮し，主として以下の改正を行った．

1) 医療機器の生物学的安全性評価が JIS T 14971 又は ISO 14971 のリスクマネジメントプロセスにおける検証作業の一環として行われるものであることを追記した（1 項，4 項の 1），10 項の 1））．

2) ISO 10993-1 及び JIS T 0993-1 に規定された定義，用語及び評価の進め方との整合を図った（2 項の 2），2 項の 5），4 項の 2），4 項の 3），5 項，図 1，表 1）．

3) 再使用可能な医療機器（2 項の 4）），ナノマテリアル（5 項の 1）），Transitory-contacting medical device（10 項の 2）），生分解性評価（10 項の 4）），生殖発生毒性（10 項の 5））及びがん原性（10 項の 6））の評価における注意事項を記載した．

4) 試験は原則 GLP に従って実施することを追記した（8 項）

12. 参考文献

1) 実験動物の飼養及び保管並びに苦痛の軽減に関する基準の解説（2017 年 10 月環境省）

2) U.S. Food and Drug Administration（2016）: Guidance for Industry and Food and Drug Administration Staff Use of International Standard ISO 10993-1, "Biological evaluation of medical devices-Part 1: Evaluation and testing within a risk management process"

3) International Agency for Research on Cancer（IARC）monograph chemicals

4) OECD Guidelines for the Testing of Chemicals, Section 4: Health Effects Test No. 453（2018）: Combined Chronic Toxicity/Carcinogenicity Studies

5) ICH M7 "Assessment and Control of DNA Reactive（Mutagenic）Impurities in Pharmaceuticals to Limit Potential Carcinogenic Risk"（June 2014）

6) JECFA: Evaluation of Certain Food Additives and Contaminants-Forty-fourth report of the Joint FAO/WHO Expert Consultation on Food Additives, 1995

7) FDA: Food Additives: Threshold of Regulation for Substances Used in Food Contact Articles; Final Rule, 21 CFR Part 170.39

leachable substances" to "Toxicological risk assessment of medical device constituents" and ISO/TC 194/WG 11 is being revised.

In relation to this, the concept of "Threshold of Toxicological Concern (TTC)" was advocated. TTC represents the chemicals other than the product itself and in terms of all the chemicals contained in the product regardless of being intended or not, the exposure threshold which indicates an apparent health risk when it is less than the threshold. Guideline for assessment and control of impurities in pharmaceuticals[5] and acceptable exposure threshold for flavor materials and indirect additives in food[6, 7] employ TTC as the grounds. On the other hand, ISO/TS 21726 was issued for a field of medical devices.

11.　Points changed from MHLW Notification, YAKUSHOKUKI-HATSU 0301 No. 20

The followings were mainly revised in view of harmonization with ISO 10993-1: 2018 and corresponding JIS T 0993-1.

1)　It was added that biological safety evaluation of medical devices is a part of the verification work in the risk management process of JIS T 14971 or ISO 14971 (1., 4.1) and 10.1)).

2)　It promoted consistency with the definitions provided in ISO 10993-1 and JIS T 0993-1 and terminologies and evaluation procedures (2.2), 2.5), 4.2), 4.3), 5., figure 1 and Table 1).

3)　For reusable medical devices (2.4)), nanomaterials (5.1)), Transitory-contacting medical device (10.2)), biodegradation evaluation (10.4)) and evaluation of Reproductive and developmental toxicity (10.5)) and carcinogenicity (10.6)), notes were described.

4)　It was added that tests were generally conducted in accordance with GLP (8.).

12.　References

1)　Explanation for Standards relating to the Care and Keeping and Reducing Pain of Laboratory Animals (the Ministry of the Environment, October 2017)

2)　U.S. Food and Drug Administration (2016): Guidance for Industry and Food and Drug Administration Staff Use of International Standard ISO 10993-1, "Biological evaluation of medical devices-Part 1: Evaluation and testing within a risk management process"

3)　International Agency for Research on Cancer (IARC) monograph chemicals

4)　OECD Guidelines for the Testing of Chemicals, Section 4: Health Effects Test No. 453 (2018): Combined Chronic Toxicity/Carcinogenicity Studies

5)　ICH M7 "Assessment and Control of DNA Reactive (Mutagenic) Impurities in Pharmaceuticals to Limit Potential Carcinogenic Risk" (June 2014)

6)　JECFA: Evaluation of Certain Food Additives and Contaminants-Forty-fourth report of the Joint FAO/WHO Expert Consultation on Food Additives, 1995

7)　FDA: Food Additives: Threshold of Regulation for Substances Used in Food Contact Articles; Final Rule, 21 CFR Part 170.39

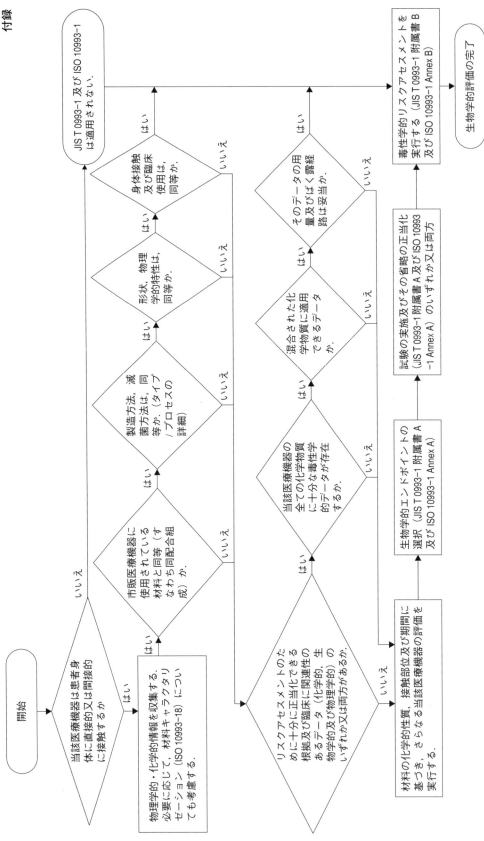

図1 　リスクマネジメントプロセスの一環として実施する医療機器の生物学的評価の体系的手引き

Appendix

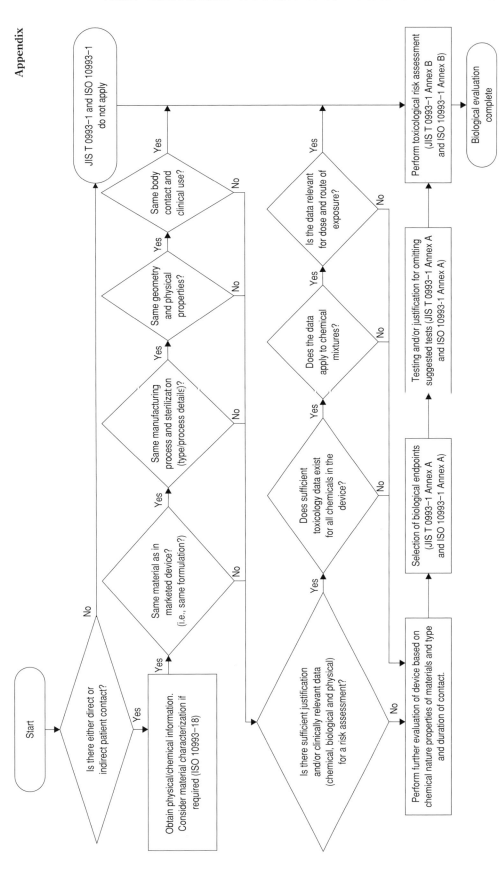

Fig. 1 Summary of the systematic approach to a biological evaluation of medical devices as part of a risk management process

表1　考慮すべき評価項目

　下表は評価が推奨される生物学的安全性評価項目を示したものであり，必ずしも試験実施を要求するものではない．既承認 / 認証の医療機器との同等性や既存化学物質の安全性情報からの評価など，適切にリスク評価を行い，評価不要と判断する場合その理由を明確にすることが必要である．逆に当該カテゴリの医療機器として印がない項目であっても，リスク評価に基づき必要と判断された場合には評価を実施すべきである．

医療機器分類	部位	接触期間	物理学的・化学的情報	細胞毒性	感作性	刺激性/皮内反応	材料由来の発熱性 a	急性全身毒性 b	亜急性全身毒性 b	亜慢性全身毒性 b	慢性全身毒性 b	埋植 b,c	血液適合性	遺伝毒性 d	がん原性 d	生殖発生毒性 d,e	生分解性 f
非接触医療機器																	
表面接触医療機器	皮膚	A	要 g	E h	E	E											
		B	要	E	E	E											
		C	要	E	E	E											
	粘膜	A	要	E	E	E											
		B	要	E	E	E		E	E			E					
		C	要	E	E	E		E	E	E	E	E		E			
	損傷表面	A	要	E	E	E	E										
		B	要	E	E	E	E	E	E			E					
		C	要	E	E	E	E	E	E	E	E	E		E	E		
体内と体外とを連結する医療機器	血液流路間接的	A	要	E	E	E							E				
		B	要	E	E	E							E				
		C	要	E	E	E		E	E	E	E	E	E	E			
	組織 / 骨 / 歯質 i	A	要	E	E	E											
		B	要	E	E	E			E			E		E			
		C	要	E	E	E			E	E	E	E		E	E		
	循環血液	A	要	E	E	E							E	E j			
		B	要	E	E	E			E				E				
		C	要	E	E	E		E	E	E	E	E	E	E			
インプラント	組織 / 骨 i	A	要	E	E	E						E					
		B	要	E	E	E			E			E		E			
		C	要	E	E	E			E	E	E	E		E	E		
	血液	A	要	E	E	E						E	E				
		B	要	E	E	E			E			E	E	E			
		C	要	E	E	E	E	E	E	E	E	E	E	E			

注記
a　ISO 10993-11 Annex F 参照
b　十分な動物数や評価項目が含まれるなど，適切な評価が行われている場合，埋植試験において得られた情報から急性全身毒性，亜急性全身毒性，亜慢性全身毒性及び慢性全身毒性を評価できることもある．それ故，急性全身毒性，亜急性全身毒性，亜慢性全身毒性及び慢性全身毒性を評価するための試験は必ずしも別の試験として行う必要はない．
c　適切な埋植部位を考慮する必要がある．例えば，正常な粘膜と接触する医療機器は，理想的には正常な粘膜と接触させた試験・評価を行うとよい．
d　医療機器が発がん性，変異原性，並びに生殖毒性を有することが知られている化学物質を含む場合には，リスクアセスメントにおいて検討する．
e　新規材料，生殖 / 発生毒性を有することが公知となっている材料，生殖 / 発生毒性と関係の深い患者集団（例えば妊婦）に適用する医療機器，並びに構成材料が生殖器官に局所的に使用する可能性のある医療機器については，生殖 / 発生毒性の評価を考慮することが望ましい．
f　構成部材や構成材料が患者の体内に残留し，生体内で分解する可能性がある医療機器については，生体内分解性に関する情報を示すことが望ましい．
g　「要」はリスクアセスメントに先立って必要となる情報を意味する．
h　「E」はリスクアセスメントにおいて評価すべきエンドポイントを意味する．リスクアセスメントには，既知の毒性情報を用いた評価，エンドポイントに示された生物学的安全性試験の実施，試験を省略する場合にはその妥当性を説明することが含まれる．医療用途として未使用の新規材料が使用されている場合で，かつ，文献などで毒性情報が得られない場合には，「E」と記されていないエンドポイントについても評価の対象に加える必要がある．医療機器の特性によっては，示されたエンドポイント以外も評価対象とすることが適切な場合があるとともに，それとは逆に示されたエンドポイントよりも少ない項目が適切なこともある．
i　組織液や皮下も組織に含める．間接的接触のみを伴うガス回路に用いる医療機器や部材については，その機器に固有の規格（ISO 18562 -1）を参照すること．
j　体外循環装置に使用される全ての医療機器

Appendix

Table 1   Endpoints to be addressed in a biological risk assessment

The following Table shows recommended endpoints for biological safety evaluation. It is not necessarily required to conduct all of these tests. Risk should be properly evaluated in relation to the equivalency with previously approved/certified medical devices, evaluation based on safety information of existing chemicals, etc. It is important to clearly state the reasons if evaluation is considered unnecessary. In contrast, endpoints not marked for the medical device category should be evaluated when risk assessment suggests that it may be necessary.

Contact duration (cumulative): A: Limited (≤24 h) B: Prolonged (>24 h to 30 d) C: Long-term (>30 d)			Physical and/or chemical information	Cytotoxicity	Sensitization	Irritation or intracutaneous reactivity	Material mediated pyrogenicity[a]	Acute systemic toxicity[b]	Subacute systemic toxicity[b]	Subchronic systemic toxicity[b]	Chronic systemic toxicity[b]	Implantation effects[b,c]	Hemocompatibility	Genotoxicity[d]	Carcinogenicity[d]	Reproductive/developmental toxicity[d,e]	Degradation[f]
Non-contact medical devices																	
Surface medical device	Intact skin	A	X[g]	E[h]	E	E											
		B	X	E	E	E											
		C	X	E	E	E											
	Mucosal membrane	A	X	E	E	E											
		B	X	E	E	E		E	E			E					
		C	X	E	E	E		E	E	E	E	E			E		
	Breached or compromised surface	A	X	E	E	E	E	E									
		B	X	E	E	E	E	E	E			E					
		C	X	E	E	E	E	E	E	E	E	E		E	E		
Externally communicating medical device	Blood path, indirect	A	X	E	E	E	E	E					E				
		B	X	E	E	E	E	E	E				E				
		C	X	E	E	E	E	E	E	E	E	E	E	E	E		
	Tissue/bone/dentin[i]	A	X	E	E	E	E	E									
		B	X	E	E	E	E	E	E			E		E			
		C	X	E	E	E	E	E	E	E	E	E		E	E		
	Circulating blood	A	X	E	E	E	E	E					E	E[j]			
		B	X	E	E	E	E	E	E			E	E	E			
		C	X	E	E	E	E	E	E	E	E	E	E	E	E		
Implant medical device	Tissue/bone[i]	A	X	E	E	E	E	E									
		B	X	E	E	E	E	E	E			E		E			
		C	X	E	E	E	E	E	E	E	E	E		E	E		
	Blood	A	X	E	E	E	E	E				E	E	E			
		B	X	E	E	E	E	E	E			E	E	E			
		C	X	E	E	E	E	E	E	E	E	E	E	E	E		

Notes:

a   Refer to ISO 10993-11, Annex F

b   Information obtained from comprehensive implantation assessments that include acute systemic toxicity, subacute systemic toxicity, subchronic systemic toxicity and/or chronic systemic toxicity may be appropriate if sufficient animals and timepoints are included and assessed. It is not always necessary to perform separate studies for acute, subacute, subchronic and chronic toxicity.

c   Relevant implantation sites should be considered. For instance, medical devices in contact with intact mucosal membranes should ideally be studied/considered in contact with intact mucosal membranes.

d   If the medical device can contain substances known to be carcinogenic, mutagenic and/or toxic to reproduction, this should be considered in the risk assessment.

e   Reproductive and developmental toxicity should be addressed for novel materials, materials with a known reproductive or developmental toxicity, medical devices with relevant target populations (e.g. pregnant women), and/or medical devices where there is the potential for local presence of device materials in the reproductive organs.

f   Degradation information should be provided for any medical devices, medical device components or materials remaining within the patient, that have the potential for degradation.

g   "X" means prerequisite information needed for a risk assessment.

h   "E" means endpoints to be evaluated in the risk assessment (either through the use of existing data, additional endpoint-specific testing, or a rationale for why assessment of the endpoint does not require an additional data set). If a medical device is manufactured from novel materials, not previously used in medical device applications, and no toxicology data exists in the literature, additional endpoints beyond those marked "E" in this table should be considered. For particular medical devices, there is a possibility that it will be appropriate to include additional or fewer endpoints than indicated.

i   Tissue includes tissue fluids and subcutaneous spaces. For gas pathway devices or components with only indirect tissue contact, see device specific standards for biocompatibility information relevant to these medical devices (ISO 18562-1).

j   For all medical devices used in extracorporeal circuits.

医療機器の生物学的安全性試験法ガイダンス

目次

Guidance on Test Methods for Biological Safety Evaluation of Medical Devices

contents

第 1 部　細胞毒性試験

1．適用範囲

　本試験法は，医療機器又は原材料の細胞毒性をほ乳類培養細胞を用いて評価するためのものである（4.1 項参照）．

　ISO 10993-5, Biological evaluation of medical devices-Part 5: Tests for *in vitro* cytotoxicity には，抽出法（Test on extracts），直接接触法（Test by direct contact），間接接触法（Test by indirect contact）が含まれている（4.2 項参照）．これらの試験法はさらに，試験に使用する細胞株の種類，試験条件，細胞毒性の指標及びその評価法などによって，多種多様となるが，ISO 10993-5 では定量的に評価可能な試験法を推奨している．またそのような試験法として 4 種類の試験法（ニュートラルレッド法，コロニー形成法，MTT 法及び XTT 法）が Annex A〜D に記載されている（4.3 項参照）．その他にも，ISO 10993-5 が引用する「Guidance Document on Using *In Vitro* Data to Estimate *In Vivo* Starting Doses for Acute Toxicity, 2001. NIH Publication No. 01-4500」では，MTT 法，XTT 法と並び MTS 法が記載されている．ここでは，ISO 10993-5 に記載されている試験法の中から，感度の高い試験法であるコロニー形成法について，抽出法による場合と組織との直接接触による影響を評価できる直接接触法による場合について紹介する（4.4 項参照）．

　なお，医療機器の接触組織を勘案した時，適切な感度・再現性又は用量依存性が示されれば，ISO 10993-5 に準拠した他の方法で試験を実施してもよい．

2．引用規格

2.1　ISO 10993-5: 2009, Biological evaluation of medical devices-Part 5: Tests for *in vitro* cytotoxicity

3．コロニー形成法による細胞毒性試験

3.1　目的

　本試験は，試験試料（最終製品又は原材料）の試験液（抽出液）又は試験試料そのものと細胞を接触させて培養することにより，試験試料から溶出する物質の細胞毒性を確認するための試験である．

3.2　試験の要約

　播種した細胞を試験試料の試験液（抽出液）で処理，又は，試験試料上に直接細胞を播種し，所定の期間培養後のコロニー形成能をコントロールと比較して評価する．

3.3　試験試料（test sample）及び対照試料（control sample）の取扱い

3.3.1　試験試料

　試験試料が抽出液や液体（4.5 項参照）の場合は，適切な溶媒や培養液で希釈して試験する．必要であれば，溶媒のみを培地で適切な濃度まで希釈して試験し，使用した溶媒の影響を明らかにする．

Part 1   Cytotoxicity Test

1.   Scope

The test methods described in this guidance are designed to evaluate the cytotoxicity of medical devices or the raw materials of medical devices using cultured mammalian cells (see 4.1).

ISO 10993-5 (Biological evaluation of medical devices-Part 5: Tests for *in vitro* cytotoxicity) describes a test on extracts, a test by direct contact, and a test by indirect contact (see 4.2). These respective tests vary depending on the cell lines, test conditions, cytotoxicity parameters, and methods of assessment used. ISO 10993-5 recommends the use of quantitative methods and also present 4 quantitative test methods (neutral red uptake test, colony formation test, MTT test, and XTT test) in the Annex A to D (see 4.3). Furthermore, "Guidance Document on Using *In Vitro* Data to Estimate *In Vivo* Starting Doses for Acute Toxicity, 2001. NIH Publication No. 01-4500" cited in ISO 10993-5 describes MTS test as well as MTT and XTT tests. This guidance describes colony formation tests, a test on extracts and a test by direct contact, which can evaluate effects of direct contact with the tissues (see 4.4). The colony formation test is the highly sensitive method among tests recommended by ISO 10993-5.

The other methods specified in ISO 10993-5 can be used to conduct a cytotoxicity test when they demonstrate appropriate sensitivity, reproducibility, or dose-dependency relevant to the nature of body contact during use of the medical device.

2.   Normative reference

2.1   ISO 10993-5: 2009, Biological evaluation of medical devices-Part 5: Tests for *in vitro* cytotoxicity

3.   Cytotoxicity test using colony formation method

3.1   Objective

The objective of this test is to confirm the cytotoxicity of substances eluting from the test sample (the final product or a raw material) by culturing cells in contact with a test solution (liquid extract) of the test sample or with the test sample itself.

3.2   Summary of the test

Inoculated cells are treated with a test solution (liquid extract) of the test sample or cells are directly plated on a test sample, then cells are cultured for a defined period. Colony-forming ability of the test sample is compare with that of control to evaluate cytotoxicity of the test sample.

3.3   Handling of test and control samples

3.3.1   Test sample

A liquid extract of the test sample or a liquid test sample (see 4.5) should be diluted in the appropriate vehicle or culture medium. If necessary, the vehicle can also be diluted with culture medium to clarify the impact of the vehicle alone in the test.

3.3.2　対照試料

1)　陰性対照材料（negative reference material）

陰性対照材料は，ここで示した方法に従って試験した時，規定された基準値を満たす材料であり，以下のものが入手可能である．

抽出法用：高密度ポリエチレンシート（検定済みのもの，4.6項参照）

直接接触法用：接着細胞用プラスチック製カバースリップ又はシート（試験成立条件を満たす材料，4.6項参照）

2)　陽性対照材料（positive reference material）

陽性対照材料は，ここで示した方法に従って試験した時，中程度の細胞毒性を示す陽性対照材料A及び弱い細胞毒性を示す陽性対照材料Bの2種類であり，以下のものが入手可能である（検定済みのもの，4.7項参照）．

陽性対照材料A：0.1％ジエチルジチオカルバミン酸亜鉛（zinc diethyldithiocarbamate, ZDEC）含有ポリウレタンフィルム

陽性対照材料B：0.25％ジブチルジチオカルバミン酸亜鉛（zinc dibutyldithiocarbamate, ZDBC）含有ポリウレタンフィルム

3)　陽性対照物質（positive control substance）

細胞の感度及び精度を明らかにするために使用する物質である．以下のものが入手可能である．原料化学物質の細胞毒性試験を実施する場合には，陽性対照物質として用いる．

陽性対照物質：ZDBC

3.4　滅菌

試験試料は，最終製品と同じ方法で滅菌する．滅菌方法が定まっていない場合には，生化学的又は物理化学的特性などを考慮し，適切な滅菌処理を行う．

エチレンオキサイドガス滅菌をした場合には，エチレンオキサイド又はエチレンクロルヒドリンが残留しないように十分ばっ気した後，試験に使用する．

臨床使用時に滅菌を必要としない試験試料は，無菌的に取り扱う．しかし，微生物による汚染が生じた試験結果は誤った試験評価に繋がることから，そのような汚染を避けるためには滅菌するのが妥当である．ただし，滅菌操作によって材料が変化しない方法を選択すべきである．

滅菌後の試料は，無菌的に取り扱う．

3.5　細胞株及びその取扱い

3.5.1　細胞株

以下に示した細胞株を使用する．他の細胞株及び初代培養細胞を使用する場合は，その細胞での検出感度を陽性対照物質によって判断し，一定レベルの感度及び精度があることを確認する必要がある（4.8項参照）．

①　L929細胞：ATCC CCL 1（NCTC clone 929）

②　Balb/3T3 clone A31細胞：JCRB9005又はATCC CCL 163

③　V79細胞：JCRB0603

試験に用いる細胞については，コロニー形成能（3.6.6項参照）が良好であることを確認する．

3.3.2   Control sample

1) Negative reference materials

Material which, when tested in accordance with this guidance, meets the defined standard values. The following are recommended:

Test on extracts: high-density polyethylene sheet (a material previously validated. see 4.6)

Test by direct contact: plastic cover slips or sheets for adherent cell culture (a material which satisfy the acceptance criteria. see 4.6)

2) Positive reference materials

Positive reference materials A and B which, when tested in accordance with this guidance, respectively show moderate and weak cytotoxicity. The following are recommended (a material previously validated. see 4.7).

Positive reference material A: polyurethane film containing 0.1 % zinc diethyldithiocarbamate (ZDEC)

Positive reference material B: polyurethane film containing 0.25 % zinc dibutyldithiocarbamate (ZDBC)

3) Positive control substance

Substance used to demonstrate cell response and accuracy. The substance listed below is recommended. When chemical substances are used as test samples for cytotoxicity tests, the positive control substance should be included in the test.

Positive control substance: ZDBC

3.4   Sterilization

The test sample should be sterilized in the same manner as the final product. If no sterilization method has been established, the test sample should be sterilized by a method appropriate for the test sample based on the biochemical or physicochemical properties of the test sample.

When ethylene oxide gas sterilization is performed, aerate thoroughly before initiation of the test in order to avoid residue of ethylene oxide or ethylene chlorohydrin.

Test samples that do not require sterilization before clinical use should be aseptically handled. However, these samples can also be sterilized to avoid microbial contamination because the contamination can lead to a false assessment of cytotoxicity. The sterilization method chosen should not change the properties of the test samples.

Handle all sterilized samples aseptically.

3.5   Cell lines and handling

3.5.1   Cell lines

The cells lines shown below can be used. When other cell lines or primary cell cultures are used, it should be confirmed that they have the required level of sensitivity and accuracy based on the results of response of the cells to the positive control substance (see 4.8).

[1]   L929 cell: ATCC CCL 1 (NCTC clone 929)

[2]   Balb/3T3 clone A31 cell: JCRB9005 or ATCC CCL 163

[3]   V79 cell: JCRB0603

Verify that the cells used in the test have adequate colony-forming ability (see 3.6.6).

3.5.2　培養液（培地）

　上記細胞を維持・継代する場合は牛胎児血清を 10 vol％添加した Eagle の Minimum Essential Medium（MEM10 培地）を使用する．細胞に影響を及ぼさない濃度で抗生物質を添加してもよい．

3.5.3　細胞の取扱い

1) 　微生物による汚染を防ぐため，全て無菌的に操作する．
2) 　溶液などは，細胞と接触させる前に，あらかじめ 37℃付近に温めておく．
3) 　培養容器内で細胞が単層で増殖し，飽和に近い状態の時，トリプシン処理などにより細胞を剥がして均一な細胞懸濁液とし，細胞株に最も適した細胞濃度あるいは継代比率に従って，新しい培養容器に植え込む．
4) 　培養液の交換及び継代は，使用する細胞株に適切な間隔で行う．
5) 　細胞株は，市販の細胞凍結保存液又は凍結保護剤を含む培養液中で凍結保存する．－80℃以下の超低温槽では短期間（1年間程度）保存は可能であるが，長期間保存は液体窒素保存容器中とする．
6) 　細胞の履歴を記録する．
7) 　凍結保存細胞は，凍結時のロットごとにマイコプラズマ汚染の有無をチェックする．

3.6　抽出法によるコロニー形成法

3.6.1　抽出溶媒

　試験試料の化学的性状を考慮して抽出溶媒を選択することが原則であるが，ほ乳動物培養細胞を用いる細胞毒性試験では，5 ないし 10 vol％の血清を含む培養液を使用する（4.9 項参照）．なぜなら，血清含有培養液は極性物質と非極性物質の両方を抽出できると同時に細胞の増殖にも必須のためである．

　試験試料によっては，極性物質（例えば，イオン性物質）を抽出する場合など血清を含まない培養液の選択も考慮する必要がある．その他，生理食塩液，精製水又はジメチルスルホキシド（DMSO）などがこの試験の適切な抽出溶媒に含まれるが，細胞へのばく露量を考慮して抽出溶媒を選択する（4.10 項参照）．血清含有培養液以外の抽出溶媒を選択した場合には，その理由を報告書に記載する．

3.6.2　抽出条件

　医療機器の使用条件や性状を考慮して抽出条件を選択すべきであるが，抽出溶媒として培養液を使用する細胞毒性試験では，37±1℃の 24±2 時間抽出が一般的な抽出条件である．

　なお，正常皮膚あるいは粘膜の表面にのみ短時間しか接触しない医療機器（累積接触期間が4時間未満）については，4時間以上 24 時間未満で抽出した試験液での試験も可能である．一般的な抽出条件以外での試験を選択する場合は，医療機器の使用状態を十分に考慮し，細胞毒性に関する安全性を適切に評価できる適切な抽出条件で試験を実施する．またその理由を報告書に記載する．

3.5.2   Culture medium

Use Eagle's minimum essential medium (MEM10 medium) containing fetal bovine serum (10 %v/v) to maintain and subculture the above cells. Antibiotics may be added to the media at a concentration that they do not adversely affect the cells.

3.5.3   Cell handling

1) Handle cells in an aseptic manner to prevent microbial contamination.
2) Warm solutions to about 37 ℃ before contact with the cells.
3) Prior to complete confluency, prepare a uniform cell suspension by using trypsin or a similar reagent to detach cells for splitting. Inoculate cells into a new culture vessel at a cell density or a split ratio optimal for each cell line.
4) Perform medium exchange and subculture at an interval appropriate for the cell line used.
5) In commercially available freezing medium or a culture medium containing an anti-freezing agent, cells may be stored in an ultra-low temperature freezer (−80 ℃ or below) for up to one year. Cells should be stored in a liquid nitrogen tank for longer storage.
6) Record the cell history.
7) Check each lot of cryopreserved cells for mycoplasma contamination.

3.6   Colony formation test on extracts
3.6.1   Extraction vehicle

In principle, an appropriate extraction vehicle considering the chemical characteristics of the test sample should be selected. In a cytotoxicity test using cultured mammalian cells, use of culture medium with 5 or 10 % (v/v) serum is should be used for extraction because of its ability to support cellular growth as well as extract both polar and non-polar substances (see 4.9).

In addition to culture medium with serum, use of medium without serum should be considered in order to specifically extract polar substances (e.g. ionic compounds). Other suitable vehicles such as physiological saline, purified water, dimethyl sulfoxide (DMSO), etc. should be selected with consideration given to the final cellular exposure concentration of extractables (see 4.10). When an extraction vehicle other than culture medium with serum is used, the reason for the choice shall be justified and documented in the test report.

3.6.2   Extraction conditions

The extraction conditions shall be selected considering the nature and use of the final product. In a cytotoxicity test using a culture medium as the extraction vehicle, the recommended conditions are normally 24 ± 2 hours at 37 ± 1 ℃. For medical devices that are in short-term contact (no greater than 4 hours cumulative contact duration) with intact skin or mucosa, this may include extraction times of less than 24 hours but no less than 4 hours. When other extraction conditions than the recommended condition are used, consider the use conditions of the device and use extraction conditions that could evaluate cytotoxicity appropriately. The reason for the chosen extraction condition shall be justified and documented in the test report.

3.6.3　抽出操作

1) 可能であれば，試験試料を切断（約2×15 mm程度の大きさ）する．特別な表面処理をした試験試料は，細切しないものについて試験を実施する．

2) 試験試料は，スクリューキャップ付き滅菌ガラス容器又はプラスチック管に入れ，1g又は厚みを考慮した細切前の実表面積60 cm²に対して抽出溶媒を10 mLの割合で加え，軽く栓をする．必要に応じて，付録1の規定を参照しても差し支えない．

3) 培養液を用いる場合には，そのpHが中性域（培地の色で判断）であることを確認後，37±1℃で，静置又は攪拌して抽出する（通常は24±2時間）．なお，抽出液のpHが酸性又は塩基性を示し，かつ細胞毒性が認められた場合，緩衝作用の強い培養液などを用いた追加試験によりpHの影響を確認し，評価の補助とすることが可能である．

4) 対照材料については，1g又は表裏表面積60 cm²に対して血清含有培養液を10 mLの割合で加え，37±1℃で，静置又は攪拌して24±2時間抽出する（4.8項参照）．

5) 抽出容器から，抽出液のみを取り出す（100％抽出液）．100％抽出液をろ過，遠心，あるいは試験液を試験に適用する前に他の方法による何らかの処理を行った場合には，その詳細及び妥当性を報告書に記載する．

3.6.4　試験液調製

1) 抽出溶媒として血清含有培養液を用いた場合には，100％抽出液を100％試験液とし，さらに培養液で，原則として3倍以下の割合で段階希釈し，試験系に適用する複数濃度の試験液を調製する．

2) 血清含有培養液以外の抽出溶媒を用いた場合には，100％抽出液を抽出溶媒で段階希釈してそれらを培養液に添加するか，又は，100％抽出液を培養液に添加して等量の抽出溶媒を含む培養液で段階希釈して，複数濃度の試験液を調製する．
なお，希釈は，原則として3倍以下の割合とする．

3.6.5　試験操作

1) 継代した細胞からトリプシン処理などにより単離細胞を調製し，培養液に懸濁する．

2) 直径60 mmシャーレには100～200個（培地4～6 mL），35 mmシャーレには50～100個（1～3 mL），12ウェル又は24ウェルプレートのウェルには40～50個（0.5～2 mL）の細胞を播種する．

3) 細胞を播種したシャーレ又はプレートを37℃の炭酸ガス培養器内に入れ，4～24時間静置し，細胞をシャーレ又はウェル底面に接着させる．

4) 培養液を除き，各試験液をシャーレ又はウェルに加える．加える液量は，細胞播種時の培養液量と同様とする．

5) 新鮮な培養液を加えたシャーレ又はウェルをコントロール群とする．

6) 抽出溶媒として血清含有培養液以外の溶媒を用いたときには，コントロール群とは別に，溶媒対照群として抽出液と等量となるよう抽出溶媒のみを培養液に加えた

3.6.3　Extraction procedure

1) If possible, cut the test sample into small pieces (about 2 mm by 15 mm). This is not required for test samples with a special surface treatment.

2) Place the test sample in a sterilized glass container or plastic tube with a screw cap. Add 10 mL of an extraction vehicle per 1 g or 60 cm^2 (actual surface area before cutting, with consideration for thickness) of the test sample, and cap loosely. If necessary, extraction conditions in Attachment 1 can be chosen.

3) Confirm in the culture medium that the pH is within the neutral region (by the color), and stand or agitate the container or tube at 37 ± 1 ℃ for extraction (normally for 24 ± 2 hours). If the pH of the extract is acidic or basic and the cytotoxic result is obtained, additional testing to confirm the effects of pH using a culture medium with a strong buffering effect, etc. may be helpful to evaluate cytotoxic effects of the test sample.

4) For reference materials, add 10 mL of the culture medium with serum per 1 g or 60 cm^2 (the combined surface area of both sides), then stand or agitate for extraction at 37 ± 1 ℃ for 24 ± 2 hours (see 4.8).

5) Transfer only the extract from the container or tube (100 % extract). If the 100 % extract is filtered, centrifuged or test solutions are processed by other methods prior to being applied to the cells, these details shall be recorded in the final report along with a rationale for the additional steps.

3.6.4　Preparation of the test solutions

1) When culture medium with serum is used as an extraction vehicle, the 100 % extract is used as the 100 % test solution. The 100 % test solution is diluted with the culture medium at 3-fold or less by serial dilution to prepare multiple concentrations of test solutions for test.

2) When culture medium with serum is not used as an extraction vehicle, multiple concentrations of test solutions for test are prepared as follows. The 100 % extract is serially diluted with the extraction vehicle and the diluted extracts are added to culture media to make test solutions, or alternatively, the 100 % extract is added to culture medium to make the original test solution and the solution is serially diluted with culture medium containing an equal volume of extraction vehicle to the 100 % extract. Dilution is conducted at 3-fold or less.

3.6.5　Test procedures

1) Detach subcultured cells from the culture vessel by trypsin treatment etc. and suspend them in the culture medium.

2) Inoculate 100 to 200 cells (4 to 6 mL of the culture medium) into a 60 mm dish in diameter, 50 to 100 cells (1 to 3 mL) into a 35 mm dish in diameter, or 40 to 50 cells (0.5 to 2 mL) into a well of 12- or 24-well plate.

3) Place the inoculated dishes or plates into a CO_2 incubator (37 ℃) and culture for 4 to 24 hours to allow the cells to adhere to the bottom of the dishes or wells.

4) Remove the culture medium, and add the test solutions to the dishes or wells. Volume of test solution is equal to that of the culture medium added for cell inoculating.

5) As a control group, fresh culture medium is added to dishes or wells.

6) When culture medium with serum is not used as an extraction vehicle, in addition to a control group, as a vehicle control group, an equal volume of extraction vehicle to the extract is added to dishes or wells.

7) Also add the negative and positive reference material test solutions to the dishes or wells as the same manner as above.

シャーレ又はウェルを設ける.
7)　陰性対照材料及び陽性対照材料の試験液についても同様に加える.
8)　各濃度の試験液について, 少なくとも3つのシャーレ又はウェルを使用する.
9)　試験液を加えたシャーレ又はプレートは, 直ちに炭酸ガス培養器に入れ, 静置して培養する.
10)　培養期間は, 使用する細胞株により異なるが, コントロール群における染色した個々のコロニー（50個以上の細胞集団）が明確に区別できるまで培養する（4.11項参照）.
11)　培養終了後, 培養液を捨てる. 適切な固定液を加えて固定する. 必要があれば, 固定前に平衡塩類溶液で洗う.
12)　固定後, ギムザ染色液など（4.12項参照）を加え, コロニーを染色する.
13)　染色後, 染色液を捨て, 水洗して乾燥させる.

3.6.6　観察

1)　各シャーレ又は各ウェル内の染色されたコロニー数を数える. コロニーは, 肉眼又は適切な顕微鏡で観察し, 細胞が50個以上集まっている集団について数える. 迅速な判定法として, コロニーカウンターを用いたコロニー数測定も可能である. その際は, 機械での測定結果の精度など結果の信頼性が確保されていることを確認する.
2)　コントロール群に播種した細胞数と実際に形成されたコロニー数からコロニー形成能（形成したコロニー数/播種した細胞数）を求める. コントロール群（溶媒対照群がある場合には溶媒対照群）でのコロニー数の平均値を100%として, 試験液で形成された平均コロニー数を百分率（%）, すなわちコロニー形成率で示す.
3)　実験結果は, 縦軸がコロニー形成率（コントロール群又は溶媒対照群のコロニー数の平均値を100%とする）を, 横軸が試験液の濃度（対数）を示すグラフ上にプロットする. グラフより, コロニー形成率を50%阻害する試験液の濃度（%）を求めIC_{50}値とする.
4)　統計理論式から得られるIC_{50}値を, コンピュータで計算することもできる.
5)　IC_{50}値を細胞毒性強度の指標とする.

3.6.7　試験成立条件

以下に記載する内容を満たした試験において, 試験試料の細胞毒性を正しく評価できる.
1)　コントロール群及び溶媒対照群のいずれか又は両方でのコロニー形成能が良好である.
2)　陰性対照材料での100%抽出液で形成されたコロニー数は, コントロール群のコロニー数と同程度である.
3)　陽性対照材料A及び陽性対照材料Bをここで示した方法に従って試験した時, 陽性対照材料の試験液の濃度とコロニー形成率との間に各々用量反応関係を認め, さらに, 得られたIC_{50}値は陽性対照材料A及び陽性対照材料Bにおいて各々下記の値を満たす（4.8, 4.13項参照）.
陽性対照材料AのIC_{50}値：7%未満
陽性対照材料BのIC_{50}値：80%未満

8) Use at least 3 replicates at each concentration.

9) Place the dishes or plates into a CO_2 incubator immediately after the test solutions are added and culture under static conditions.

10) The culturing period depends on the cell line used. Culture until individual colonies (formed by 50 or more cells) in the control group can be easily differentiated (see 4.11).

11) Discard the medium after completion of culturing. Add suitable fixative to fix the cells. If necessary, wash the cells with balanced saline solution before fixing.

12) After fixing, stain the colonies using a staining solution such as Giemsa's stain (see 4.12).

13) After staining, discard the staining solution, wash the culture vessels with water and then dry them.

3.6.6 Observation

1) Count the number of stained colonies in each dish or well. Only count the colonies formed by 50 or more cells using a suitable microscope or with the naked eye. A colony counter may be used for efficient counting. Confirm the reliability of the counts obtained with the colony counter (e.g. accuracy).

2) Calculate the colony-forming ability in the control group by dividing the number of counted colonies by the number of inoculated cells. Calculate relative plating efficiency: the percentage of mean number of colonies in each test solution relative to the mean number of colonies in the control group (or the vehicle control group, if applicable).

3) Plot the obtained data on a graph showing relative plating efficiency (%) to the mean number of colonies in the control group or the vehicle control group on the ordinate and the concentration of the test solution (log number) on the abscissa. From the graph, determine the 50 % inhibition concentration of the test solution (IC_{50}) at which the relative plating efficiency is inhibited until 50 %.

4) The IC_{50} value may be calculated on a computer using the theoretical formula.

5) The IC_{50} value is the index of cytotoxic potential.

3.6.7 Acceptance criteria of the test

The cytotoxicity of a test sample can be appropriately assessed when the following criteria are met;

1) The control group and/or the vehicle control group shows adequate colony-forming ability.

2) The number of colonies in the negative reference material group at 100 % concentration is comparable to that in the control group.

3) When the positive reference material A and positive reference material B are tested in accordance with this part of the guidance, the positive reference materials should show a dose-response relationship between the decrease in the relative plating efficiencies and the increase in the concentrations of the test solution. Also, the IC_{50} value for positive reference material A and positive reference material B (see 4.8 and 4.13) meet the following criteria.

    IC_{50} of positive reference material A: < 7 %

    IC_{50} of positive reference material B: < 80 %

4)　必要に応じて，陽性対照物質（ZDBC）の細胞毒性強度（IC_{50} 値）を調べ，試験系の検出感度及び精度評価の参考とする（4.8 項参照）．

3.6.8　評価

試験試料の 100 ％抽出液処理群のコロニー形成率が 70 ％未満の場合，細胞毒性作用有りと評価する（4.14 項参照）．その他の基準値を採用した場合には，その妥当性を報告書に記載する．

3.7　直接接触法によるコロニー形成法（4.4 項参照）

3.7.1　試料調製

1)　試験に使用する 12 ウェル又は 24 ウェルプレートの形状に合うように，円板の試験試料及び対照材料（陰性対照材料及び陽性対照材料 B）を作製し，可能な場合には，重量及び表面積を測定する．
2)　未滅菌の試験試料及び対照材料については，その使用目的に合った滅菌処理を施す．

3.7.2　試験操作

1)　細胞株は V79 細胞を，培養液は MEM10 培地を用いる．
2)　試験試料，陰性対照材料及び陽性対照材料 B を，ウェルによく密着させる．
3)　12 ウェルプレートのウェルには 40〜50 個（培地 1 〜 2 mL），24 ウェルプレートのウェルには 40〜50 個（培地 0.5〜 1 mL）の細胞を播種する．
4)　細胞をウェルに直接播種した群をコントロール群とする．
5)　細胞を播種したプレートを 37 ℃の炭酸ガス培養器内に入れ，6 〜 7 日間静置して培養する．
6)　培養終了後，培地を捨てる．試験試料に適した固定液で固定する．必要があれば，固定前に平衡塩類溶液で洗う．
7)　固定後，ギムザ染色液など（4.12 項参照）を加え，コロニーを染色する．
8)　コロニーが良く染色されていることを確認後，染色液を捨て，水洗・乾燥させる．
9)　各ウェルのコロニー数を数える．

3.7.3　観察

1)　コントロール群のコロニー数の平均値を 100 ％とする．
2)　試験試料上に直接播種した細胞のコロニー数を数え，その平均値からコントロール群のコロニー数に対する割合（％），すなわちコロニー形成率を求める．
3)　同様に，陰性対照材料及び陽性対照材料 B のコロニー形成率（％）を求める．

3.7.4　試験成立条件

1)　コントロール群でのコロニー形成能が良好である．
2)　以下に記載する内容を満たした試験において，試験試料の直接接触法での細胞毒性を正しく評価できる．

4) If necessary, determine the cytotoxic potential (IC_{50}) of the positive control substance (ZDBC) as a reference for the assessment of the sensitivity and accuracy of the test system (see 4.8).

3.6.8 Evaluation of the test sample

The relative plating efficiency of less than 70 % at 100 % concentration of the test sample is considered a cytotoxic effect (see 4.14). Other criteria shall be justified and documented.

3.7 Colony formation test by direct contact (see 4.4)

3.7.1 Sample preparation

1) Prepare a disk-shaped test sample and control samples (negative reference material and positive reference material B) to suite the well size of the 12- or 24-well plate used in the test. If possible, weigh the samples and measure their surface area.
2) Sterilize non-sterilized test sample and control samples in a manner suitable for the specific conditions of use.

3.7.2 Test procedures

1) Use V79 cells and MEM10 medium.
2) Place the test sample, negative reference material, and positive reference material B tightly in individual wells. Each piece should be fitted tightly within the well.
3) Inoculate 40 to 50 cells (1 to 2 mL of the culture medium) into the wells of a 12-well plate or 40 to 50 cells (0.5 to 1 mL of the culture medium) into the wells of a 24-well plate.
4) As the control group, cells are inoculated into the wells directly.
5) Place the plates in a CO_2 incubator (37 ℃), and culture for 6 to 7 days.
6) Discard the medium after completion of culturing. Fix the cells with a suitable fixative. If necessary, wash the cells with balanced saline solution before fixing.
7) After fixing, stain the colonies using a stain such as Giemsa's stain (see 4.12).
8) Confirm that the colonies are well stained, discard the staining solution, wash the plates with water and then dry them.
9) Count the number of colonies in each well.

3.7.3 Observation

1) The mean number of colonies in the control group is used for calculation of relative plating efficiency (%).
2) Count the number of colonies formed in the wells with the test sample, and calculate the relative plating efficiency: the percentage of mean number of colonies in test sample relative to the mean number of colonies in the control group.
3) Calculate the relative plating efficiency for the negative reference material and positive reference material B.

3.7.4 Acceptance criteria of the test

1) The control group shows adequate colony-forming ability.
2) The cytotoxicity of a test sample can be accurately assessed in a test by direct contact when the following criteria are met;

　　　陰性対照材料でのコロニー形成率：80 % 以上

　　　陽性対照材料 B でのコロニー形成率：10 % 以下

3)　必要に応じて陽性対照物質（ZDBC）の細胞毒性強度（IC_{50} 値）を調べ，試験系の検出感度及び精度評価の参考とする．

3.7.5　評価

　　試験試料上に直接播種した細胞のコロニー形成率が 30 % 未満でその試験試料の抽出法におけるコロニー形成率が 70 % 未満の場合には，細胞毒性作用有りと評価する（4.13 項参照）．ただし，試験試料上に直接播種した細胞のコロニー形成率が 30 % 未満で，抽出法におけるコロニー形成率が 70 % を超える場合には，試験試料の抽出を 72 時間行った抽出液で試験を実施し，その結果も考慮して評価する．なお，コロニー形成率低下の原因を特定できれば，必ずしも 72 時間抽出した試験液での試験を実施する必要はない．

3.8　試験報告書

　　試験報告書には，少なくとも以下の事項を記載する．

1)　試験実施機関及び試験責任者

2)　試験実施期間

3)　試験試料（最終製品又は原材料）を特定する要素

　　（例：医療機器の名称，製造販売業者名，製造番号，原材料名など）

4)　使用した対照材料（陰性対照材料，陽性対照材料又は陽性対照物質）

5)　試験試料の試験への適用方法（滅菌した場合は，その方法を含む）

　　（例：採取重量又は面積，細切の方法，滅菌方法など）

6)　試験液の調製（抽出前後の 100 % 抽出液の変化の有無を含む）

7)　使用した細胞株

8)　使用した培地（使用した抗生物質の種類及び含量）

9)　使用した細胞及びコントロール群のコロニー形成能（形成したコロニー数 / 播種した細胞数）

10)　試験結果

　　抽出法による場合：

　　　　試験試料，陰性対照材料及び陽性対照材料での個々のデータ及びその計算値（平均値，標準偏差）の表，データをプロットしたグラフ，IC_{50} 値

　　直接接触法による場合：

　　　　試験試料，陰性対照材料及び陽性対照材料でのコロニー形成率と写真（プレート全体と 1 個のコロニーの状態が判定可能な写真）

　　原料化学物質の場合：

　　　　試験試料，陽性対照物質での個々のデータ及びその計算値（平均値，標準偏差）の表，データをプロットしたグラフ，IC_{50} 値

11)　結果の評価と考察

12)　参考文献

Relative plating efficiency in the negative reference material: $\geq 80\,\%$

Relative plating efficiency in the positive reference material B: $\leq 10\,\%$

3) If necessary, determine the cytotoxic potential (IC_{50}) of the positive control substance (ZDBC) as a reference for assessment of the sensitivity and accuracy of the test system.

3.7.5 Evaluation of the test sample

When the relative plating efficiencies in a test by direct contact and a test on extracts are less than 30 % and less than 70 %, respectively, the test sample is evaluated to be cytotoxic (see 4.13). If the relative plating efficiencies in a test by direct contact and a test on extracts are less than 30 % and more than 70 %, respectively, repeat the test on extract using a liquid extract of the test sample for 72-hour and incorporate the results in the cytotoxicity assessment. This additional testing is not necessarily required if the cause of the decrease in colony formation is identified.

3.8 Test report

The test report should, at a minimum, include the following items.

1) Test facilities and the study director
2) Test period
3) Factors identifying the test sample (final products or raw materials)
   (e.g. name of the medical device, manufacturer, batch number, and raw materials);
4) Control samples (negative reference material, positive reference material, or positive control substance) used
5) Details of the test sample preparation used in the test (if applicable, include the sterilization method used)
   (e.g. sample weight or surface area used, cutting size and sterilization method)
6) Preparation of test solution (include change in the 100 % extract after extraction)
7) Cell line used
8) Culture medium (and the type and amount of any antibiotics used) used
9) Colony-forming ability of the control group (number of colonies formed / number of inoculated cells) in the test condition
10) Test results
    Results of the test on extracts:
    Tabulation of individual and calculated values (mean and standard deviation) for the test sample, negative reference material, and positive reference material, graph in which data is plotted and IC_{50} values.
    Results of the test by direct contact:
    Relative plating efficiency and micrographs (that show the entire plate and allow differentiation of individual colonies) of the test sample, negative reference material, and positive reference material
    Results of the test of a chemical substance:
    Tabulation of individual and calculated values (mean and standard deviation) for the test sample, and positive control substance, graph in which data is plotted and IC_{50} values.
11) Evaluation of the results and discussion
12) References

4. 参考情報

4.1 細胞毒性試験の位置づけ

　細胞毒性試験は感度の高い試験系であり，*in vivo* での毒性作用の可能性を検索するために，全てのカテゴリーの医療機器の生物学的安全性評価項目となっている．

　本試験系は，動物レベルでの毒性試験結果を，より単純な実験系として，細胞レベルで明らかにしようとするものであり，主に，毒性発現メカニズムを明らかにするための手段として，初代培養細胞や樹立細胞株を用いて研究されてきた．しかし，通常試験に使用されている細胞株の場合には，生体臓器を構成する細胞とは異なる感受性をもっており，*in vivo* での有害作用とは完全には相関しないことも常に考慮しておくことが重要である．

　その一方で，従来からある方法のみにとらわれることなく，科学的根拠に基づいた精度の高いデータを得るための代替試験法を取り入れて評価することも重要である．

4.2 細胞毒性試験における試験試料の適用方法の違いとその特徴

　医療機器又は原材料の細胞毒性試験には，材料の抽出液を用いる方法と，材料と細胞との直接接触及び間接接触による方法とがある．

　直接接触による方法には，細胞の上に材料を載せる方法と逆に材料の上に細胞を播種する方法がある．細胞の上に材料を載せる方法は，材料の物理的重みなどによる細胞の傷害が伴う可能性がある．一方，材料の上に細胞を播種する場合には，細胞が付着しにくい材料の場合には，細胞毒性を評価しにくい．それぞれ欠点があるが，材料からの溶出成分と細胞とが即反応するため，不安定な化合物例えば過酸化物などの毒性を検知するのには優れており，細胞毒性の検出感度は一般的に高いと考えられている．

　材料と細胞との間接接触による方法には，寒天重層法やミリポアフィルター重層法，ならびにセルカルチャーインサート法がある．これらは，細胞と材料との間に寒天やフィルターが存在する．寒天は脂溶性の化合物は拡散しにくく検出感度が低く，半定量的評価法である．ミリポアフィルター重層法は寒天重層法の改良型であり，寒天重層法と同様に *in situ* で重合する材料（例：コンポジットレジン）の試験としては有用であるが，細胞毒性の検出感度は低く，眼粘膜刺激を示す材料でも陽性とならないことがあるので，眼粘膜に直接接触する医療機器へ適用するには不適切である．一方，セルカルチャーインサート法はウェル底面に材料を置き，その上にセルカルチャーインサートを置き，そのフィルター上に細胞を播種することにより，感度よく細胞毒性作用を評価することが可能で，直接接触法の結果を補足する試験として利用できる．

　血清含有培養液による抽出液を用いる抽出法は最も一般的に行われている方法である．抽出液を試験する時の細胞密度や判定方法により，検出感度や精度が異なるが，採用する試験法の妥当性を明らかにすることができれば，どの方法で試験を行ってもよい．

4.3 掲載試験法選択背景

　ISO 10993-5 で Annex A〜D にニュートラルレッド法，コロニー形成法，MTT 法及び XTT 法が紹介されているが，これらの方法は細胞毒性作用を定量的に評価する方法で

4. Reference information

4.1 Position of the cytotoxicity test

The cytotoxicity test is a highly sensitive test system and listed as a biological evaluation test of medical devices in all categories in order to evaluate possibility of *in vivo* toxic effects.

A cytotoxicity test system attempts to identify *in vivo* toxicity at a cellular level. Cytotoxicity tests have been conducted using primary cell cultures and established cell lines to study the mechanism of toxicity. It is important to know, however, that cell lines commonly used in cytotoxicity tests have different sensitivities from the cells of living organs and that toxicities observed in these cell lines are not completely correlated with adverse effects observed *in vivo*.

At the same time, without adhering to conventional methods, adopting alternative test methods to obtain accurate data for evidence-based assessment are acceptable.

4.2 Characteristics of methods appling test samples in cytotoxicity test

Test methods used in the evaluation of the cytotoxicity of medical devices or raw materials of medical devices are largely divided into the following: extract test, direct-contact test, and indirect-contact test.

Direct-contact tests involve either placing a test material directly on cells or seeding cells onto the material. Methods that place a test material onto cells may damage the cells due to the weight of the material. On the other hand, those methods that seed cells onto the test material are not suitable when the material does not allow easy cell adhesion. While both have their disadvantages, the direct-contact methods are suitable for detecting toxicity of unstable compounds such as peroxides because the eluting components and cells react immediately. They are therefore generally thought to have a high level of sensitivity for cytotoxicity.

Indirect-contact methods include agar diffusion, Millipore filter diffusion, and cell culture insert tests. In these methods, agar or a filter is between the cells and the test material. Lipophilic compounds do not diffuse well in agar, so the sensitivity of agar diffusion test is low for such compounds. Agar diffusion test only allows semi-quantitative evaluation. Millipore filter diffusion test is a modification of agar diffusion test. Just like agar diffusion test, Millipore filter diffusion test is useful for testing materials that can be polymerized *in situ* (e.g. composite resin). However, the sensitivity of Millipore filter diffusion test for cytotoxicity is low, and it sometimes fails to detect cytotoxicity even with a material that causes eye mucosal irritation. Therefore, the Millipore filter diffusion test is not suitable for testing medical devices that directly contact the eye mucosa. The cell culture insert method is conducted by seeding cells onto a cell culture insert placed on the test material at the bottom of the well. The method is highly sensitive for cytotoxic effects and can supplement the results of a test by direct contact.

Tests on extracts using a culture medium with serum are the most commonly used method. The sensitivity and accuracy of a test method also depends on the cell density and the determination method of cytotoxicity. Any of test methods may be used provided that the reliability of the method is demonstrated.

4.3 Rationale for the test methods included

The neutral red uptake test, colony formation test, MTT test, and XTT test are described in Annex A to D of ISO 10993-5. These methods allow quantitative cytotoxicity assess-

ある．ニュートラルレッド法及びコロニー形成法については，国際バリデーション試験や国際 round-robin 試験で化学物質や医療機器の検出に適していることが示されており，MTT 法及び XTT 法は定量的方法として広く使用されている方法である．

　本ガイダンスでは，医療機器の安全性評価を目的とすることから，検出感度が高く，特殊な測定機器がなくても，定量的に判定できる方法を導入することを念頭に入れ，コロニー形成法を掲載した．

4.4　直接接触法の実施とその注意点

　直接接触法による細胞毒性試験は，抽出法による細胞毒性試験の実施に加えて，抽出時に失活することが予想される材料及び眼粘膜に接触する材料について実施する．試験が困難な材料でも，眼粘膜に接触する材料や，刺激への感受性が敏感な組織に使用する材料については，直接接触法に相当する感度で細胞毒性の評価を実施する．なお，直接接触法は，細胞が付着しにくい材料の場合には見かけ上コロニー形成能が低下することや，抽出条件や処理条件が抽出法と必ずしも同じではないことから，その評価が困難な場合がある．そのような場合には，半円板の試験試料を用いる方法や，セルカルチャーインサートのフィルター膜に細胞を播種し，直接接触法と同様の条件で試験を実施して試験試料の細胞毒性作用を評価する方法もある．

4.5　原料化学物質の試験

　試験試料から溶出する物質の細胞毒性を確認するために，原料化学物質の細胞毒性試験を実施することも想定される．また細胞の感度及び精度を明らかにするために標準物質の細胞毒性試験が行われる．その場合，このガイダンスの抽出溶媒を溶媒として化学物質の原液（溶液又は懸濁液）を調製し，この原液を 100 ％抽出液と読み換えることによって同様の方法で試験が可能である．なお，化学物質の場合の最終処理濃度として OECD テストガイドライン 432 及び OECD ガイダンスドキュメント No. 129 では 1 mg/mL，OECD テストガイドライン 473，476，487，490 では 10 mmol/L，2 mg/mL 又は 2 μl/mL のいずれかの最も低い濃度が採用されている．なお，混合物のような場合には 5 mg/mL が推奨されるかもしれない．

4.6　陰性対照材料及び陽性対照材料の入手先情報

　直接接触法の陰性対照材料を除く対照材料については，下記の機関で検定された材料が頒布されている．

　　（一財）　食品薬品安全センター　秦野研究所　対照材料担当
　　　　　　電話　0463-82-4751，FAX　0463-82-9627
　　　　　　e-mail：rm.office@fdsc.or.jp

　24 ウェルプレート用のプラスチック製カバースリップ（セルデスク LF1），これまで直接接触用の陰性対照材料として推奨されていた組織培養用プラスチックシート及び陽性対照材料 B を用いて 3 機関による共同実験が 2019 年 4 月～2019 年 6 月に行われ，以下のような直接接触法の結果が得られている（試験条件：24 ウェルプレート，V79 細胞 50 個播種 / ウェル，3 ウェル / 試料，繰り返し数 n = 3）．

ment. International validation studies and international round–robin tests have demonstrated that the neutral red test and the colony formation test are suitable for detection of cytotoxicity in chemicals and medical devices. The MTT and XTT assays are common quantitative methods of cytotoxicity assessment.

This guidance is aimed at introducing methods for assessment of the safety of medical devices. The colony formation test is included as it is highly sensitive and allows quantitative assessment without special measuring instruments.

4.4   Criteria and precautions for conducting a test by direct contact

In addition to cytotoxicity assessment by a test on extracts, a test by direct contact should be carried out for materials expected to lose activity during extraction and materials that directly contact the eye mucosa. If the test by direct contact is not suitable for, or difficult to apply to, a material that directly contacts with the eye mucosa or other tissues that are sensitive to irritation, other test methods having equivalent sensitivity to the direct contact by test should be used. The colony–forming ability of a test by direct contact can decrease for materials to which cells do not adhere well. Also, the extraction and treatment conditions for a material in a test by direct contact may not be always the same as those for the test on extracts. These characteristics can make cytotoxicity evaluation difficult. When this is the case, the test may be performed using a half disk–shaped test sample, or by seeding cells onto the filter of a cell culture insert, under the same conditions as those of the test by direct contact.

4.5   A test of chemical substances

To evaluate the cytotoxicity of substances leached from test samples, cytotoxicity of chemicals may also need to be tested. To demonstrate cell response and accuracy of cells in cytotoxicity tests, the control substance is used. In these cases, a cytotoxicity test is possible to perform in the same manner as this guidance by replacing 100 % extracts with stock solutions of test substances. The stock solutions (or suspensions) are prepared using extraction vehicles in this guidance. In OECD Test Guideline No. 432 and OECD Guidance Document No. 129, 1 mg/mL is applied as the maximum final treatment concentration for chemicals, while in OECD Test Guideline Nos. 473, 476, 487 and 490, the lowest concentration, either 10 mmol/L, 2 mg/mL or 2 μL/mL is applied. For mixtures, 5 mg/mL may be recommended.

4.6   Supplier of negative and positive reference materials

Previously validated reference materials are supplied by the following institution, except for negative reference materials used in a test by direct contact:

Person in charge of Reference Materials
Hatano Research Institute, Food and Drug Safety Center
Tel: +81–463–82–4751, Fax: +81–463–82–9627
Email: rm.office@fdsc.or.jp

Collaborative study was performed in 3 testing facilities from April to June 2019 using three materials, a plastic coverslip used in 24–well plate (Cell Desk LF1), a plastic sheet for tissue culturing that has been a recommended negative reference material for a test by direct contact, a positive reference material B. The results are shown below (test conditions: 24–well plate; V79 cells; 50 cells per well; 3 wells per sample; number of repetitions, n = 3).

Cell Desk LF1 may be easily moved in a well because Cell Desk LF1 is smaller than posi-

　なお，セルデスクLF1は，陽性対照材料Bより小さく，ウェル内で動きやすい．固定・染色・カウントの際には，物理的影響によるコロニー損傷に注意する必要がある．

試験施設	コロニー形成率（％）±SD		
	セルデスク LF1	組織培養用プラスチックシート	陽性対照材料 B
A	99.9 ± 3.3	98.5 ± 3.0	0.0 ± 0.0
B	104.3 ± 7.7	97.7 ± 12.3	0.0 ± 0.0
C	96.4 ± 2.7	98.3 ± 8.8	0.0 ± 0.0

SD：標準偏差

4.7　陽性対照材料

　実験系の適切性及び検出感度を判定する物差しとして，弱い細胞毒性を示す陽性対照材料Bと中程度の細胞毒性を示す陽性対照材料Aを採用した．2種の陽性対照材料を導入した目的は，①試験法や細胞の相違，実験室間の変動があっても，これらの陽性対照材料と比較することで試験試料の細胞毒性強度の相対的位置を知る，②その相対的位置から組織刺激性の程度を予測する，ことにある．

　抽出条件が異なる試験試料の結果であっても，試験試料の細胞毒性強度を陽性対照材料の結果と比較することにより，試験試料の組織刺激性の程度の予測が可能となる．

4.8　陽性対照物質及び陽性対照材料の IC_{50} 値

　L929細胞，Balb/3T3 clone A31細胞（MEM10培地を使用），及びV79細胞（M05培地を使用：4.9項参照）を用いた時の IC_{50} 値の幅を参考のため記す．

陽性対照	IC_{50} 値の幅		
	L929 細胞	Balb/3T3 細胞	V79 細胞
ZDBC（μg/mL）	2.5～5.5	0.2～0.4	1.0～4.0[*]
陽性対照材料 A（％）	2～5	2～6	1～3[*]
陽性対照材料 B（％）	50～60	15～25	50～60[*]

[*]MEM10培地使用時のV79細胞における陽性対照物質（ZDBC），陽性対照材料A及びBの IC_{50} 値は，M05培地使用時に比べて，弱い細胞毒性を示す（例えば，ZDBC：4～8 μg/mL，陽性対照材料A：3～8 %，陽性対照材料B：>100 %）．

　またISO/TC 194/WG5が2005～2006年に実施した国際round-robin試験で行われた試験法間の比較結果は以下のとおりであった．

陽性対照	IC_{50} 値の幅（平均）	
	コロニー形成法 （V79 細胞）	NR 法 （Balb/3T3 細胞）
陽性対照材料 A（％）	0.36～1.6（0.57）	7.0～26（6.7）
陽性対照材料 B（％）	24～80（55.9）	32～93（89.4）

　以上の結果は，0.1 g/mLの抽出割合で抽出した対照材料の結果であり，この抽出割合

tive reference material B. Therefore, precautions should be taken not to physically damage any colony during fixation, staining and counting.

Testing facility	Relative plating efficiency (%) ± SD		
	Cell Desk LF1	Plastic sheet for tissue culture	Positive reference material B
A	99.9 ± 3.3	98.5 ± 3.0	0.0 ± 0.0
B	104.3 ± 7.7	97.7 ± 12.3	0.0 ± 0.0
C	96.4 ± 2.7	98.3 ± 8.8	0.0 ± 0.0

SD: Standard deviation

4.7   Positive reference materials

The weakly-cytotoxic positive reference material B and moderately-cytotoxic positive reference material A are introduced as measures of test system reliability and sensitivity. Two positive reference materials are presented because, firstly, comparison of them allows assessment of the cytotoxicities of the materials in relative terms even when differences in test methods and cells or interlaboratory variations exist, and secondly, the relative cytotoxicity of the materials to positive reference materials enables estimation of tissue irritability.

Even if the test sample is extracted under different conditions, tissue irritability of the test sample may be estimated by comparing the cytotoxicity level of the test sample with that of the positive reference materials.

4.8 IC_{50} of positive control substance and positive reference materials

The ranges for IC_{50} values in L929 cells, Balb/3T3 clone A31 cells (with MEM10 culture medium), and V79 cells (with M05 culture medium: see 4.9) are presented below for reference.

Positive control	IC_{50}		
	L929 cell	Balb/3T3 cell	V79 cell
ZDBC (μg/mL)	2.5–5.5	0.2–0.4	1.0–4.0[*]
Positive reference material A (%)	2–5	2–6	1–3[*]
Positive reference material B (%)	50–60	15–25	50–60[*]

[*]The IC_{50} of the positive control substance (ZDBC) and positive reference materials A and B are lower (weaker cytotoxicity) when MEM10 medium is used with V79 cells than when M05 medium is used (i.e., IC_{50} of ZDBC, positive reference material A, and positive reference material B is 4 to 8 μg/mL, 3 to 8 %, and >100 %, respectively).

The results of the international round-robin test, which ISO/TC 194/WG5 conducted for a comparison of test methods in 2005 and 2006, are as follows.

Positive control	IC_{50} (mean)	
	Colony formation test (V79 cell)	Neutral red test (Balb/3T3 cell)
Positive reference material A (%)	0.36–1.6 (0.57)	7.0–26 (6.7)
Positive reference material B (%)	24–80 (55.9)	32–93 (89.4)

The table above references the results of extracts of reference materials at an extraction

でのコロニー形成法が ISO 10993-5 の Annex B に掲載されている．またコロニー形成法は感度の高い試験法であることから，本ガイダンスでは，試験試料の抽出割合を 0.1 g/mL 又は 6 cm^2/mL とした．

4.9　抽出に用いる培養液

　L929 細胞及び Balb/3T3 細胞については，MEM10 培地を抽出溶媒として使用する．V79 細胞を用いる抽出法による試験では，M05 培地を使用すると陽性対照物質及び陽性対照材料に対する感度が高くなる（4.8 項参照）．同等の感度を示すならば MEM10 培地も使用可能である．

　M05 培地の調製法を以下に示した．

　Eagle の MEM で Earle の平衡塩類溶液を含む培地に，MEM 非必須アミノ酸，ピルビン酸ナトリウム（0.11 g/L）及び牛胎児血清（5 vol%）を加える．細胞に影響を及ぼさない濃度で抗生物質を添加してもよい．

　5 〜 10 ％血清含有培養液を用いて 6 cm^2/mL で，37 ℃，24 時間抽出した陽性対照材料 B の溶液を，USP 24 〈87〉 Biological reactivity tests, *In vitro*（以下，Elution Test）に従って試験を実施すると，スコア 4 を示し，細胞毒性は不合格（細胞毒性有り）となるが，同材料を無血清 MEM 培地で抽出した場合には，スコア 2 を示し，細胞毒性は合格判定となる．

　蒸留水を用いて 6 cm^2/mL で，37 ℃，24 時間抽出した陽性対照材料の溶液を Elution Test で評価すると，陽性対照材料 A 及び B ともにスコア 0 を示し，材料中に含まれる細胞毒性を検知できない．さらに，蒸留水を用いて，50 ℃で 72 時間，70 ℃で 24 時間，121 ℃で 1 時間抽出した溶液について，Elution Test で試験した結果，陽性対照材料 A 及び B ともに，細胞毒性を検知することはできなかった．

　蒸留水や無血清培地では，オリゴマーや添加剤のような物質は溶出されにくいこと，また化合物によっては高温で分解されることが検知できない原因として考えられる．したがって，通常は，血清を 5 〜 10 ％含有する培地で抽出した溶液を細胞毒性試験用抽出液として試験する．なお，血清又はタンパクがある種の溶出物に結合することがあることを認識しておく必要がある．

4.10　培養液以外の抽出溶媒

　培養液以外の抽出溶媒として，生理食塩液や精製水を用いた場合には，試験系に添加できる量は限られる（通常，10 vol％が最大量である）．抽出可能な溶出物の検出力を高めるには，試験系に添加する試験液の量を多くする必要がある．そのための方法として，2 〜 5 倍濃い濃度の培養液で精製水抽出液を希釈して試験する方法もある．また DMSO を抽出溶媒とすることも考えられるが，DMSO は 0.5 vol％以上の濃度では試験系において細胞毒性作用があるため，試験系への添加量は 0.5 vol％程度までとなる．したがって，血清含有培養液よりも希釈率が高くなるため DMSO で抽出可能な溶出物の濃度は必ずしも高いとは言えない．このように，培養液以外の抽出溶媒を選択する場合には，抽出可能な溶出物の細胞への最終的なばく露量を考慮して決める必要がある．

ratio of 0.1 g/mL. The colony formation test performed at an extraction ratio of 0.1 g/mL is described in Annex B of ISO 10993-5. Because the colony formation test is highly sensitive for cytotoxicity, this guidance recommends an extraction ratio of 0.1 g/mL or 6 cm^2/mL for a test sample.

4.9   Culture medium for extraction

MEM10 medium is recommended as the extraction vehicle with L929 and Balb/3T3 cells. In the test on extracts using V79 cells, M05 medium can increase sensitivity for the positive control substance and positive reference materials (see 4.8). MEM10 medium may also be used, if MEM10 shows the same sensitivity as M05 medium.

The procedure for preparation of M05 medium is given below.

Add MEM nonessential amino acids, sodium pyruvate (0.11 g/L), L-glutamine (0.292 g/L), sodium bicarbonate (2.2 g/L), and fetal bovine serum (5 %v:v) to Eagle's MEM containing Earle's balanced saline solution. Antibiotics may be included in the medium provided that they do not adversely affect the cells.

When positive reference material B was extracted with a culture medium containing 5 to 10 % serum (6 cm^2/mL, for 24 hours at 37 ℃) and tested in accordance with USP 24 ⟨87⟩ Biological reactivity tests, *In vitro* (hereinafter referred to as Elution Test), the extract showed a cytotoxicity grade of 4, which is outside the acceptable cytotoxicity limit. When the same material was extracted using in MEM medium without serum, the cytotoxicity grade was 2, which is within the acceptable limit.

When the Elution Test was used to evaluate the positive reference materials by extracting with distilled water (6 cm^2/mL, for 24 hours at 37 ℃), both the positive reference materials A and B produced a grade of 0, indicating that the test did not detect any cytotoxicity. When the materials were extracted using distilled water for 72 hours at 50 ℃, 24 hours at 70 ℃, and 1 hour at 121 ℃, the Elution Test again failed to detect cytotoxicity in either positive reference material A or B.

The reasons the test failed to detect cytotoxicity were mostly likely because substances such as oligomers and excipients do not elute well in distilled water or serum-free media and because some compounds degrade at high temperatures. Therefore, a test on extracts should generally use a test solution obtained by extracting the test material in a culture medium containing 5 to 10 % serum.

It is important to recognize that serum/proteins are known to bind, to some extent, extractables.

4.10   Extraction vehicles other than culture medium

When physiological saline and purified water is used as the extraction vehicle, it can only be added up to a certain limit (normally 10 % by volume) to a culture medium. It is necessary to use a larger amount of test solution in the test system to increase the detectability of extractable components. Extract with purified water may also be diluted with a 2 to 5 times concentrated culture medium to achieve this. DMSO can also be used as the extraction vehicle, but DMSO may only be added up to 0.5 % by volume as DMSO is cytotoxic at greater than 0.5 % (volume fraction). The cellular exposure concentration of extractables in DMSO will be lower due to the greater dilution as compared to extraction in culture medium with serum. Therefore, consideration should be given to the final amount of exposure of extractables to the cells when selecting anything other than culture medium as the extraction vehicle.

4.11　コロニー形成までの培養期間

　肉眼で判断できるコロニーを形成させるまでの培養期間は，細胞株の種類によって異なる．一般的には，Balb/3T3 clone A31 細胞は 9〜11 日間，L929 細胞は 7〜9 日間，V79 細胞は 6〜7 日間が目安である．しかしながら，コロニーのサイズや形態は，細胞の増殖率に依存することから，試験条件，特に試験に使用する血清のロットによる影響が大きい．したがって，試験施設ごとに試験条件を検討し最適な培養期間を決定するとよい．

4.12　染色液

　コロニーの染色は，一般的には市販のギムザ染色液を使用直前にリン酸緩衝液（M/15，pH 6.4）で 10〜50 倍に希釈して使用する．染色時間は，コロニーがはっきりと染色される時間で十分である．また染色の目的は，コロニーの判別を容易にすることであるから，クリスタルバイオレットなどで染色してもよい．

4.13　細胞毒性強度と組織刺激性との相関

　細胞毒性強度を示す IC_{50}（％）値と種々の生体組織での刺激性強度との関係を図1（原典の参考文献 3）の図を，参考文献 4）及び 5）を参考に一部改変）に示す．ZDEC を種々の濃度で含む対照材料をこのガイダンスに従って抽出し，Balb/3T3 clone A31 細胞を用いたコロニー形成法で IC_{50} 値を求めた．一方，対照材料をコンタクトレンズにコーティングし，ウサギ眼への装用試験，対照材料のウサギ筋肉内埋植試験，及び健常皮膚へのパッチ試験を行い，IC_{50} 値と in vivo 刺激性強度との関係を明らかにした．その結果，同じ細胞毒性強度を示す材料では，眼粘膜が最も感受性が高く，IC_{50} 値 35 ％近辺以下を示す材料を装用すると眼刺激性を生じた．筋肉組織に対しては，IC_{50} 値が 5 ％近辺以下の材料で炎症反応がおきた．一方，健常皮膚では，0.1 ％の IC_{50} 値を示す強い対照材料でも皮膚刺激性は認められなかった．このように対照材料を用いると組織間の感受性の違いも明らかになる．

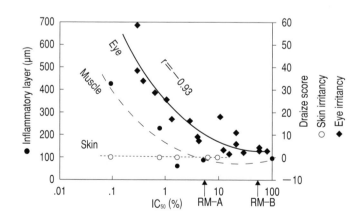

図1　材料の細胞毒性強度と異なる組織での刺激性との関係

4.11 Incubation period required for formation of colonies

The period of incubation sufficient for macroscopic colony formation varies with the cell line used. Normally, it is roughly 9 to 11 days with Balb/3T3 clone A31 cells, 7 to 9 days with L929 cells, and 6 to 7 days with V79 cells. However, as colony sizes and morphology also depend on the growth rate, the optimal incubation period varies with test conditions, particularly with the serum used. Therefore, the suitable incubation period should be determined at each laboratory after validation testing of the test conditions.

4.12 Staining solution

Normally, colonies are stained with commercially available Giemsa's stain diluted with phosphate buffer (M/15, pH 6.4) 10 to 50 times immediately before use. The cells are stained until the colonies are clearly stained. Crystal violet solution also may be used for staining as staining is aimed at achieving better differentiation of colonies.

4.13 Correlation between cytotoxicity and tissue irritability

Figure 1 (this figure originated in the reference No. 3 has been partially modified referring to reference No. 4 and 5) shows the correlation between IC_{50} values (%), an index of cytotoxicity, and irritancy in tissues. A reference material containing different concentrations of ZDEC was extracted in accordance with this guidance, and the IC_{50} values were calculated in a colony formation test using Balb/3T3 cells. Also, eye irritation test using the reference material-coated contact lenses, muscular implantation test and skin irritation test using the reference material were conducted in rabbits to investigate the correlation between IC_{50} values and *in vivo* irritancy. These tests showed that the eye mucosa was most sensitive to cytotoxic effects and that a coated lens having cytotoxic effects of an IC_{50} of about 35 % or less was irritant in the eye mucosa. Inflammatory response was observed in the muscle tissue when a reference material having cytotoxic effects of an IC_{50} of about 5 % or less was implanted. In healthy skin no irritation was observed even with a reference material having cytotoxic effects of an IC_{50} of 0.1 %. Using the reference materials can therefore clarify differences in sensitivity to cytotoxic effects between tissues.

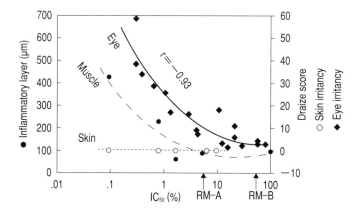

Fig. 1 Relationship between cytotoxic potential of materials and irritation in different tissues

細胞毒性強度（IC_{50} 値）	予測される生物学的反応
コロニー形成率の低下（70 ％未満）が認められたが，100 ％以上	非常に弱い細胞毒性が示された[#]．
陽性対照材料 B より弱い	弱い細胞毒性が示された． 弱い眼粘膜刺激が起こり得る．
陽性対照材料 A と B の中間	中程度の細胞毒性が示された． 粘膜組織に対しても炎症反応がおきる場合がある．
陽性対照材料 A より強い	強い細胞毒性が示された． 筋肉組織に対して炎症反応がおきる可能性が高い．

[#]：抽出法によるコロニー形成法で 100 ％以上の IC_{50} 値を示す場合でも Draize score 4 以下の眼粘膜刺激性を示す場合があることを認識する必要がある．

4.14　結果の評価

　　細胞毒性試験の結果は，他の生物学的安全性試験結果や医療機器の使用目的などを考慮して評価すべきである．細胞毒性作用有りという結果が得られた場合には，血清の濃度や血清不含の培養液を用いた抽出法による追加試験や原因物質の特定などの他の試験を実施することを検討する．何らかの細胞毒性作用が考えられる場合においても，それは生体内における毒性の可能性を示唆する結果ではあるが，必ずしも医療機器として不適切であるということを意味するわけではない．

5．薬食機発 0301 第 20 号からの変更点

1)　記載内容の大きな変更は無いが，前回の改訂で ISO 10993-5 との整合性を考慮したことにより，不明確となっていた以下の点について明確にした．
- ・抽出溶媒として血清含有培養液を用いること
- ・対照材料の抽出溶媒は血清含有培養液を用い，原則，37 ± 1 ℃で 24 ± 2 時間抽出すること
- ・血清含有培養液以外の抽出溶媒を用いる時はコントロール群とは別に溶媒対照群を設けること

2)　抽出操作について，ISO 10993-12 との整合性を考慮し，容易に攪拌抽出ができるように，炭酸ガス培養器での抽出に限定せず，抽出温度と抽出時間の記載とした．

3)　原料化学物質の試験法について，参考情報に加えた．それにともない以下の点も変更した．
- ・ZDBC を原料化学物質の細胞毒性試験を実施する場合の陽性対照物質として使用することを記載した．
- ・試験報告書の陽性対照物質（ZDBC）関連の記載を変更した．

6．参考文献

1)　日本組織培養学会編：細胞トキシコロジー試験法，朝倉書店（1991）
2)　大野忠夫編著：動物実験代替法マニュアル，培養細胞を用いた理論と応用，共立出版（1994）
3)　中村晃忠：医用材料の細胞毒性試験における標準材料，組織培養 22：228-233

Degree of cytotoxicity (IC_{50})	Expected biological response
$\geq 100\ \%$, however, decreasing of the relative plating efficiency (less than 70 %)	Very weak cytotoxicity[#].
Weaker than positive reference material B	Weak cytotoxicity. Weak irritation of the eye mucosa may occur.
Between positive reference materials A and B	Moderate cytotoxicity. Inflammatory response may occur in mucosal tissues.
Stronger than positive reference material A	Strong cytotoxicity. Inflammatory response likely to occur in the muscle tissue.

#: It should be noted that a material showing an IC_{50} of 100 % or higher in a colony formation test (test on extracts) can cause eye mucosal irritation of up to 4 on the Draize score.

4.14 Assessment of results

Cytotoxicity data shall be assessed in relation to other biocompatibility data and the intended use of the product. If there is a cytotoxic effect, further evaluation can be performed, for example, additional tests (presence/absence of serum, changing of the level of serum in the culture medium) and chemical characterization of leachable components etc. Any cytotoxic effect can be of concern. However, it is primarily an indication of potential for *in vivo* toxicity and the device cannot necessarily be determined to be unsuitable for a given clinical application based solely on cytotoxicity data.

5. Points changed from MHLW Notification, YAKUSHOKUKI-HATSU 0301 No. 20

1) No major changes have been made to the contents. The following matters that had become unclear by harmonization with ISO 10993-5 in the previous version have been clarified.
   - Use of culture medium with serum as an extraction vehicle
   - Use of culture medium with serum as an extraction vehicle for reference materials, and in principle, to extract at $37 \pm 1\ ℃$ for 24 ± 2 hours
   - When culture medium with serum is not used as an extraction vehicle, establish a vehicle control group in addition to the control group

2) Considering harmonization with ISO 10993-12, extraction conditions described only extraction temperature and time in order to apply extraction not only by standing in a CO_2 incubator but also by agitation.

3) Testing methods for chemical substances have been added to the general information, and the following changes were made along with that addition:
   - Use of ZDBC as a positive control substance when testing cytotoxicity of chemical substances.
   - Changes have been made to the descriptions of the positive control substance (ZDBC) in the test report.

6. References

1) The Japanese Tissue Culture Association, ed.: Cytotoxicology test methods. Asakura Publishing Co., Ltd. (1991)
2) Ohno, T.: Manual of alternative animal testing methods-theory and application of tests using cultured cells. Kyoritsu Shuppan Co., Ltd. (1994)
3) Nakamura, A.: Standard reference materials for cytotoxicity tests of biomaterials. Tissue

（1996）

4)　厚生省薬務局医療機器開発課監修：医療用具及び医療材料の基礎的な生物学的試験のガイドライン 1995 解説，薬事日報社（1996）

5)　日本薬剤師研修センター：医薬品 GLP ガイドブック，薬事日報社（2008）

6)　Nakamura, A., Ikarashi, Y., Tsuchiya, T., Kaniwa, M.-A., Sato, M., Toyoda, K., Takahashi M.: Correlations among chemical constituents, cytotoxicities and tissue responses: in the case of natural rubber latex materials. Biomaterials 11, 92–94 (1990)

7)　Ikarashi, Y., Toyoda, K., Ohsawa, N., Uchima, T., Tsuchiya, T., Kaniwa, M.-A., Sato, M., Takahashi, M., Nakamura, A.: Comparative studies by cell culture and *in vivo* implantation test on the toxicity of natural rubber latex materials. J. Biomed. Master. Res. 26, 339–356 (1992)

8)　Tsuchiya, T., Ikarashi, Y., Hata, H., Toyoda, K., Takahashi, M., Uchima, T., Tanaka, N., Sasaki, K., Nakamura, A.: Comparative studies of the toxicity of standard reference materials in various cytotoxicity tests and *in vivo* implantation tests. J. Applied Biomaterials 4, 153–156 (1993)

9)　Tsuchiya, T., Arai, T., Ohhashi, J., Imai, K., Kojima, H., Miyamoto, S., Hata, H., Ikarashi, Y., Toyoda, K., Takahashi M., Nakamura, A.: Rabbit eye irritation caused by wearing toxic contact lenses and their cytotoxicities: *In vivo/in vitro* correlation study using standard reference materials. J. Biomed. Mater. Res. 27, 885-893 (1993)

10)　Tsuchiya, T., Ikarashi, Y., Arai, T., Ohhashi, J., Isama, K., Nakamura, A.: *In vivo* toxic tissue/biomaterials responses: Correlation with cytotoxic potential but not cell attachment. Clinical Materials 16, 1–8 (1994)

11)　Tsuchiya, T.: Studies on the standardization of cytotoxicity tests and new standard reference materials useful for evaluating the safety of biomaterials. J. Biomaterials Applications 9, 138–157 (1994)

12)　Ohno, T. *et al.*: Validation study on five cytotoxicity assays by JSAAE-1. Overview of the study and analyses of validations of ED50 value. Alternatives to Animal Testing & Experimentation (AATEX) 5, 1–38 (1998)

13)　Tanaka, N. *et al.*：Validation study on five cytotoxicity assays by JSAAE-IV. Details of colony formation assay. AATEX 5, 74–86 (1998)

14)　Isama, K., Matsuika, A., Haishima, Y., Tsuchiya, T.: Proliferation and differentiation of normal human osteoblasts on dental Au-Ag-Pd casting alloy: Comparison with cytotoxicity using fibroblast L929 and V79 cells. Mater. Trans. 119, 61-64 (2001)

Culture 22, 228–233 (1996)

4) Medical Device Development Division, Pharmaceutical Affairs Bureau, Ministry of Health and Welfare, Supervision: Guidelines for basic biological tests of medical materials and devices 1995 –Guide Book, Yakuji Nippo Ltd. (1996)

5) Japan Pharmacists Education Center: GLP Guide Book, Yakuji Nippo Ltd. (2008)

6) Nakamura, A., Ikarashi, Y., Tsuchiya, T., Kaniwa, M.-A., Sato, M., Toyoda, K., Takahashi M.: Correlations among chemical constituents, cytotoxicities and tissue responses: in the case of natural rubber latex materials. Biomaterials 11, 92–94 (1990)

7) Ikarashi, Y., Toyoda, K., Ohsawa, N., Uchima, T., Tsuchiya, T., Kaniwa, M.-A., Sato, M., Takahashi, M., Nakamura, A.: Comparative studies by cell culture and in vivo implantation test on the toxicity of natural rubber latex materials. J. Biomed. Master. Res. 26, 339 –356 (1992)

8) Tsuchiya, T., Ikarashi, Y., Hata, H., Toyoda, K., Takahashi, M., Uchima, T., Tanaka, N., Sasaki, K., Nakamura, A.: Comparative studies of the toxicity of standard reference materials in various cytotoxicity tests and in vivo implantation tests. J. Applied Biomaterials 4, 153–156 (1993)

9) Tsuchiya, T., Arai, T., Ohhashi, J., Imai, K., Kojima, H., Miyamoto, S., Hata, H., Ikarashi, Y., Toyoda, K., Takahashi M., Nakamura, A.: Rabbit eye irritation caused by wearing toxic contact lenses and their cytotoxicities: In vivo/in vitro correlation study using standard reference materials. J. Biomed. Mater. Res. 27, 885–893 (1993)

10) Tsuchiya, T., Ikarashi, Y., Arai, T., Ohhashi, J., Isama, K., Nakamura, A.: In vivo toxic tissue/biomaterials responses: Correlation with cytotoxic potential but not cell attachment. Clinical Materials 16, 1–8 (1994)

11) Tsuchiya, T.: Studies on the standardization of cytotoxicity tests and new standard reference materials useful for evaluating the safety of biomaterials. J. Biomaterials Applications 9, 138–157 (1994)

12) Ohno, T. et al.: Validation study on five cytotoxicity assays by JSAAE-1. Overview of the study and analyses of validations of ED_{50} value. Alternatives to Animal Testing & Experimentation (AATEX) 5, 1–38 (1998)

13) Tanaka, N. et al.: Validation study on five cytotoxicity assays by JSAAE-IV. Details of colony formation assay. AATEX 5, 74–86 (1998)

14) Isama, K., Matsuoka, A., Haishima, Y., Tsuchiya, T.: Proliferation and differentiation of normal human osteoblasts on dental Au-Ag-Pd casting alloy: Comparison with cytotoxicity using fibroblast L929 and V79 cells. Mater. Trans. 119, 61–64 (2001)

第 2 部　感作性試験

1．適用範囲

　本試験は，医療機器又は原材料が遅延型アレルギー反応の一つである感作性を引き起こす可能性を評価するためのものである．ここでは，モルモットを用いる試験法として Maximization Test（別名：Guinea pig maximization test: GPMT）と Adjuvant and Patch Test（A&P，別名：scratched skin method）の 2 種と，マウス局所リンパ節試験（Local Lymph Node Assay: LLNA）を記載した．

　なお，この試験は，即時型アレルギー（抗原性）を検出する目的のものではない．

2．引用規格

　ISO 10993-10: 2010, Biological evaluation of medical devices-Part 10: Tests for irritation and skin sensitization

3．試験試料と試験法の選択

3.1　原則

　試験の具体的手技は，引用規格及び他の公的規格を参考にする．上述の 3 試験法は，適切な抽出液や試験試料を用いて試験を実施する場合には感度は同等とみなされ，リスク評価に用いることが可能である．

　新規原材料を使用している医療機器，使用方法や設計仕様が新規である機器，又は使用期間の変更（短期から長期），用途の変更（表面接触からインプラント）の場合には，特に試験試料の作製及び試験法の選択には十分留意してリスク評価を行う必要がある．以下に代表的な試験法の特徴を示した．

1）　GPMT：感作性試験として確立された方法．試験試料（最終製品又は原材料）あるいは試験試料からの抽出物が皮内投与可能な溶媒に溶解するか，又は均一に分散する場合（フロッキングなどを起こさず注射針を通過する場合）に用いられる．GPMT の特性として，偽陽性が多いこと，色素の評価が困難であることが知られている．

2）　A&P：試験試料からの抽出物が皮内投与可能な溶媒に溶解あるいは分散しない場合（フロッキングなどを起こして注射針を通過しない場合）に用いられる．また医療機器の臨床使用方法が貼付の場合には，GPMT に優先して実施されることがある．A&P では，貼付物の粒子サイズや形状による刺激性が結果に影響することがある．

3）　LLNA：単一化学物質を対象に，GPMT の代替法として国際的に認められている．現在，化学物質に対しては動物愛護の観点も含め，優先される試験となりつつある．LLNA の特性として，偽陰性や偽陽性物質の存在，ある種の金属や高分子化合物といった皮膚に浸透しないものでは正確な評価は難しいことが知られている．同様に，水系媒体では評価が困難な場合がある．また刺激により LLNA が陽性反応を示す可能性のあることも認識しておかなければならない．試験試料は溶液，懸濁液，ゲル若しくはペーストなど，マウスの耳に適用できる性状でなければならない．

　以上のとおり，各試験法にはメリット，デメリットが存在し，いずれの試験法も万能でないことを理解し，適切な試験法を選択することが重要である．試験試料は，適切な媒体に溶解して適用することが原則であるが，生体に適用しても評価に影響するような

Part 2   Sensitization Test

1.   Scope

These tests are designed to assess potential of a medical device or a raw material to induce sensitization, which is one of delayed-type allergic reactions. In this part, the Maximization Test (also referred to as the Guinea pig maximization test: GPMT) and the Adjuvant and Patch Test (A & P, also referred to as Scratched Skin Method), and the Murine Local Lymph Node Assay (LLNA) are described.

These tests are not intended to detect immediate-type hypersensitivity (antigenicity).

2.   Normative reference

ISO 10993-10: 2010, Biological evaluation of medical devices-Part 10: Tests for irritation and skin sensitization

3.   Selection of the test sample and method

3.1   General principles

The actual techniques of the tests should be referred to the normative reference and other official guidance standards. The three test methods mentioned above are regarded to show comparable sensitivity when they are implemented using suitable extracts or test samples and may be applied to evaluation of risks.

It is required to evaluate risks by careful preparation of a test sample and selection of a test method for medical devices with a novel raw material, devices with a new usage or design specification that changes the duration of use (from limited to a long term), or when the intended use changes (from surface contact type to implant type). Major properties of the test methods are described below.

1) GPMT: The test method established as a sensitization test. It is used when a test sample (final product or raw materials) or its extracts is soluble or dispersed uniformly (passable through an injection needle without flocking) in a solvent injectable intradermally. It is known that the GPMT is prone to false-positives and evaluation of pigments is difficult.

2) A&P: The method is used when extracts of a test sample is not soluble or dispersed uniformly (not passing an injection needle due to flocking) in a solvent injectable intradermally. When clinical usage of a medical device is topical application, A&P can be used, instead of the GPMT. In A&P, irritation due to the particle size or shape of a patch may affect the results.

3) LLNA: The method is internationally accepted for testing single chemicals as a stand-alone alternative to GPMT. At present, this is becoming a preferred assay for chemicals including the standpoint of animal welfare. LLNA is characteristically known for false negatives, false positives and difficulty of accurate evaluation of certain metals and high molecular weight substances, which do not penetrate the skin. Likewise, evaluation may be difficult for the test sample in polar solvents. One should be aware that irritation can also result in positive lymph node responses. The test sample shall be solution, suspension, gel or paste such that it can be applied to the ears of the mice.

It is important to understand that each test method is not universal as it has merits and demerits as mentioned above and select a suitable test method. In principle, a test sample

刺激性あるいは感作性を示さない媒体を選択することが肝要である．必要に応じて事前に刺激性あるいは感作性を確認し，刺激性あるいは感作性を示す可能性がある溶媒を用いる場合には，判定時に陰性対照群の反応などを十分に考慮することが望ましい．適切な媒体が見つからない場合は，懸濁液での投与も考慮すべきである．また最終的に選択した媒体が全身毒性又は局所刺激性を示すものである場合は，その毒性を勘案して試験法を選択することが必要である．

3.2　試験試料・試験液の調製と試験法の選択

試験試料の生化学的又は物理化学的特性は試験法の選択に重要である．「基本的考え方」に則り，1．既知の知見を確認し，2．化学的特性評価を行い，3．医療機器のクラス分類，4．原材料の新規性などを十分に評価し，生物学的安全性試験実施の要否を判断しなくてはならない．試験試料と試験法の選択に関しては図1に概要をフローチャートとして示した．その詳細を以下に記載する．

3.2.1　水又はアルコールに溶解するもの

水又はアルコールに溶解するものについては，蒸留水（生理食塩液）又は適切なアルコールに溶解してGPMTにより評価する．あるいは適切なアルコール又はジメチルスルホキシド（DMSO）に溶解してLLNAにより評価する．

3.2.2　金属又はセラミックス

材料を構成する金属のイオンとしての感作性が，適切な感作性試験によって既に確認されている場合は，あらためて試験を実施する必要はない．十分な感作性のデータがない金属元素種が材料に含まれる場合は，当該金属のイオン溶液について，感作性の強さを評価する．例えば，一旦，酸（希塩酸など）による過酷条件で抽出後，中和して（水酸化ナトリウムなどによる中和）pHを中性付近にした（この時金属イオンの一部又は大部分は通常水酸化物などとして沈殿する）金属イオンと金属沈殿物微粒子から成る懸濁液を用いて，感作性の強さを評価することも可能である．

3.2.3　低分子有機化合物

低分子有機化合物については，試験結果の判定に影響を与えない適切な溶媒に溶解又は均一に分散させてGPMT若しくはLLNAにより評価する．GPMTの溶媒としては，植物油，DMSO又は蒸留水が使用可能であるが，これらに溶解せずアセトンなどの有機溶媒に溶解する場合は，有機溶媒に溶解させた後，その溶液に植物油又はDMSOを混ぜながら有機溶媒を揮散させて分散させることも可能である．LLNAでは，アセトン：オリブ油＝4：1（AOO）の混液が用いられることが多い．またアセトン，エタノールなどの有機溶媒に溶解する場合は，有機溶媒をそのまま媒体として用いることも可能である．

3.2.4　高分子化合物

高分子化合物については，原則として抽出率の最も高い有機溶媒による抽出物の溶液を試験液としてGPMT若しくはLLNAにより評価する．この場合の抽出溶媒及び試験

dissolved in an appropriate vehicle should be applied. It is important to select a vehicle that does not exhibit irritation or sensitivity that could affect the evaluation when applied to the body. Irritation or sensitivity should be checked in advance if required. When using a solvent that possibly exhibits irritation or sensitization, it is desirable to sufficiently consider the responses observed in the negative control group during evaluation. Use of a suspension should also be considered when no appropriate vehicle is found. Moreover, the test method should be selected taking the toxicity of the vehicle being chosen into consideration when the chosen vehicle exhibits systemic toxicity or local irritation.

3.2 Preparation of test sample/test solution and selection of the test methods

Biochemical or physicochemical properties of the test sample are important for selecting a test method. In accordance with the "Basic Principles", the necessity of a biological safety test should be judged through full evaluation of 1. confirmation of known findings, 2. chemical characterization, 3. classification of the medical device and 4. novelty of raw materials, etc. Selection of the test sample and test methods is outlined as a flow chart in Fig. 1. The details are described in the following.

3.2.1 Water or alcohol-soluble test samples

Test samples soluble in water or alcohol are dissolved in distilled water (physiological saline) or a suitable alcohol for evaluation by GPMT. Or they may be dissolved in a suitable alcohol or DMSO for evaluation by LLNA.

3.2.2 Metals or ceramics

It is not required to conduct a test when sensitization of a metal ion constituting a raw material has been confirmed already by a suitable sensitization test. When the materials include a metal element not provided with adequate sensitization data, sensitization potential of an ionic solution of the metal should be evaluated. For example, it is possible to evaluate sensitization potential of a suspension consisting of metallic ion and metallic precipitates obtained by extraction under a severe condition with acids (such as dilute hydrochloric acid) and neutralizing (with sodium hydroxide, etc.) to a neutral pH (a part or most of metallic ions are precipitated as hydroxides).

3.2.3 Low-molecular organic compounds

Low-molecular organic compounds are dissolved or dispersed uniformly in a suitable solvent not affecting judgment of the test results and sensitization is assessed by the GPMT or LLNA. While vegetable oil, DMSO and distilled water are usable as a solvent for GPMT, low-molecular organic compounds not soluble in those solvents, but an organic solvent such as acetone may be dissolved in an organic solvent, which is then mixed and dispersed in a vegetable oil or DMSO while volatizing the organic solvent. In LLNA, a commonly used vehicle is an acetone-olive oil (AOO) 4:1 mixture. When the test sample is dissolved in an organic solvent such as acetone or ethanol, the organic solvent itself may be used as a vehicle.

3.2.4 High-molecular weight compounds (Polymers)

For high-molecular weight compounds, in principle, sensitization is assessed by the GPMT or LLNA using an extract with an organic solvent yielding the highest amount of residue

液の調製については，以下の点に留意すること．なお，新規原材料が用いられていない医療機器で，単回かつ一時的接触（24 時間以内）医療機器あるいはクラス I や II など比較的生体への侵襲が小さくリスク管理が容易な医療機器については，有機溶媒以外の抽出液を用いた試験によるリスク評価も可能である．

　　抽出溶媒は，ISO 10993-10 Annex E，E.2.1 に記載されている溶媒及び抽出条件を参考に，抽出率の最も高い溶媒を選択する．

　　有機溶媒としては，通例，メタノール又はアセトンを用いる．ただし，以下の場合は他の適切な有機溶媒を選ぶ．①溶媒中で試験試料が溶解したり，原形をとどめないほど変形・変質するような場合，又は，②メタノール，アセトンによる抽出では十分な量の抽出物が得られない場合．抽出溶媒の次候補としては，2-プロパノール / シクロヘキサン混液（1：1），n-ヘキサンが挙げられる．

　　抽出は，ISO 10993-10 Annex E に準じて行う．細切することで特に問題がなければ試験試料を細切しその重量の 10 倍から 20 倍容量の溶媒を加え，室温で攪拌又は振とうして行う．抽出時間は 24 時間から 72 時間とする．

　　有機溶媒抽出液からの試験液の調製方法には，以下の二とおりが考えられる．すなわち，必要な量の抽出物が得られる場合（第 1 法）と，得られない場合（第 2 法）である．

1)　第 1 法（抽出物【残留物】を用いる方法）

　　抽出液からロータリーエバポレーターを用いて 30 ℃以下で溶媒を留去して残留物を得，この残留物を植物油，DMSO，蒸留水，アセトン又はエタノールに溶解又は均一に分散させて試験液とする．有機溶媒分散液に植物油を添加して，抽出物を植物油に置換して均一に分散させる方法もある．局所適用濃度は，感作の成否の重要な因子であることから，投与濃度は結果に悪影響を与えない範囲で可能な限り高くすることが望ましい．したがって，抽出物の投与濃度は一般的に 10 ％を目安とし，実際に試験に使用した濃度の設定理由を説明すること．

2)　第 2 法（抽出液を用いる方法）

　　ロータリーエバポレーターなどを用いて溶媒留去後，適切な他の溶媒を試験試料 1 g 当たり 1 mL の割合で添加し，溶解又は均一に分散し 100 ％試験液とする．100 g 以上の重量を有する大型の医療機器などの場合の最終濃度は，10 g から 100 g 当たり 1 mL に濃縮調製することも考慮する．

　　第 1 法，第 2 法とも抽出操作ごとに抽出率を求め，抽出量に大きなばらつきのないことを確認しておく．抽出率は，抽出物の重量を直接測定して求めるか，抽出後の試験試料の重量を測定して求める．

　　備考：「必要な量の抽出物が得られる場合」とは，通例試験試料から得られる抽出物量が試験試料の重量の 0.5 ％以上を目安とする．ただし，1 回に用いる医療機器（最終製品）の重量が 0.5 g 未満の小さな医療機器の場合は 1 ％以上を目安とする．また事前に検討して求めた抽出率は，試験液の調製方法を選択する際の目安である．実際の試験液調製時には，調製量の違いなどから，誤差を生じる場合のあることを考慮する．

as the test solution. In this case, the extraction solvent and test solution should be prepared in consideration of the following points. For medical devices without novel raw materials intended for a single use and limited body contact (within 24 hours) as well as Class I or II medical devices, which are relatively less invasive and thus require simple risk management, the risk may be assessed using the test results derived from an extract other than organic solvents.

A solvent yielding the highest amount of residues is chosen as the extraction solvent by referring to solvents and extracting conditions described in ISO 10993−10 Annex E, E.2.1. In general, methanol and acetone are the recommended organic solvents for extraction. However, other suitable organic solvents should be selected if (1) the test sample dissolves or is deformed/denatured beyond recognition, or (2) a sufficient amount of residues is not obtained with methanol or acetone. N−hexane or a 1:1 mixture of cyclohexane and 2−propanol can be used as an alternative extraction solvent.

Extraction is performed in accordance with ISO 10993−10 Annex E. The test sample is cut into small pieces, if it doesn't happen any problem, mixed with 10 to 20 volumes of a solvent to the weight of the sample, and agitated or shaken at room temperature. The extraction period is for 24 to 72 hours.

There are two methods for preparing the test solution from the organic solvent extract. Method 1 is applicable when a sufficient amount of residues is obtained, while Method 2 is applicable when the amount of residues obtained by extraction of a test sample is not sufficient.

1) Method 1 (method using extracts [residue])

The extract is evaporated at 30 ℃ or lower using a rotary evaporator to evaporate the solvent and the residue is dissolved or dispersed uniformly in a vegetable oil, DMSO, distilled water, acetone or ethanol, which is then used as the test solution. Another method is the addition of vegetable oil to an organic solvent dispersion, so that the organic solvent is replaced with vegetable oil for uniform dispersion of the residue. Concentration for local application is a critical factor in affecting the success of sensitization and the concentration of the test article is desirable to be as high as possible within the range not affecting the results adversely. Therefore, the concentration of the extracts is generally on the level of 10 %, and the basis for setting the concentration used in the test should be explained.

2) Method 2 (method using extract solution)

After removing the solvent using a rotary evaporator etc., add 1 mL of another suitable solvent per 1 g of test sample, and dissolve or uniformly disperse to make a 100 % test solution. Take into consideration that the final concentration of a large medical device weighing 100 g or more should be prepared by evaporating to 1 mL/10 g or 100 g.

For both Methods 1 and 2, in parallel to each extraction procedure of the test sample, determine the percent yield of the residues and ensure that variation of the extracted amount is not large. The percent yield of the residues is obtained by directly measuring the weight of the residue or measuring the weight of the test sample after extraction.

Note: "A case that the sufficient amounts of residues can be obtained" is generally a case that the amount of residues obtained from the test sample is at least 0.5 % of the weight of it. However, when the weight of the medical device (final product) used at one time is less than 0.5 g, it is 1 % or more of the weight of the test sample. The percent yield of the residues being determined in advance is a guide for selecting a test solution preparation method. Take into consideration that percent yield may be varied

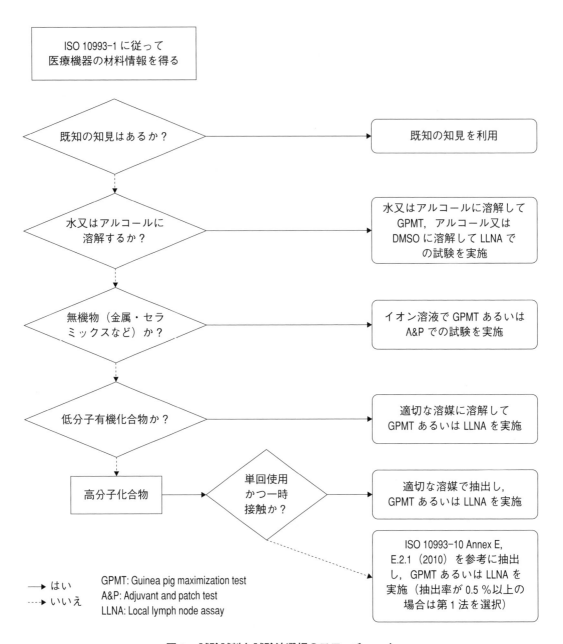

図1 試験試料と試験法選択のフローチャート

due to a difference in the amount of preparation, etc. when a test solution is actually prepared.

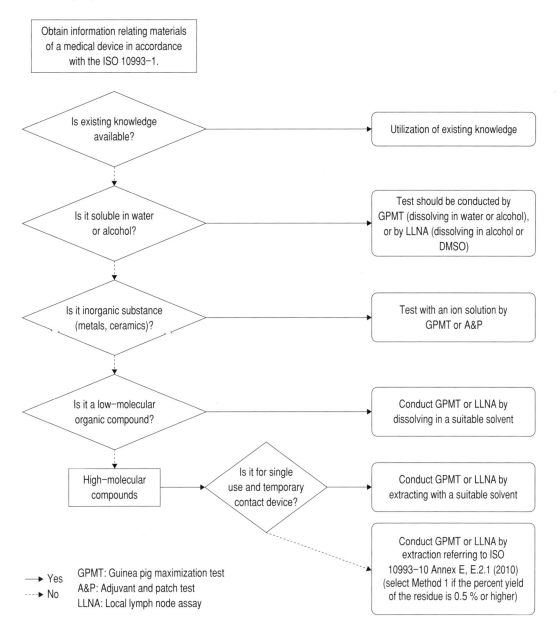

Fig. 1 Flow chart for selecting the test sample and the test method

4．GPMT

4.1　試験法

4.1.1　試験動物と動物数

　　体重 400 g 前後の健康な若齢白色モルモット（通常 1 ～ 3 カ月齢）を使用する．雄ないし雌の動物を使用することが可能であるが，雌を使用する場合は妊娠していない未経産の動物を使用する．

　　動物数は，試験群 10 匹，対照群は最低 5 匹とする．感作性評価が困難な場合には，再惹起あるいは動物数を増やすなどの対応が必要である．また動物は無作為に各群に振り分けるようにする．

4.1.2　群構成及び陽性対照物質

　　試験群と陰性対照群，陽性対照群を設定する．惹起濃度を複数設定できる場合には試験群を 1 群とし，陰性，陽性対照群の 3 群設定する．また試験液を希釈あるいは濃縮して感作濃度を複数設定できる場合には試験群を最低 3 群設定し，用量依存性を評価する方法もある．生理食塩液抽出液のように，濃縮処理などが困難でかつ抽出液の原液で感作することで十分に安全性を評価できると判断される場合も，試験群を 1 群とし，陰性，陽性対照群の 3 群での試験も可能である．

　　陽性対照物質は，試験動物の感度及び感作性の強さの比較に必要であり，次のような物質が用いられている．p-フェニレンジアミン（CAS No. 106-50-3），1-クロロ-2,4-ジニトロベンゼン（CAS No. 97-00-7），重クロム酸カリウム（CAS No. 77781-50-9），硫酸ネオマイシン（CAS No. 1405-10-3），硫酸ニッケル（CAS No. 7786-81-4）．その他，文献で知られた感作性物質も使用可能である．

4.1.3　感作

1)　一次感作

　　あらかじめ刈毛したモルモットの肩甲骨上部皮膚（約 2 × 4 cm）に，以下のものを図 2 に示すように左右対称に 0.1 mL ずつ皮内注射する．

　(a)　生理食塩液あるいは蒸留水と Freund 完全アジュバント（FCA）の 1：1 の油中水型（W/O），乳化物（E-FCA）

　(b)　各試料液（試験液，陽性対照液，陰性対照（溶媒）液）

　(c)　(b)の試料液（有機溶媒などの濃縮可能な抽出溶媒を使用した場合は(b)の 2 倍濃度）と FCA との等量混合物（乳化が難しい場合はあらかじめ媒体と FCA の乳化物を調製後，試料液と等量混合し乳化する方法，あるいは，FCA に被験物質を溶解あるいは懸濁後，生理食塩液あるいは蒸留水と等量混合し乳化する方法もある．）

2)　二次感作

　　皮内注射後 7 ± 1 日目に，皮内注射部位（刈毛した肩甲骨上部皮膚部，図 2）にラウリル硫酸ナトリウム（ワセリン中 10 ％）を塗布する．ただし，試料液に刺激性がある場合，この操作は不要である．翌日，ラウリル硫酸ナトリウム（ワセリン中 10 ％）の残留が認められた場合はそれを拭き取った後，同一部位に試料液(b) 0.2 mL を 48 ± 2 時間閉塞貼付する．

4. GPMT

4.1 Test methods

4.1.1 Test animals and number of animals

Healthy young white guinea pigs (usually 1 to 3 months old), each weighing about 400 g shall be used. Either male or female animals may be used. If female animals are used, they shall be nulliparous and not pregnant.

Treat 10 animals with the test sample and use a minimum of 5 animals as a control group. When evaluation of sensitization is controversial, it is necessary to re-challenge those animals or retest with increasing the number of animals. Randomly allocate the animals to respective groups.

4.1.2 Group composition and positive control substances

Test group(s), negative control groups and positive control groups shall be prepared. If multiple concentrations can be set for the challenge procedure, one test group and each group for negative control and positive control (total three groups) shall be prepared. If more than one concentration can be set for the induction procedure by dilution or concentration of the test solution, it is possible to evaluate dose dependence by providing at least 3 test groups. The test may be performed with one test group and each group for negative and positive controls (total three groups) when concentration of the test solution is difficult such as a case of extract with physiological saline and the safety can be thoroughly evaluated by induction using the undiluted extract.

A positive control substance is necessary for comparison of sensitivity and sensitization potential of test animals and following substances are used: p phenylene diamine (CAS No. 106-50-3), 1-chloro-2,4-dinitrobenzene (CAS No. 97-00-7), potassium dichromate (CAS No. 77781-50-9), neomycin sulfate (CAS No. 1405-10-3) and nickel sulfate (CAS No. 7786 -81-4). In addition, sensitizers listed in literatures may be used.

4.1.3 Induction

1) Primary induction

The following substances prepared should be intradermally injected at a dose of 0.1 mL at 6 symmetrical sites as shown in Fig. 2 on the clipped skin area (approximately 2×4 cm) of the upper back of the guinea pig.

(a) A water in oil (W/O) emulsion of physiological saline or distilled water and Freund complete adjuvant (FCA) at 1:1 (E-FCA)

(b) Each sample solution (test solution, positive control solution or negative control solution [solvent])

(c) Emulsified mixture of the test solution (at a concentration 2 times that of the test solution in (b) if an extraction solvent that can be concentrated is used, such as an organic solvent) and FCA at 1:1 (If emulsification is unfeasible, it can be done by preparing an emulsified mixture of the vehicle and FCA in advance and then mixing with equal amounts of test solution, or by dissolving or suspending the test substance with FCA and then mixing with an equal amount of physiological saline or distilled water).

2) Secondary induction

On 7 ± 1 days after the intradermal injection, sodium lauryl sulfate (10 % in Vaseline) is applied on the intradermal injection sites (clipped skin area on the upper back Fig. 2). The sample is demonstrating an irritancy potential, this procedure can be omitted. If the residue of sodium lauryl sulfate (10 % in Vaseline) is observed on the following day, wipe the residue and apply a closed patch of 0.2 mL of the sample solution (b) on the same sites for 48 ± 2 hours.

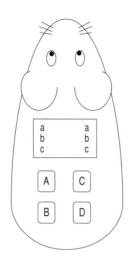

図2　皮内注射及び貼付による感作誘導部位と
　　　惹起貼付部位
　　　a，b及びcは皮内注射部位，□□□は
　　　貼付部位（2 cm×4 cm）を示す．□は
　　　惹起部位を示す。

4.1.4　惹起

　閉塞貼付後14±1日目に，試料液を適切な溶媒に溶解あるいは混合したもの及びその段階希釈した試料液をあらかじめ刈毛した背部又は側腹部に適用する．試験群には，溶媒のみ（0 %液）も適用し，判定の参考にする．

　惹起に用いる濃度は，予備試験で刺激性を示さなかった最高濃度から段階的に希釈したもの各0.1 mLを個々のモルモットの皮膚に適用する（図2）．試料液が生理食塩液及び植物油抽出液では，段階希釈をせずに抽出原液のみで惹起することも可能である．適用は，閉塞貼付あるいは開放塗布で行う．原料化学物質あるいは金属材料を試験する場合であって，それらが水溶性の場合は水溶液を用いてもかまわない．

　植物油（オリブ油，綿実油及びゴマ油など）は刺激性あるいは感作性を示すことがあるので，陰性対照群の反応などを十分考慮して判定すること．

4.1.5　皮膚反応の判定

　閉塞貼付の場合は，24±2時間後に貼付物を取り去り，その24±2及び48±2時間後に皮膚反応を通常の判定基準に従って採点し，以下のように表示する．通常の判定基準とは，表1に示した評点などをさす．

　開放塗布の場合は，塗布後24±2，48±2，72±2時間の皮膚反応を採点する．

　なお，平均評価点が約1.0になる惹起濃度から，およその最低感作濃度を推定することができる[1]．

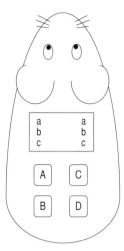

Fig. 2　**Induction sites and challenge sites by intradermal injection and patch application**
a, b and c show intradermal injection sites, and the area surrounded by a rectangle shows the application site (2×4 cm).
The areas surrounded by squares show the challenge sites.

4.1.4　Challenge

On 14±1 days after the application of the closed patch, apply the sample solution dissolved or mixed in a suitable solvent and the serial dilutions of these solutions on the hair clipped back or flank area. Apply the solvent (0 % test sample solution) alone in the test group for reference of judgment.

Apply 0.1 mL each of the solutions prepared by serial dilution of the sample solution from the highest concentration not exhibiting irritation in the preliminary test to the skin of individual guinea pigs (Fig. 2). If an extract with physiological saline or vegetable oil is used as the test solution, the challenge procedure can be done with undiluted extract (no serial dilution). Application is conducted by closed patch or open application. An aqueous solution may be used for testing a chemical raw material or metallic material that is soluble in water.

Since a vegetable oil (olive oil, cotton seed oil, sesame oil, etc.) may exhibit irritation or sensitization, the result should be evaluated with thorough consideration of the reaction in the negative control group.

4.1.5　Assessment of skin reactions

In case of a closed patch, remove the patch after 24±2 hours and score skin reactions at 24±2 and 48±2 hours after the removal in accordance with the general evaluation criteria of skin reactions shown and present the results as follows. The general assessment criteria means the criteria as shown in Table 1.

In case of open application, score skin reactions at 24±2, 48±2 and 72±2 hours after application.

The minimum induction concentration may be estimated from the challenge concentration that gives the mean score of about 1.0[1].

表1　皮膚反応の評点付け（ISO 10993-10, 7 Magnusson and Kligman scale）

視認できる変化なし	0
非常に軽度なあるいはパッチ状紅斑	1
中程度で一体化した紅斑	2
高度紅斑及びあるいは浮腫	3

4.2　試験報告書

試験報告書には，少なくとも以下の事項を記載する．

1)　試験実施機関及び試験責任者
2)　試験実施期間
3)　試験試料（最終製品又は原材料）を特定する要素
　　（例：医療機器の名称，製造販売業者名，製造番号，材料，滅菌方法，形状，物理学的特性など）
4)　使用した対照物質（陽性対照物質）
　　（例：対照物質名，入手先，製造番号など）
5)　試験液の調製方法
　　（抽出方法，抽出率を含む）
6)　試験動物の種と系統，数，週齢，性別
7)　試験方法
8)　実験開始時及び終了時の個別体重
9)　個々の動物の皮膚反応結果及び総括表
10)　結果の評価と考察
11)　参考文献

　　採点結果は下表に例示するごとく，惹起濃度，陽性率，平均評価点などが見やすいものを作成する．

Table 1　Scoring system for skin reaction (source: Table 4 Magnusson and Kligman scale shown in Section 7 of ISO 10993-10)

No visible change	0
Discrete or patchy erythema	1
Moderate and confluent erythema	2
Intense erythema and/or swelling	3

4.2　Test report

The test report shall include the following details at the minimum:

1) Name of the testing agency and study director
2) Test period
3) Factors to identify the test sample (medical device or its raw materials)
   (e.g., name of the medical device, name of the marketing authorization holder, manufacturing number, materials, sterilization process, shape, physical properties, etc.)
4) Control materials (positive control substances)
   (e.g. name of the control substance, supplier, manufacturing number, etc.)
5) Method employed in preparing the test solution (including the extraction method and the percent yield of the residue)
6) Species and strain, number, age by weeks and sex of test animals
7) Test methods
8) Individual body weights at the start and the end of experiment
9) Results of skin reactions in individual animals and summary table
10) Evaluation of results and discussion
11) References

Summary tables for the results of scoring should be prepared so that challenge concentrations, positive rates, mean scores are easily understood as exemplified in the following tables.

第1法の総括表の例（抽出率 0.5 ％）

感作濃度	惹起濃度 (％)	観察時間 (hr)[*1]	評価	
			陽性率[*2]	平均評価点[*3]
10 ％[*4]	10	24	100	2.4
		48	100	3
	1	24	80	1.6
		48	90	2
	0.1	24	20	0.2
		48	20	0.2
	0.01	24	0	0
		48	0	0
	0	24	0	0
		48	0	0

*1　観察時間は，貼付物除去後 24 時間と 48 時間
*2　（陽性動物数 / 当該群の動物数）×100
*3　当該群における Magnusson and Kligman scale などによる反応評価点の総計 / 動物総数
*4　抽出物の重量を測定し，投与用媒体に希釈して調製

第2法の総括表の例（抽出率 0.1 ％）

感作濃度	惹起濃度 (％)	観察時間 (hr)[*1]	評価	
			陽性率[*2]	平均評価点[*3]
100 ％[*4]	100	24	100	3
		48	100	3
	50	24	100	2
		48	100	2
	25	24	100	1.2
		48	100	1
	12.5	24	100	1
		48	0	0
	0	24	0	0
		48	0	0

*1　観察時間は，貼付物除去後 24 時間と 48 時間
*2　（陽性動物数 / 当該群の動物数）×100
*3　当該群における Magnusson and Kligman scale などによる反応評価点の総計 / 動物総数
*4　抽出液を濃縮した後，適切な投与用溶媒で元の試験試料 1 g 当り 1 mL 溶液にする．

Example of summary table of Method 1 (the percent yield of the residue: 0.5 %)

Induction concentration	Challenge concentration (%)	Observation period (hr)[1]	Evaluation	
			Positivity rate[2]	Mean evaluation score[3]
10 %[4]	10	24	100	2.4
		48	100	3
	1	24	80	1.6
		48	90	2
	0.1	24	20	0.2
		48	20	0.2
	0.01	24	0	0
		48	0	0
	0	24	0	0
		48	0	0

[1] Observe the skin reactions at 24 and 48 hours after patch removal.
[2] (Number of animals giving positive reactions/Number of animals in the group) × 100
[3] Total score of reactions evaluated by the Magnusson and Kligman scale, etc. in the group/total number of animals
[4] Prepared by measuring the weight of the residue and diluting with the dosing vehicle

Example of summary table of Method 2 (the percent yield of the residue: 0.1 %)

Induction concentration	Challenge concentration (%)	Observation period (hr)[1]	Evaluation	
			Positivity rate[2]	Mean evaluation score[3]
100 %[4]	100	24	100	3
		48	100	3
	50	24	100	2
		48	100	2
	25	24	100	1.2
		48	100	1
	12.5	24	100	1
		48	0	0
	0	24	0	0
		48	0	0

[1] Observe the skin reactions at 24 and 48 hours after patch removal.
[2] (Number of animals giving positive reactions/Number of animals in the group) × 100
[3] Total score of reactions evaluated by the Magnusson and Kligman scale, etc. in the group/total number of animals
[4] After concentrating the extract, it shall be made 1 mL per 1 g of original test sample by an appropriate vehicle for administration.

5．A&P

5.1　試験法

5.1.1　試験動物と動物数

　　4.1.1 と同様に動物を選択し，準備する．

5.1.2　群構成及び陽性対照物質

　　試験群と陰性対照群，陽性対照群を設定する．惹起濃度を複数設定できる場合には試験群を 1 群とし，陰性，陽性対照群の 3 群設定する．また試験液を希釈あるいは濃縮して感作濃度を複数設定できる場合には試験群を最低 3 群設定し，用量依存性を評価する方法もある．最終製品で直接感作することで十分に安全性を評価できると判断される場合も，試験群を 1 群とし，陰性，陽性対照群の 3 群での試験も可能である．

　　陽性対照物質は，4.1.2 に従って適切な物質を選択する．

5.1.3　感作

1) あらかじめ刈毛したモルモットの肩甲骨上部皮膚（約 2 × 4 cm）の 4 隅に，4.1.3 (a) E-FCA を 0.1 mL ずつ皮内注射する．
2) E-FCA 注射部位に注射針を用いて＃型の傷をつける．その部位に試料約 0.1 mL を 24 ± 2 時間閉塞貼付する．揮発性の有機溶媒による試験液で試験する場合は，開放適用してもよい．最終製品を直接適用する場合は，1.5×1.5 cm 大の四角形あるいは直径 1.5 cm 大の円形に整形したものを貼付する．
3) 1 日 1 回，計 3 回連続して 2) の操作を繰り返す．
4) 感作開始 7 ± 1 日後に，皮内注射部位（刈毛した肩甲骨上部皮膚部）にラウリル硫酸ナトリウム（ワセリン中 10 %）を塗布する．
5) 翌日，ラウリル硫酸ナトリウム（ワセリン中 10 %）を拭き取った後，同一部位に試料 0.2 mL あるいは 2 × 4 cm 大の四角形に整形したものを 48 ± 2 時間閉塞貼付する．

5.1.4　惹起

　　閉塞貼付後 14 ± 1 日目に，試料液を適切な溶媒に溶解あるいは混合したもの及びその段階希釈した試料液，最終製品を直接適用する場合は，1.5×1.5 cm 大の四角形あるいは直径 1.5 cm 大の円形に整形したものを貼付する．貼付部位は 4.1.4 項と同様とする．試験群には，溶媒のみ（0 %液）も適用し，判定の参考にする．媒体を用いない場合は，無処置部位を確保する．

5.1.5　評価

　　惹起後，4.1.5 に従って評価する．

5.2　試験報告書

　　4.2 項参照．

5. A&P

5.1 Test methods

5.1.1 Test animals and number of animals

The animals shall be selected and prepared in the same manner as in Section 4.1.1.

5.1.2 Group composition and positive control substances

Test group, negative control group and positive control group shall be prepared. If multiple concentrations can be set for the challenge procedure, one test group and each group for negative control and positive control (total three groups) shall be prepared. If multiple concentrations can be set for the induction phase by diluting or concentrating the test solution, it is possible to evaluate dose dependence by having at least 3 test groups. When it is judged that safety can be sufficiently evaluated by sensitizing directly with final product, it is also possible to perform the test consisting of three test groups; one test group, one positive control group and one negative control group.

Appropriate positive control substances shall be selected in accordance with Section 4.1.2.

5.1.3 Sensitization

1) Inject intradermally 0.1 mL of 4.1.3(a) E−FCA at 4 corners of the shaven intrascapular skin (approximately 2×4 cm) of the upper back of guinea pigs.
2) Scratch the injection site of E−FCA in # shape with an injection needle. Apply a closed patch containing approximately 0.1 mL of the sample at the site for $24 + 2$ hours. A test solution in a volatile organic solvent may be applied in an open state. Use a patch cut into a square shape (1.5×1.5 cm) or a round shape (1.5 cm in diameter) when directly applying the final product.
3) Repeat the procedure in Step (2) once daily for 3 consecutive days.
4) On Day 7 ± 1 after the start of the sensitization phase, apply sodium lauryl sulfate (10 % in Vaseline) to the intradermal injection sites (shaven intrascapular skin).
5) Wipe with sodium lauryl sulfate (10 % in Vaseline) the following day, and apply a closed patch containing 0.2 mL of the sample or a 2×4 cm square patch at the same site for 48 ± 2 hours.

5.1.4 Challenge

On Day 14 ± 1 after the application of the closed patch, apply the sample solution dissolved or mixed in a suitable solvent, the serial dilutions of these solutions or a patch cut into a square shape (1.5×1.5 cm) or a round shape (1.5 cm in diameter) when directly applying the final product. Application sites shall be the same as those described in Section 4.1.4. Apply the solvent (0 % solution) alone in the test group for reference of judgment. If any vehicle is not used, set an untreated site.

5.1.5 Evaluation

After the challenge phase, evaluate the test results in accordance with Section 4.1.5.

5.2 Test report

See Section 4.2.

6．LLNA

6.1　試験法

6.1.1　試験動物と動物数

　CBA/Ca 若しくは CBA/J 系統の健康な雌性マウスを使用する．マウスは非妊娠，未経産で，8～12 週齢を用いる．動物数は試験群，対照群ともに 1 群最低 5 匹を使用し，個体別の反応を測定することが望ましい．

6.1.2　群構成及び陽性対照物質

　試験試料が濃縮あるいは希釈により用量を変化させて投与可能な場合には，試験群を 3 群，陰性，陽性対照群を各 1 群設定することが望ましい．陽性対照物質は 4.1.2 を参考にして適切なものを選択する．

6.1.3　感作

　初回投与時にマウスの体重を個別に記録する．適切な媒体で調製された試験試料を 3 日間連続でマウスの両耳の背部に 25 μL 塗布する．3 回の投与は可能な範囲で同等な時間帯に行うことが望ましい．

6.1.4　放射性物質の投与

　初回投与から 6 日後マウスの体重を個体別に測定，記録した後，最後の感作投与から 72 ± 2 時間後に，細胞増殖確認用のラベル化合物を静脈内に投与する．すべての群のマウスに 20 μCi（740 kBq）の ^{3}H-メチルチミジンを含有するリン酸緩衝生理食塩液（PBS）250 μL を尾静脈から投与する．

6.1.5　測定試料の調製

　標識化合物の投与 5 ±0.75 時間後，マウスを安楽死させ，耳介リンパ節を採取する．個別にマウスの両耳のリンパ節をプールする．調製した単離細胞は，遠心分離により 2 回洗浄を行い，PBS に再懸濁する．細胞を 5 w/v％トリクロロ酢酸（TCA）中，4 ± 2℃ で 18 ± 1 時間沈殿させる．最後の遠心分離後，ペレットを 1 mL の TCA に再懸濁し，^{3}H の計測をシンチレーションカウンタで行う．

6.1.6　放射活性測定

　マウス 1 匹当たりのカウント毎分（cpm）でリンパ節の細胞中の放射活性レベルを測定する．cpm を壊変毎分（dpm）に換算する．

6.1.7　反応性評価

　陰性対照群の平均 dpm に対する試験群の平均 dpm の比を Stimulation Index（SI）で表し，3 以上の SI を示した物質を感作性陽性とみなす．必要に応じて統計学的考察を行う．

　陽性対照の SI は 3 以上でなければならない．

6. LLNA

6.1 Test methods

6.1.1 Test animals and number of animals

Healthy female CBA/Ca or CBA/J mice, which shall be nulliparous and not pregnant and aged 8 to 12 weeks. It is desirable to use at least 5 animals in each test group and in the control groups and evaluate reactions in individual animals.

6.1.2 Group composition and positive control substances

If administration is possible by changing dose levels by concentration or dilution of the test sample, provide three test groups and one group each for negative control and positive control. Select a suitable positive control substance referring to Section 4.1.2.

6.1.3 Sensitization

Record the body weights of individual mice at the time of initial administration. Apply 25 μL each of the test sample prepared in a suitable vehicle on the back of both ears for 3 consecutive days. Preferably, perform the 3 administrations at the same time frame as much as possible.

6.1.4 Administration of radioactive substances

After measuring and recording the body weight of individual mice on Day 6 after the initial administration, administer intravenously the labeled compound for detection of cellular growth at 72 ± 2 hours after the last administration. Inject 250 μL of phosphate–buffered physiological saline (PBS) containing 20 μCi (740 kBq) of ^{3}H–methylthymidine into the caudal vein.

6.1.5 Preparation of measurement samples

At 5 ± 0.75 hours after administration of the labeled compound, euthanize mice and collect auricular lymph nodes. Pool lymph nodes sampled from both ears of each mouse. Wash isolated cells twice by centrifugation, and resuspend in PBS. Precipitate the cells in 5 % (w/v) trichloroacetic acid (TCA) at 4 ± 2 ℃ for 18 ± 1 hour. After the final centrifugation, resuspend the pellet in 1 mL of TCA, and measure ^{3}H by a scintillation counter.

6.1.6 Measurement of radioactivity

Determine radioactivity level in cells in lymph nodes by count per minute (cpm) per animal. Convert cpm to disintegration per minute (dpm).

6.1.7 Evaluation of reactivity

Present the ratio of the mean dpm in the test group to that in the negative control group as Stimulation Index (SI) and regard the substances giving SI of 3 or higher as positive sensitizing substances. Statistical analysis and its discussion are performed if needed.
The SI of a positive control must be 3 or higher.

6.2　試験報告書

試験報告書には，少なくとも以下の事項を記載する．

1)　試験実施機関及び試験責任者
2)　試験実施期間
3)　試験試料（最終製品又は原材料）を特定する要素
　　（例：医療機器の名称，製造販売業者名，製造番号，材料，滅菌方法，形状，物理学的特性など）
4)　使用した対照物質（陽性対照物質）
　　（例：対照物質名，入手先，製造番号など）
5)　試験液の調製方法
6)　試験動物の種と系統，数，週齢，性別
7)　試験方法
8)　実験開始時及び終了時の個別体重及び一般状態
9)　個別の放射活性値及び総括表
10)　結果の評価と考察
11)　参考文献

7．参考情報

7.1　薬食機発 0301 第 20 号からの変更点

薬食機発 0301 第 20 号は，事務連絡医療機器審査 No. 36 を踏襲して作成された．今回，薬食機発 0301 第 20 号を改訂するに当たり，原則は踏襲した．その上で今までより表現を明確化し，合わせて ISO 10993-10 との整合性を高め，主として以下の改訂を行った．

1)　GPMT の試験方法の記載を ISO 10993-10 の記載に合わせ，原則として同じ操作手順・評価基準で試験が実施できることを示した．
2)　フローチャートの流れを整理し，見やすくした．

7.2　試験法の選択

GPMT と A&P については多くの経験により，通常の試験試料では，GPMT の感度が高いものの，試験試料の形状によっては A&P が適していることが示されている[2]．LLNA は単一化学物質については，GPMT 及び臨床試験との相関性が認められているが，医療機器の分野ではまだ十分なデータが得られていない．しかし，ISO 10993-10 では，化学物質の試験結果を外挿して医療機器でも十分に感作性を評価できると判断しており，またモデル物質を作製し，その抽出液で試験を行った場合，LLNA でも GPMT と同様の結果が得られたという報告[3]があり，抽出液による試験でも同等性が示されている．LLNA で注意すべき点は，抽出媒体の選択である．特に LLNA は耳に塗布して感作する試験であるため，塗布による感作が十分に行われなければ感度は低下する．そのため，媒体としては生理食塩液などの水系は不適切であり，刺激性の少ないアセトンなどの有機溶媒が適切である．OECD Test Guideline No. 429 で投与媒体として多く利用されているアセトン / オリブ油混液（4：1）での抽出も可能である．他の媒体を選択することも可能であるが，媒体による刺激性について確認しておく必要がある．

以上の点に留意して試験法を選択する場合には，いずれの試験法を用いても感作性を評価することが可能であると判断した．

6.2   Test report

The test report shall include the following items at the minimum:

1) Name of the testing agency and study director
2) Test period
3) Elements identifying the test sample (the final products or raw materials)
   (e.g., name of the medical device, name of manufacturer, manufacturing number, materials, sterilization process, shape, physiological properties, etc.)
4) Control materials (positive control substances)
   (e.g. name of the control substance, supplier, manufacturing number, etc.)
5) Method employed in preparing the test solution
6) Species and strains, number, age in weeks and sex of test animals
7) Test methods
8) Individual body weights and general conditions at the start and the end of experiment
9) Radioactivity in individual animals and summary table
10) Evaluation of results and discussion
11) References

7.   Reference information

7.1   Points changed from MHLW Notification, YAKUSHOKUKI-HATSU 0301 No. 20

YAKUSHOKUKI-HATSU 0301 No. 20 was drawn up on the basis of Jimurenraku No. 36. In revising the YAKUSHOKUKI-HATSU 0301 No. 20 this time, the principles were incorporated. In addition, expressions were further clarified and consistency with ISO 10993-10 was enhanced. The main revisions made are as follows:

1) Description of GPMT test procedures was made consistent with that in ISO 10993-10 to indicate that in principle, the same procedures and evaluation criteria can be used for testing.
2) Flow of the flow chart was arranged to make it easier to see.

7.2   Selection of test methods

Concerning GPMT and A&P, it has been shown by many experiences that the GPMT is more sensitive to general test samples whereas A&P is favorable depending on the shape of the test sample[2]. LLNA has been shown to correlate with GPMT and clinical studies for a single chemical but not sufficient data are available in the field of medical devices. However, in ISO 10993-10, extrapolating the data obtained with a chemical substance was deemed to be sufficient for evaluating the sensitization of a medical device. In addition, it has been reported that the same results were obtained with the extract of a model substance by LLNA and GPMT[3], and equivalence has also been shown in the test using the extract. In LLNA, an extraction vehicle should be selected carefully. As LLNA in particularly is the test to sensitize animals by application of a test sample on ears, the sensitivity decreases when induction by application is insufficient. Therefore, polar vehicles such as physiological saline are inappropriate and organic solvents such as acetone with little irritation are preferred. A mixture of acetone and olive oil (4:1), which is often used as a dosing vehicle in OECD Test Guideline No. 429, can be used for extraction. Other vehicles may be used; however, the irritation of the vehicle must be confirmed.

In consideration of the above points, it was judged possible to evaluate sensitization potential by any of the test methods selected.

7.3　抽出率による試験法の選択

ポリマー製品など，有機溶媒抽出で試験を実施する場合，予備検討として，抽出率を確認しておくことが望ましい．またその抽出物を用い，投与用媒体の検討を行うことも重要である．抽出溶媒は，メタノール，アセトン，2-プロパノール/シクロヘキサン混液（1：1），あるいはn-ヘキサンが一般的に用いられている．これらのうち，メタノールは感作性が知られているので，メタノール抽出物の試験では，投与用媒体にはメタノールを用いない方がよい．

7.4　試験液の調製溶媒について

抽出方法はISO 10993-12に述べられている．試験液の調製溶媒は，抽出物を可溶化し，皮膚透過性を高めることなどを考慮して選択すべきである．

GPMTでは，試験試料を溶解させて投与した方が，検出感度が高まることが知られている．通常，生理食塩液，水，植物油（オリブ油，綿実油及びゴマ油など），DMSO，アセトンなどが汎用されている．DMSO及びアセトンについては，皮内注射によって壊死が生じるために試験の感度が下がることも予想されるが，ごく局所にとどまるような影響で，全身に対する毒性がない場合は，物質を溶解して投与した方が感度は上がることが多い．

LLNAでは，一般的に原料化学物質の溶媒として，アセトン/オリブ油混液（4：1）が用いられている．親水性試料あるいは耳介の皮膚に十分に付着しない液体の試料などは耳介に十分付着するよう塗布方法を工夫すべきである．例えばカルボキシメチルセルロースや水酸化エチルセルロース（0.5 w/v％）のような懸濁液を添加する方法もある．一部の水溶性の化学物質に対しては，DMSOやN,N-ジメチルホルムアミド，エタノールなどが界面活性剤 Pluronic® L92より好ましい．他の溶媒も投与用媒体として使用できるが，抽出媒体への添加や溶媒成分の変更による影響を十分に検証し，記録しなければならない．この影響は陽性対照物質として一般的に用いられる弱若しくは中等度の感作性物質を使用した実験によって検証可能である．さらに，陽性対照物質を試験試料に添加して行う試験によって，調製された抽出液が媒体などによる妨害を受けることなく十分に感作性物質の存在を検出できることを実証することが可能である．

7.5　試験動物について

試験動物の選択に当たっては感受性の高い動物を用いることが原則である．

GPMTやA&Pではいずれもモルモットが用いられている．モルモットが選ばれたのは，感作性反応の感度の良さに加えて，外観的に紅斑及び浮腫を形成し，種々の化学物質においてヒトに類似した反応を示すことが知られており，さらに，豊富な背景データの蓄積があることが主たる理由である．動物の体重は重要な要因であり，あまり小さい（200 g以下）と操作がやりにくく，あまり大きい（600 g以上）と反応性が鈍くなるため，実験開始時の体重が400 g前後の，健康な若齢白色モルモット（通常1～3カ月齢）を用いるのが望ましい．雄ないし雌の動物を使用することが可能であるが，雌を使用する場合は妊娠していない未経産の動物を使用する．

LLNAではDBA/2, B6C3F1, BALB/cなどの系統でも使用可能であるとの報告はあるが，実際に用いる場合にはCBA系統と感度が同等であることを確認する必要がある．各試験で使用するマウスは同一週齢（1週間以内のもの）とする．感度が雌と同等であるこ

7.3 Selection of test methods by the percent yield of residues

When performing sensitization testing with residues of a device, such as polymer resins extracted in organic solvent, a preliminary test should be performed to determine the percent yield of residues. It is also important to determine the vehicle for administration of the residues. Methanol, acetone, a mixture of cyclohexane and 2-propanol (1:1) or N-hexane are generally employed as extraction solvents. Among them, methanol is known for its sensitization potential, therefore, for the test with extracts obtained by methanol extraction, it is not preferable to use methanol as a vehicle for administration.

7.4 Solvents for preparation of test solutions

The extraction methods are described in the ISO 10993-12. Solvents for preparation of the test solution should be selected to solubilize the residues and enhance permeability.

In GPMT, it has been known to improve the sensitivity by administering the test sample being dissolved in a vehicle. Physiological saline, water, vegetable oils (olive oil, cotton seed oil, sesame oil, etc.), DMSO, acetone, etc. are used frequently. With DMSO and acetone, due to necrosis induced by the intradermal injection, the sensitivity of the test is expected to decrease. However, when the effect is limited to a very local area and produces no systemic toxicity, sensitivity is usually elevated when a substance is dissolved and then administered.

In LLNA, a commonly used solvent for chemical substances is an acetone olive oil (AOO) 4:1 mixture. For a hydrophilic sample or a liquid sample not fully adhering to the skin of ear lobes, the application method should be devised to make sufficient adhesion to ear lobes. For example, a suspension such as carboxymethyl cellulose and hydroxyethyl cellulose (0.5 % (w/v)) may be added. For some water-soluble chemicals, use of DMSO, *N,N*-dimethylformamide, and ethanol is preferred to surfactant Pluronic® L92. Other solvents may be used as a dosing vehicle provided that the effects of adding to the extraction solvent and the effects due to a change in solvent components are thoroughly investigated and recorded. Such effects can be verified in an experiment conducted using a weak or moderate sensitizer used generally as a positive control substance. In addition, it is possible to demonstrate in a test conducted by the addition of a positive control substance to the test sample that the extract prepared can show presence of a sensitizer adequately without interference of the vehicle, etc.

7.5 Test animals

In selecting test animals, in principle, those with high sensitivity should be used. GPMT and A&P both employ guinea pigs. Selection of guinea pigs is based on good sensitivity in sensitization reactions, reactions such as external formation of erythema and edema to various chemicals resembling those in man, as well as accumulation of abundant background data. The body weight of animals is an important factor since handling of very small animals is difficult and sensitivity is reduced in very large animals (600 g or more). Therefore, it is favorable to use young healthy white guinea pigs (generally aged 1 to 3 months) with the body weight of about 400 g at the start of experiment. Either male or female animals may be used. If female animals are used, they shall be nulliparous and not pregnant.

In LLNA, use of DBA/2, B6C3F1 or BALB/c mice has been reported but it is necessary to confirm that the sensitivity is comparable to that of CBA strain when they are actually used in the test. Mice of the same age by weeks (within 1 week) should be used in each of the tests. Males may be used if they show comparable sensitivity to that in females.

As for the number of groups, an extract from a medical device is often used in the test and

とを示すことができれば，雄を使用してもよい.

　群数に関しては，医療機器では，試験に用いる試料は抽出液になることが多いので，1用量のみしか設定できない場合もあるが，抽出液を濃縮乾固後に再溶解することで用量を複数設定できる場合には3群程度設定し，用量依存性を確認することが望ましい．陽性対照群も試験ごとに設定することが望ましい．LLNA では特に媒体の刺激性が反応に大きく影響することから，試験試料と同じ媒体を使用できる物質を選択すべきであるが，適切な陽性対照物質が存在しない場合には，別途陽性対照用の媒体群も設定して試験を行い，それぞれの陰性対照に対する SI を求めるべきである.

7.6　LLNA の試験方法について

7.6.1　感作について

　LLNA において投与部位が乾きにくい場合にはドライヤーなどで冷風を当てて乾燥させることも可能である．感作投与物質が他の動物に影響することが予想される場合には個別飼育することを考える.

7.6.2　放射性物質の投与

　^{125}I–iododeoxyuridine の場合は，2 μCi（74 kBq）を含有する PBS を 250 μL，fluoro-deoxyuridine の場合は 10^{-5}M を含有する PBS を 250 μL 尾静脈から投与する.

7.6.3　測定試料の調製例

　リンパ節採取の際，群間の組織試料の交叉汚染に気をつけなければならない．細胞の単離はリンパ節を 200 μm のステンレスメッシュかナイロンメッシュあるいはスライドグラスのフロスト部分などを利用して優しく押しつぶして行う．遠心分離（例えば4℃，10分，190×g）により2回洗浄を行い，PBS に再懸濁する．次いで細胞を5% TCA 中，4±2℃で18±1時間沈殿させる．最後の遠心分離後，ペレットを1 mL の TCA に再懸濁し，^{3}H の計測には 10 mL のシンチレーション溶液を入れたシンチレーションバイアルに移し，シンチレーションカウンタで測定する．^{125}I の測定には直接 γ カウンターに移して測定する.

7.6.4　放射活性測定

　それぞれの結果からバックグラウンドを差し引いた後，群ごとの平均と標準偏差（個体ごとの検体採取の場合）を計算する.

7.6.5　反応性評価

　結果が判定基準値に近似している場合などは，補足的に統計処理を行うことも有用である.

7.6.6　他の LLNA

　他に放射性ラベルを使用しない代替法が存在する．医療機器の評価における正当性が示される場合には使用可能である．（例：bromodeoxyuridine（BrdU）を用いる LLNA-BrdU 法，adenosine triphosphate（ATP）を測定する LLNA-DA 法）

only one dose level may be available for testing in some cases. However, if multiple dose levels can be set by re-dissolving residues obtained by evaporating the extract, it is preferred to set about 3 groups and confirm dose dependence. It is also preferred to have a positive control group in each test. As irritation of a vehicle affect the sensitization response considerably in LLNA, either a positive control substance prepared in the same vehicle as that for the test sample is selected or, if a suitable positive control substance is not available, a vehicle group for the positive control should be set in the test to determine SI to the respective negative controls.

7.6   Test method for LLNA
7.6.1   Sensitization
In LLNA, it is acceptable to dry the administration site by blowing cold air with a dryer when drying of the administration site is slow. Individual housing should be considered when the sensitization substance is expected to influence other animals.

7.6.2   Administration of radioisotope
For ^{125}I-iododeoxyuridine, 250 μL of PBS containing 2 μCi (74 kBq) is injected into the caudal vein. For fluorodeoxyuridine, 250 μL of PBS containing 10^{-5} M is injected into the caudal vein

7.6.3   Preparation of samples
Lymph nodes should be collected paying attention to cross contamination of tissue samples among groups. Single cell preparations are prepared by gently pressing the lymph nodes through a 200 μm stainless steel wire mesh or nylon mesh, or frosted part of a slide glass. Wash the cells twice by centrifugation (e.g. $190 \times g$ for 10 minutes at 4 ℃) and resuspend in PBS. Then, precipitate the cells in 5 % TCA at 4 ± 2 ℃ for 18 ± 1 hours. After the last centrifugation, resuspended the pellets in 1 mL of TCA, transfer to a scintillation vial containing 10 mL of scintillation solution for the measurement of ^{3}H and measure by a scintillation counter. For the measurement of ^{125}I, transfer the solution directly to a γ counter.

7.6.4   Measurement of radioactivity
Subtract the background value from each result and calculate the mean and standard deviation (in case of sampling from individual animals) in each group.

7.6.5   Evaluation of reactivity
It is useful to perform statistical analysis supplementary if the results are close to the evaluation criteria.

7.6.6   Other LLNAs
Alternative methods not using radiolabeling are also available. These may be used when their justification to use in evaluation of a medical device is demonstrated (e.g. LLNA-BrdU method using bromodeoxyuridine [BrdU] and LLNA-DA method using adenosine triphosphate [ATP]).

7.7　皮膚反応の採点基準について

　モルモットの場合，血管拡張に基づく紅斑と，血管透過性亢進に基づく浮腫とが容易に区別できることから，皮膚反応の判定基準は，紅斑（erythema）の程度に浮腫（edema）の形成を加味して行っているものもある．ISO 10993-10 では，総合的に 4 段階でスコアをつけており，本ガイダンスでは Magnusson and Kligman のスコアを例示した．LLNA では評価に用いるものではないが，投与期間中の耳介の状態を観察することが重要である．刺激性が強い物質では，耳介の状態が悪化し，結果として感作性の反応が低下するおそれがあるため，試験結果の評価に重要な情報となる．

7.8　感作性の強さの評価について

　GPMT 及び A&P における皮膚反応の平均評価点は，皮膚反応（紅斑及び浮腫）の程度をスコア化し，その総点を使用動物数で割った値であり，皮膚の炎症の程度を表わす[2]．最低感作濃度は感作性が認められる最も低い感作濃度を示し，実験的に求めることは可能であるが，試験規模が膨大となり，現実的でない側面がある．最低感作濃度は最高感作濃度群における MRl 惹起濃度（皮膚の平均評価点がおよそ 1.0 を示すところの最も低い惹起濃度）とほぼ同程度であることが明らかにされている[1]ことから，MRl 惹起濃度からおおよその最低感作濃度を類推することが可能である．ただし，Magnusson and Kligman のスコアに従った最高スコアが 3 点の評価法と薬食機発 0301 第 20 号以前に掲載されていた 8 点の評価法では，計算値が異なる場合があるので，評価法の異なるものを比較する際には注意が必要である．LLNA では用量依存性が認められた場合，求められた SI を基に SI が 3 を示す濃度（EC3）を算出し，この EC3 濃度を既存の感作性物質と比較することにより，感作性の強さを評価することが可能である[3]．

7.9　*in vivo* 感作性試験の代替法について

　現在，OECD テストガイドラインには，複数の *in vitro* 感作性試験法が収載されている．これらは，単純化学物質の評価においては，十分な科学的根拠のあることが示されている．ISO/TC 194 の WG では，医療機器の生物学的安全性評価に感作性試験代替法の導入を目指して，ISO 10993-10 の Annex に試験法の概要を記載した．

8．引用文献

1）　Nakamura, A., Momma, J., Sekiguchi, H., Noda, T., Yamano, T., Kaniwa, M.-A., Kojima, S., Tsuda, M., Kurokawa, Y.: A new protocol and criteria for quantitative determination of sensitization potencies of chemicals by guinea pig maximization test. Contact Dermatitis 31, 72-85 (1994)

2）　Sato, Y., Katsumura, Y., Ichikawa, H., Kobayashi, T., Kozuka, T., Morikawa, F., Ohta, S.: A modified technique of guinea pig testing to identify delayed hypersensitivity allergens. Contact Dermatitis 7, 225-237 (1981)

3）　Organization for Economic Cooperation and Development (OECD), Guideline for the testing of chemicals No. 429, Skin sensitization: Local lymph node assay, OECD Publications (2010)

7.7 Scoring criteria for skin reactions

In the case of guinea pigs, erythema caused by vasodilation is easily distinguished from edema caused by accelerated vascular permeability, and therefore evaluation criteria for skin reactions are often set by the addition of edema formation to the severity of erythema. Comprehensive skin reactions are scored in 4 scales in ISO 10993-10. In this guidance, the Magnusson and Kligman scoring system is cited as an example. In the LLNA, it is important to observe the state of ear auricles during the administration period though it is not used in the evaluation. Such observation provides important information in the evaluation since a highly irritable substance may aggravate the condition of ear auricles resulting in a decrease in sensitization reaction.

7.8 Evaluation of sensitization potential

The mean evaluation score for the skin reactions in GPMT and A&P is calculated by scoring severity of skin reactions (erythema and edema) and dividing the total score by the number of animals used and it indicates the degree of skin inflammation[2]. The minimum induction concentration shows the lowest concentration that induces sensitization and can be determined experimentally but it requires a massive test scale and is not practical. Since the minimum induction concentration has been shown to be comparable to MR1 challenge concentration (the lowest challenge concentration that gives the mean evaluation score of about 1.0 in the skin) in the highest induction concentration group[1], it is possible to estimate an approximate minimum induction concentration from the MR1 challenge concentration. However, calculated metrics based on the Magnusson and Kligman scoring system, which has a highest score of 3, may differ from the evaluation method demonstrated earlier than the issuance of PFSB/ELD/OMDE Notification No. 0301-20, which has a highest score of 8. Precautions should be taken when comparing data derived from different evaluation scoring systems. In the LLNA, the concentration that gives SI of 3 (EC3) is calculated based on the SI determined when dose dependence is observed, and sensitization potential can be evaluated by comparing the EC3 concentration with existing sensitizers[3].

7.9 Alternatives to the *in vivo* sensitization test

Several *in vitro* sensitization tests are listed in the current OECD Test Guidelines. Sufficient scientific basis has been demonstrated for these tests in the evaluation of simple chemical substances. Brief descriptions of test methods have been added to the Annexes of ISO 10993-10 by the ISO/TC 194/WG with the aim of introducing alternative methods to the sensitization test for the biological safety evaluation of medical devices.

8. References cited

1) Nakamura, A., Momma, J., Sekiguchi, H., Noda, T., Yamano, T., Kaniwa, M.-A., Kojima, S., Tsuda, M., Kurokawa, Y.: A new protocol and criteria for quantitative determination of sensitization potencies of chemicals by guinea pig maximization test. Contact Dermatitis 31, 72-85 (1994)

2) Sato, Y., Katsumura, Y., Ichikawa, H., Kobayashi, T., Kozuka, T., Morikawa, F., Ohta, S.: A modified technique of guinea pig testing to identify delayed hypersensitivity allergens. Contact Dermatitis 7, 225-237 (1981)

3) Organization for Economic Cooperation and Development (OECD), Guideline for the testing of chemicals No. 429, Skin sensitization: Local lymph node assay, OECD Publications (2010)

9. 参考文献

1) van Ketal, W.G., Tan-lim, K.N: Contact dermatitis from ethanol. Contact Dermatitis 1, 7-10 (1975)

2) Stotts, J., Ely, W.J.: Induction of human skin sensitization to ethanol. J. Invest. Dermat. 69, 219-222 (1977)

3) Kero, M., Hannuksela, M.: Guinea pig maximization test open epicutaneous test and chamber test in induction of delayed contact hypersensitivity. Contact Dermatitis 6, 341-344 (1980)

4) Goodwin, B.F.J., Crevel, R.W.R., Johnson, A.W.: A comparison of three guinea-pig sensitization procedures for the detection of 19 reported human contact sensitizers. Contact Dermatitis 7, 248-258 (1981)

5) Ikarashi, Y., Tsuchiya, T., Nakamura, A.: Detection of contact sensitivity of metal salts using the murine local lymph node assay. Toxicol. Lett. 62, 53-61 (1992)

6) Ikarashi, Y., Momma, J., Tsuchiya T., Nakamura, A.: Evaluation of skin sensitization potential of nickel, chromium, titanium and zirconium salts using guinea-pigs and mice. Biomaterials 17, 2103-2108 (1996)

7) Ikarashi, Y., Kaniwa, M., Tsuchiya, T.: Sensitization potential of gold sodium thiosulfate in mice and guinea pigs. Biomaterials 23, 4907-4914 (2002)

8) Ikarashi, Y., Tsuchiya, T., Toyoda, K., Kobayashi, E., Doi, H., Yoneyama, T., Hamanaka H.: Tissue reactions and sensitivity to iron-chromium alloys. Mater. Trans. 43, 3065-3071 (2002)

9) Lee, J.K., Park, J.H., Park, S.H. *et al.*, A nonradioisotopic endpoint for measurement of lymph node cell proliferation in a murine allergic contact dermatitis model, using bromodeoxyuridine immunohistochemistry. J. Pharmacol. Toxicol. Methods 48, 53-61 (2002)

10) Tsuchiya, T., Ikarashi, Y., Uchima, T., Doi, H. Nakamura, A., Ohshima, Y., Fujimaki, M., Toyoda, K., Kobayashi, E., Yoneyama, T., Hamanaka, H.: A method to monitor corrosion of chromium-iron alloys by monitoring the chromium ion concentration in urine. Mater. Trans. 43, 3058-3064 (2002)

11) Cockshott, A., Evns, P., Ryans, C.A. *et al.*, The local lymph node assay in practice: a current regulatory perspective. Human Exp. Toxicol. 25, 387-394 (2006)

12) Gerberick, G.F., Ryan, C.A., Dearman, R.J., Kimber, I.: Local lymph node assay (LLNA) for detection of sensitization capacity of chemicals. Methods 41, 54-60 (2007)

13) ASTM Standard F 2148-07: Standard Practice for Evaluation of Delayed Contact Hypersensitivity Using the Murine Local Lymph Node Assay (LLNA)

9.   References

1)   van Ketal, W.G., Tan-lim, K.N: Contact dermatitis from ethanol. Contact Dermatitis 1, 7 –10 (1975)

2)   Stotts, J., Ely, W.J.: Induction of human skin sensitization to ethanol. J. Invest. Dermat. 69, 219-222 (1977)

3)   Kero, M., Hannuksela, M.: Guinea pig maximization test open epicutaneous test and chamber test in induction of delayed contact hypersensitivity. Contact Dermatitis 6, 341-344 (1980)

4)   Goodwin, B.F.J., Crevel, R.W.R., Johnson, A.W.: A comparison of three guinea-pig sensitization procedures for the detection of 19 reported human contact sensitizers. Contact Dermatitis 7, 248-258 (1981)

5)   Ikarashi, Y., Tsuchiya, T., Nakamura, A.: Detection of contact sensitivity of metal salts using the murine local lymph node assay. Toxicol. Lett. 62, 53-61 (1992)

6)   Ikarashi, Y., Momma, J., Tsuchiya T., Nakamura, A.: Evaluation of skin sensitization potential of nickel, chromium, titanium and zirconium salts using guinea-pigs and mice. Biomaterials 17, 2103-2108 (1996)

7)   Ikarashi, Y., Kaniwa, M., Tsuchiya, T.: Sensitization potential of gold sodium thiosulfate in mice and guinea pigs. Biomaterials 23, 4907-4914 (2002)

8)   Ikarashi, Y., Tsuchiya, T., Toyoda, K., Kobayashi, E., Doi, H., Yoneyama, T., Hamanaka H.: Tissue reactions and sensitivity to iron-chromium alloys. Mater. Trans. 43, 3065-3071 (2002)

9)   Lee, J.K., Park, J.H., Park, S.H. *et al.*, A nonradioisotopic endpoint for measurement of lymph node cell proliferation in a murine allergic contact dermatitis model, using bromodeoxyuridine immunohistochemistry. J. Pharmacol. Toxicol. Methods 48, 53-61 (2002)

10)   Tsuchiya, T., Ikarashi, Y., Uchima, T., Doi, H. Nakamura, A., Ohshima, Y., Fujimaki, M., Toyoda, K., Kobayashi, E., Yoneyama, T., Hamanaka, H.: A method to monitor corrosion of chromium-iron alloys by monitoring the chromium ion concentration in urine. Mater. Trans. 43, 3058-3064 (2002)

11)   Cockshott, A., Evans, P., Ryan, C.A. *et al.*, The local lymph node assay in practice: a current regulatory perspective. Human Exp. Toxicol. 25, 387-394 (2006)

12)   Gerberick, G.F., Ryan, C.A., Dearman, R.J., Kimber, L: Local lymph node assay (LLNA) for detection of sensitization capacity of chemicals. Methods 41, 54-60 (2007)

13)   ASTM Standard F 2148-07: Standard Practice for Evaluation of Delayed Contact Hypersensitivity Using the Murine Local Lymph Node Assay (LLNA)

第3部　遺伝毒性試験

1．適用範囲

　本試験は，医療機器又は原材料の遺伝毒性評価を目的としている（4.1項参照）．ISO 10993-3, Biological evaluation of medical devices-Part 3: Tests for genotoxicity, carcinogenicity and reproductive toxicity においては，遺伝子突然変異及び染色体異常を検出する試験を推奨しており，ここでは細菌を用いる復帰突然変異試験及び培養細胞を用いる染色体異常試験，小核試験又はマウスリンフォーマ TK 試験の実施を基本とする．ただし，得られた試験結果が陽性になった場合や，医療機器又は原材料の使用期間や使用条件によっては，in vivo 試験系を含む他の試験系の実施についても考慮しなければならない（4.2項参照）．

2．引用規格

2.1　ISO 10993-3: 2014, Biological evaluation of medical devices-Part 3: Tests for genotoxicity, carcinogenicity and reproductive toxicity

　ISO/TR 10993-33: 2015, Biological evaluation of medical devices-Part 33: Guidance on tests to evaluate genotoxicity-Supplement to ISO 10993-3

2.2　OECD 471, Bacterial Reverse Mutation Test

　OECD 473, In Vitro Mammalian Chromosome Aberration Test

　OECD 474, Mammalian Erythrocyte Micronucleus Test

　OECD 475, Mammalian Bone Marrow Chromosome Aberration Test

　OECD 487, In Vitro Mammalian Cell Micronucleus Test

　OECD 490, In Vitro Mammalian Cell Gene Mutation Tests Using the Thymidine Kinase Gene

2.3　平成24年9月20日付け薬食審査発0920第2号「医薬品の遺伝毒性試験及び解釈に関するガイダンスについて」

3．試験の適用

3.1　試験試料は最終製品又は原材料である．ただし，試験試料に含まれる原料化学物質，添加剤などについて遺伝毒性に関する安全性が確認されており，含まれる原料化学物質の相互作用などにより未知物質が生成される可能性が低い場合は，これら試料の試験を実施する必要はない．その場合，その科学的妥当性を明らかにする必要がある．

3.2　文献又は既存データなどにより遺伝毒性に関する安全性が確認できない場合は，ISO 10993-3 及び OECD テストガイドラインを参照し，以下の試験の実施を基本とする（4.2項参照）．

1）　細菌を用いる復帰突然変異試験

2）　培養細胞を用いる染色体異常試験，小核試験，又はマウスリンフォーマ TK 試験

Part 3 Genotoxicity Test

1. Scope

The aim of the test is to evaluate genotoxicity of medical devices or raw materials (see 4.1). In ISO 10993-3 "Biological evaluation of medical devices Part 3: Tests for genotoxicity, carcinogenicity and reproductive toxicity", tests to detect gene mutation and chromosomal aberrations are recommended. Here, the reverse mutation test with bacteria, and the chromosome aberration test with cells in culture, the *in vitro* micronucleus test, or mouse lymphoma TK test should basically be performed. However, in case of a positive test result or depending on the duration and condition of use of the medical devices or raw materials, testing in other systems including the *in vivo* systems should be considered (see 4.2).

2. Normative references

2.1 ISO 10993-3: 2014, Biological evaluation of medical devices-Part 3: Tests for genotoxicity, carcinogenicity and reproductive toxicity

ISO/TR 10993-33: 2015, Biological evaluation of medical devices-Part 33: Guidance on tests to evaluate genotoxicity-Supplement to ISO 10993-3

2.2 OECD 471, Bacterial Reverse Mutation Test

OECD 473, *In Vitro* Mammalian Chromosome Aberration Test

OECD 474, Mammalian Erythrocyte Micronucleus Test

OECD 475, Mammalian Bone Marrow Chromosome Aberration Test

OECD 487, *In Vitro* Mammalian Cell Micronucleus Test

OECD 490, *In Vitro* Mammalian Cell Gene Mutation Tests Using the Thymidine Kinase Gene

2.3 MHLW Notification, YAKUSHOKUSHINSA-HATSU 0920 No. 2 Sep. 20, 2012 Guidance on the genotoxicity tests of pharmaceuticals and the interpretation

3. Application of the test

3.1 Test samples are final products or raw materials. If the safety of the raw materials, chemical substances and additives etc. contained in the test sample concerning genotoxicity has been confirmed and it is unlikely that any unknown substance is produced by interactions of the all of the component materials once finally assembled, it is not necessary to perform the test with the finished test sample. In such cases, the rationale for not performing any testing should be documented.

3.2 If no safety data is available concerning genotoxicity in the literature or from previous tests, the following tests should basically be performed according to ISO 10993-3 and OECD test guidelines (see 4.2):

1) Reverse mutation test with bacteria
2) Chromosome aberration test with cells, the *in vitro* micronucleus test, or the mouse lymphoma TK test

3.3　試験液の調製
3.3.1　有機材料の場合

　　試験試料（最終製品又は原材料）の材質，性状，溶解性などの物理化学的特性を考慮して，以下の手順により試験に適用するための試験液を調製する．

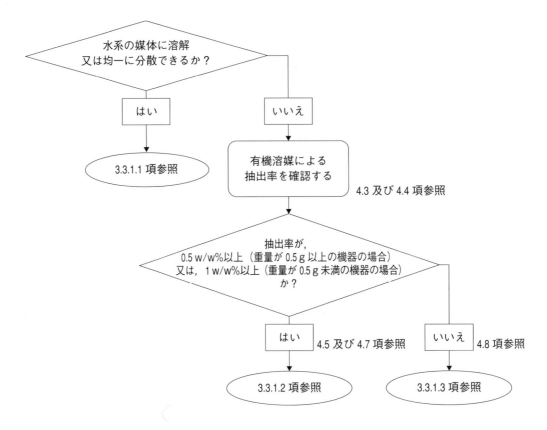

3.3.1.1　水系の媒体に溶解若しくは懸濁できる試験試料は，媒体（水・生理食塩液・血清含有培養液など）に溶解又は均一に分散して試験液とし，試験を実施する．

3.3.1.2　水系の媒体に溶解又は均一に分散できない試験試料は，有機溶媒（メタノール及びアセトン）による抽出率を確認する（4.3，4.4 項参照）．メタノール又はアセトンによって抽出物が得られる場合（4.5 項参照）は，より抽出率の高い溶媒を用い（4.6 項参照），細切した試験試料にその重量の 10 倍容量の溶媒を添加し，室温で 24 時間撹拌して抽出する．得られた有機溶媒抽出液の溶媒を留去し，必要量の抽出物を得る．抽出物は試験系に適切な媒体に溶解又は懸濁して試験液とし，試験を実施する（4.7 項参照）．

3.3 Preparation of the test solution or suspension

3.3.1 Organic materials

The test solution or suspension for testing should be prepared according to the flow chart below, considering the physico-chemical characteristics such as material, physical properties and solubility of the test sample (final products or raw materials).

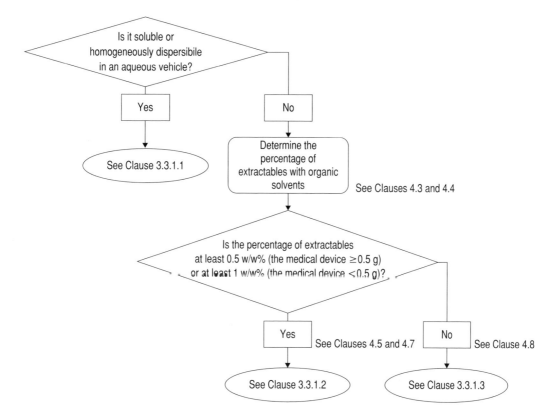

3.3.1.1 The test samples that are soluble or suspendable in an aqueous vehicle should be dissolved or dispersed homogeneously in the vehicle (water, physiological saline, culture medium with serum etc.) and then subjected to a test.

3.3.1.2 The test sample that is neither soluble nor homogeneously dispersible in an aqueous vehicle should be subjected to an extraction in an organic solvent (methanol and acetone). The percentage of extractables should be determined for each solvent (see 4.3 and 4.4). If extractables are obtained with methanol or acetone (see 4.5), the solvent with the higher percentage of extractables should be employed (see 4.6), the chopped test sample should be added with the solvent at a volume of 10 times its weight, and then extracted while stirring at room temperature for 24 h. The organic solvent of the extract obtained should be evaporated to dryness to obtain the extractables at the amount required for the test, the extractables should be dissolved or suspended in an appropriate vehicle compatible with the test system, and then subjected to the test (see 4.7).

3.3.1.3　水系の媒体に溶解又は均一に分散せず，有機溶媒でも抽出物が得られない試験試料は（4.8 項参照），復帰突然変異試験においてはジメチルスルホキシド（DMSO）による抽出液を，染色体異常試験，小核試験又はマウスリンフォーマ TK 試験においては血清含有培養液による抽出液を用いて試験を実施する（4.3 項参照）.

1)　復帰突然変異試験

　　可能な場合は試験試料を細切し，その 0.2 g に対して DMSO 1 mL（あるいは試験試料 6 cm^2 に対して DMSO 1 mL）の割合で添加し，37 ℃で振盪撹拌しながら 48 時間又は 72 時間抽出する. 必要に応じて，付録 1 の規定を参照しても差し支えない. その抽出液を試験液として，プレート当たり最高 100 μL を添加して試験を実施する.

2)　染色体異常試験，小核試験，マウスリンフォーマ TK 試験

　　可能な場合は試験試料を細切し，その 0.2 g に対して試験に用いる血清含有培養液 1 mL（あるいは試験試料 6 cm^2 に対して培養液 1 mL）の割合で添加し，37 ℃で 48 時間又は 72 時間抽出する. 必要に応じて，付録 1 の規定を参照しても差し支えない. その抽出液を 100 %抽出液とし，培養液で希釈して試験を実施する.

3.3.2　無機材料の場合

　　金属材料あるいはセラミックなどの無機材料における遺伝毒性の多くは，溶出する金属イオンの影響で評価することができる. したがって，これらの遺伝毒性試験は以下に留意する.

1)　文献あるいはこれまでの実験によって，これらの材料を構成する金属元素種のイオンの遺伝毒性に関する情報が得られる場合は，試験を実施する必要はない.

2)　構成金属元素種に関して遺伝毒性に関する十分な情報が得られない場合は，その代表的な金属イオン溶液又は材料からの抽出液について試験を実施する.

3)　遺伝毒性の最終評価を行う際には，当該金属イオンの試験試料からの溶出量も考慮する.

3.3.3　原材料化学物質の場合

　　適切な溶媒に溶解又は懸濁して試験に供する.

3.4　判定及び評価

　　本ガイダンスに従って実施した試験結果の判定は引用規格に示したガイドライン（2. 項参照）に従う. 陽性結果が得られた場合は，遺伝毒性のもつ重要性から，さらに *in vivo* 試験を含む他の遺伝毒性試験を実施することにより，ヒトへのリスク評価の一助となる場合も考えられる（4.2 項参照）. ただし，医療機器の安全性評価は，遺伝毒性の強さや濃度依存性，抽出に用いた溶媒の種類や抽出率，医療機器の接触部位や接触期間など，種々の条件を総合的に考慮して行う（4.9 項参照）.

3.3.1.3   The test sample that is neither soluble nor homogeneously dispersible in an aqueous vehicle and that does not generate extractables with organic solvents (see 4.8) should be extracted with DMSO for the bacterial reverse mutation test and with the culture medium with serum for the chromosome aberration test, the *in vitro* micronucleus test or the mouse lymphoma TK test (see 4.3). The extracts should be used for the tests according to the following methods 1) and 2).

1)   The bacterial reverse mutation test
The test sample should be chopped, if possible. Each 0.2 g (or 6 cm^2) should be added to 1 mL of DMSO and then extracted while shaking at 37 ℃ for 48 h or 72 h. If necessary, Clause 1 in Appendix may be referred to. 100 μL of the extract per plate at maximum should be added to perform the test.

2)   The chromosome aberration test, the *in vitro* micronucleus test, or the mouse lymphoma TK test
The test sample should be chopped, if possible. Each 0.2 g (or 6 cm^2) should be added to 1 mL of the culture medium with serum and then extracted at 37 ℃ for 48 h or 72 h. If necessary, Clause 1 in Appendix may be referred to. The extract designated as the 100 % extract should be diluted with the culture medium as needed and then subjected to the test.

3.3.2   In case of inorganic materials

In case of inorganic materials such as metals or ceramics, the primary genotoxicity concern in most cases is the genotoxicity due to metal ions. On this premise, genotoxicity testing of inorganic materials should be performed as follows.

1)   If genotoxicity data regarding the metal ions potentially generated by the metallic portion of the device is available in the literature, it is not necessary to perform the test panel.

2)   If the genotoxicity data concerning the constituting metal elements is insufficient, the test panel should be performed with a solution of the representative metal ion or extracts from the test sample.

3)   The amount of metal ions eluted from the test sample should be considered in the final evaluation of its genotoxicity.

3.3.3   In case of raw material chemical substances

The test sample should be dissolved or suspended in an appropriate solvent and subjected to a test.

3.4   Criteria and evaluation

The criteria to evaluate each assay performed according to this guidance are provided in guidelines in the normative references (see Clause 2). If a positive result is obtained in a test, based on the significance of genotoxicity, other genotoxicity tests including *in vivo* tests may be performed to help the risk assessment concerning the safety in humans (see 4.2). The safety evaluation of medical devices should be comprehensively conducted considering all the various conditions such as intensity and concentration–dependency of genotoxicity, type of solvent used for extraction and the percentage of extractables, and the nature and duration of body contact of the medical device (see 4.9).

3.5　試験報告書

　　試験報告書には，少なくとも以下の事項を記載する.

1) 試験実施機関及び試験責任者
2) 試験実施期間
3) 試験試料（最終製品又は原材料）を特定する要素
　　（例：医療機器の名称，製造販売業者名，製造番号，原材料名など）
4) 対照物質（背景データ）
5) 試験液の調製方法
　　例：溶媒による抽出法と抽出率，滅菌方法，抽出後の抽出液（100 %原液）の変化
　　　の有無など
6) 試験方法
　　例：菌株又は細胞
7) 試験結果
　　必要に応じて，表，図，写真を添付すること
8) 結果の評価と考察
9) 参考文献

4．参考情報

4.1　背景

　　遺伝毒性試験（genotoxicity test）は，1個の細胞に生じた DNA 傷害（DNA damage）から派生して，細胞や個体レベルで遺伝子突然変異（gene mutation）や染色体異常（chromosomal aberration）を誘発する遺伝毒性物質の検出を目的とする試験である. 遺伝毒性物質の作用は，その傷害が生体内の体細胞で起きるか，若しくは生殖細胞で起きるかにより傷害の現われ方が異なる. 各組織の体細胞において DNA 傷害が生じると，がんの原因となる場合がある. その意味で，遺伝毒性試験は発がん物質の短期スクリーニング試験の役割を果たしている. 一方，卵子や精子など生体内の生殖細胞に DNA 傷害が生じると，傷を持つ大部分の細胞は生殖細胞や胚の発生過程で淘汰を受けるが，次世代に遺伝子突然変異や染色体異常が伝わる可能性がある. また妊娠中の母体がばく露を受け，胎児の体細胞 DNA に傷害が生じた場合，奇形や身体的障害を有する新生児が産まれる可能性もある. このように，遺伝毒性物質は DNA に作用して，がんの発生や次世代に遺伝的影響を及ぼすことから，医療機器は短期的又は長期的いずれの使用条件下においても，生体に作用して遺伝毒性を示さないことが望まれる.

4.2　試験法の選択

　　一つの試験で，全ての遺伝毒性物質を検出することはできないため，通常，複数試験の組合せ（バッテリー）で実施される.

　　本ガイダンスは，原則として，遺伝毒性の主たる事象である遺伝子突然変異及び染色体異常の誘発を検出することができる試験系として，微生物（ネズミチフス菌，大腸菌）を用いる復帰突然変異試験とほ乳動物培養細胞を用いる試験（染色体異常試験，小核試験又はマウスリンフォーマ TK 試験）の二種の in vitro 試験の実施を基本としている.

　　試験種の選択に関しては，ISO 10993-3, Biological evaluation of medical devices-Part 3:

3.5 Test report

The test report should, at a minimum, include the following items.

1) Test facilities and the study director
2) Test period
3) Factors identifying the test sample (final products or raw materials)
   (name of the medical device, name of the manufacturer, the serial number, name of the raw materials, etc.)
4) Control materials and/or substances (their background data in the test)
5) Preparation method for the test solution or suspension
   (extraction method with solvent and the percentage of extractables, sterilization method, change in the extract (designated as the 100 % extract) after extraction etc.)
6) Testing methods
   (Bacterial strains or cell lines, etc.)
7) Results
   If necessary, tables, figures and photographs should be attached.
8) Evaluation of the results and discussion
9) References

4. Reference information

4.1 Background

The aim of genotoxicity tests is to detect genotoxic substances that cause gene mutation and chromosomal aberration at the cellular and individual level deriving from DNA damage developed in a single cell. Effects of genotoxic substances differ in expression of disorders depending on whether the damage is developed in the somatic cells or in the germ cells in the living body. If DNA damage has been developed in the somatic cells of various tissues, it may cause cancer. Therefore, genotoxicity tests play a role of short-term screening tests for carcinogenic substances. On the other hand, when DNA damage has been developed in the germ cells such as eggs and sperm, although most of the cells with damage undergo selection and will be eliminated during the process of development of germ cells and embryos, there is a risk that the gene mutation and chromosomal aberration may be transferred to the next generation. Furthermore, in the case where the pregnant mother has received the exposure and DNA damage has been developed in the fetal somatic cells, a risk of newborn with malformation and physical disturbance also arises. As described above, since genotoxic substances act on DNA to develop cancer or to exert genetic effects on the next generation, it is desirable that medical devices do not induce genotoxicity in the living body in either long-term or short-term use conditions.

4.2 Selection of the testing method

No single test is capable of detecting all genotoxic agents. Therefore, the usual approach is to conduct a battery of tests.

In this guidance, it is recommended to perform two *in vitro* tests, i.e., the reverse mutation test with bacteria (*Salmonella typhimurium* and *Escherichia coli*) and tests with mammalian cells in culture (the chromosome aberration test, the *in vitro* micronucleus test or the mouse lymphoma TK test). These tests can detect the major events of genotoxicity, i.e., induction of gene mutation and chromosomal aberration. In ISO 10993-3 "Biological evaluation of medical devices-Part 3: Tests for genotoxicity, carcinogenicity and reproductive toxicity", the *in vivo* tests are performed in some cases in addition to the *in vitro* tests rec-

Tests for genotoxicity, carcinogenicity and reproductive toxicity において上記の in vitro 試験に加えて in vivo 試験の実施が必要な場合も記載されており，本ガイダンスにおいても，医療機器の使用期間あるいは使用条件，得られた試験結果の科学的妥当性などを総合的に勘案して，in vivo 試験系を含む他の試験系の実施を考慮することとしている．

4.3　抽出溶媒

　試験試料から抽出物を得るための有機溶媒として，主に水溶性物質を抽出するメタノールと脂溶性物質を抽出するアセトンの 2 種類をあげた．これは試験試料から可能な限り多くの抽出物を得ることを目的とした組合せであり，インプラントのように低濃度かつ長期にわたるばく露の影響が想定される場合をも考慮したものである．有機溶媒で抽出物が得られないと判断された試験試料で，さらに DMSO が使用不可能な場合には，生理食塩液やリン酸緩衝液，血清含有培養液などでの抽出が考えられる．どのような抽出媒体を選択する場合であってもその妥当性を説明すること．

4.4　抽出率（試験試料の重量に対する試験試料から得られる抽出物量の割合）

　メタノール及びアセトンによって試験試料から得られる抽出物量に関する情報がない場合は，3.3.1.2 に従って抽出率を求める．抽出率が 0.5 w/w％以上（又は 1 w/w％以上）と，0.5 w/w％未満（又は 1 w/w％未満）の場合では，試験液の調製法が異なる．ここで，抽出率 0.5 w/w％は最終製品重量が 0.5 g 以上の医療機器に，抽出率 1 w/w％はその重量が 0.5 g 未満の医療機器に適用する．したがって抽出率をもとに試験計画を立案する必要がある．なお抽出率を調べるには，乾固した抽出物の重量を直接測定して求めるか，又は試験試料の抽出後の重量を測定して求める．

4.5　「抽出物が得られる場合」の判断

　医療機器（最終製品）の重量 0.5 g を基準として，抽出率の基準を以下のように定めた．「抽出物が得られる場合」とは，通例，抽出率が 0.5 w/w％以上（医療機器の重量が 0.5 g 以上の場合）又は抽出率が 1 w/w％以上（医療機器の重量が 0.5 g 未満の場合）の場合とする．0.5 w/w％又は 1 w/w％という抽出率の限界値は，試験に必要な抽出物量を得るための試験試料の量から設定したものである．

4.6　抽出物が得られる場合の ISO 10993-3 Annex A との違い

　有機溶媒抽出の溶媒の種類と数については，国内では以下の経緯がある．

　薬機第 99 号では，メタノール及びアセトンの 2 種の溶媒による抽出物の試験を実施することとしていたが，事務連絡医療機器審査 No. 36 では，メタノール及びアセトンの 2 種の溶媒のうち，抽出率が高い 1 溶媒からの抽出物を用いて試験を実施することに変更された．これは，薬機第 99 号発出以降に実施された 2 種の溶媒からの抽出物での

ommended above when the initial risk assessment suggests a potential risk. In this guidance, depending on the duration or condition of use of the medical device, testing other systems including the *in vivo* tests is also recommended after comprehensively considering scientific validity of the test results.

4.3 Extraction solvent

An organic solvent such as methanol or acetone should be used to extract as much extractables as possible. Methanol tends to extract mainly water–soluble substances whereas acetone tends to extract fat–soluble substances. This approach to maximize the extractables is considered important to evaluate the risk of implant devices that might expose the human body to a very low concentration of extractable substances for a long period of time. When extractables cannot be obtained with organic solvents, and for those materials for which DMSO is not suitable, extraction may be performed with physiological saline, phosphate buffer or culture medium with serum. The choice of extraction solvents should be justified and documented in the test report.

4.4 Percentage of extractables (Ratio of the amount of extractables obtained from a test sample to the weight of the test sample)

If no data concerning how much methanol and acetone extractables can be obtained is available, the percentage of extractables should be determined according to 3.3.1.2. The preparation procedure of the test solution or suspension differs depending on whether the percentage of extractables is at least 0.5 % (or 1 %) or less than 0.5 % (or 1 %). Here, the percentage of extractables of 0.5 % applies to a medical device whose final product weighs 0.5 g or more and the percentage of extractables of 1 % applies to a medical device whose final product weighs less than 0.5 g. Accordingly, the test protocol should be prepared based on the data of the percentage of extractables. There are several methods to determine the percentage of extractables, e.g. to determine the weight of dried extractables directly or to determine the weight of the remaining test sample after extraction .

4.5 Criteria for "a case where extractables can be obtained"

Taking the medical device weight of 0.5 g as a standard, the limit values for the percentage of extractables are set as follows.
"A case where extractables can be obtained" is generally a case where the amount of extractables obtained from the test sample is at least 0.5 % of the weight of the test sample (in case the medical device weighs at least 0.5 g) or at least 1 % of the weight of the test sample (in case the medical device weighs less than 0.5 g).
The limit values for the percentage of extractables, i.e., 0.5 % (in case the medical device weighs at least 0.5 g) and 1 % (in case the medical device weighs less than 0.5 g) have been established based on the amount of the test sample to obtain necessary amount of extractables for the test panel.

4.6 The difference of "a case where extractables can be obtained" between ISO 10993–3, Annex A and this guidance

The kinds and the number of organic solvents in extraction have a history below in Japan.
YAKUKI No. 99 (MHW Notification, 1995) had shown the conduct of a test with two extractables, one prepared from methanol and the other from acetone. IRYOUKIKI–SHINSA No. 36 (MHLW Memorandum, 2003) changed to the conduct of a test with one extractables prepared from a solvent (methanol or acetone) with the higher percentage of extractables.

試験結果において，両方とも陽性になるか，両方とも陰性になる場合がほとんどであったことから，より抽出率が高い溶媒1種からの抽出物の試験で現実的には問題ないであろう，と判断されたものである．

　一方，ISO 10993-3 Annex A では，日本の有機溶媒抽出の考え方を採用したが，抽出溶媒については，基本的には ISO 10993-12 の考え方を採用した．すなわち，有機材料及びそれらの製造工程で使用される添加物などは多種多様であり，原理的に，溶媒によって抽出される化学物質は異なり，生体内における溶出物のすべてを1種の溶媒で抽出できない可能性を否定できないことから，抽出できない溶出物に強い遺伝毒性物質が含まれる可能性を考慮し，ISO 10993-12 では，極性溶媒及び非極性溶媒の2種の溶媒による抽出物の試験を要求事項としている．この考えに基づき，ISO 10993-3 Annex A においても，2種の有機溶媒で抽出物が得られる場合には，2種の有機溶媒抽出物による試験が求められる．

4.7　抽出物量

　抽出物を用いて遺伝毒性試験を実施する場合に必要な抽出物の量は，試験計画によって増減はあるが，およその目安として，少なくとも復帰突然変異試験では1g，染色体異常試験では2g程度が必要である．

4.8　「抽出物が得られない場合」の判断

　「抽出物が得られない場合」とは，通例，抽出率が 0.5 w/w％ 未満（医療機器の重量が 0.5 g 以上の場合）又は抽出率が 1 w/w％ 未満（医療機器の重量が 0.5 g 未満の場合）の場合とする．ただし有機溶媒中で材料が溶解する場合，又は原形をとどめないほどに変形するような場合，抽出物は得られないものとする．

　また抽出物を用いて試験を実施せずに，原材料に含まれる原料化学物質（モノマーや添加物）の試験を実施するとともに，試験試料からの原料化学物質の溶出量を定量して評価することも可能である．

4.9　毒性学的懸念の閾値（TTC）による評価

　低濃度で存在する潜在的な毒性物質について，その許容される摂取量（Tolerable Intake: TI）を文献などで参照することができない場合，遺伝毒性のリスク評価において TTC の考え方（ISO/TS 21726: 2019）は参考となり得る．

5．薬食機発 0301 第 20 号からの変更点

1)　マウスリンフォーマ TK 試験に係わる OECD テストガイドラインが OECD 476 から分離され，新たなガイドラインとして発行された（OECD 490, 2015.7.28）ため，引用規格において OECD 476 を OECD 490 と置き換えた．
2)　引用規格を現在有効で，直接参考となるものに更新した．
3)　ISO 10993-3 及び ISO 10993-12 との整合性を図るために，抽出時間を旧ガイダンスより長い 72 時間も適切な抽出時間として追加した．
4)　ISO 10993-3: 2014 と整合性がとれていない内容や有用と考えられる内容を参考情報として追加した．

This was because of the test results below after the issue of YAKUKI No. 99. The test results with two extractables were often both positive or both negative. Testing with one extractables prepared from a solvent with the higher percentage of extractables was determined not to be a problem in practice.

On the other hand, the organic solvent extraction method performed in Japan was adopted in Annex A of ISO 10993-3, but the extraction solvent was selected according to ISO 10993-12. There are a variety of organic materials and additives used in their manufacturing processes, and in principle, chemical substances extracted from materials vary by solvent. No single solvent is capable of extracting all leached substances in human body. Therefore, considering possibility of not extracting potent genotoxic agents, ISO 10993-12 requires tests with extractables from two solvents of polar and non-polar solvent. Based on the concept above, Annex A of ISO 10993-3 also requires two extractables, one from a polar solvent and the other from a non-polar solvent, if possible.

4.7　Amount of extractables

The amount of extractables required for a genotoxicity test using extractables is, as a rough indication although it depends on the protocol, at least 1 g for the reverse mutation test and approximately 2 g for the chromosome aberration test.

4.8　Criteria for "a case where extractables cannot be obtained"

"A case where extractables cannot be obtained" is generally a case where the amount of extractables obtained from the test sample is less than 0.5 % of the weight of the test sample (in case the medical device weighs at least 0.5 g) or less than 1 % of the weight of the test sample (in case the medical device weighs less than 0.5 g). If the material is dissolved in the organic solvent or deformed beyond recognition, it is also judged that extractables cannot be obtained.

Instead of performing a test with extractables, it is also acceptable to perform a test with the raw material chemical substances (monomers, additives and so on) contained in the raw material in combination with quantitation of the amount of eluted raw material chemical substances from the test sample followed by evaluation.

4.9　Evaluation by the threshold of toxicological concern (TTC)

If the tolerable intake (TI) of potential toxic substances in low concentrations is not shown in literature etc., the concept of TTC (ISO/TS 21726: 3019) could be referred to in the risk evaluation of genotoxicity.

5.　Points changed from MHLW Notification, YAKUSHOKUKI-HATSU 0301 No. 20

1) OECD test guideline on the mouse lymphoma TK test was separated from OECD 476 and issued as a new guideline of OECD 490 on July 28, 2015. OECD 476 was replaced with OECD 490 in the normative references of this guidance.

2) The normative references are updated to those available at present and directly helpful.

3) An extraction time of 72 h was judged as appropriate and added in the text for consistency with ISO 10993-3 and ISO 10993-12.

4) Contents not consistent with ISO 10993-3: 2014 was explained (see 4.6) and a piece of useful information was added (see 4.9).

6.　参考文献

1)　石館基監修：微生物を用いる変異原性試験データ集，エル・アイ・シー，東京 (1991)

2)　日本組織培養学会編：細胞トキシコロジー試験法，朝倉書店，東京 (1991)

3)　林真：小核試験—実験法からデータの評価まで—，サイエンティスト社，東京 (1999)

4)　祖父尼俊雄監修：染色体異常試験データ集—改訂 1998 年版—，エル・アイ・シー，東京 (1999)

5)　Wever, D.J., Veldhuizen, A.G., Sanders, M.M., Schakenraad, J.M., van Horn J.R.: Cytotoxic, allergic and genotoxic activity of a nickel-titanium alloy. Biomaterials 18, 1115-1120 (1997)

6)　Honma, M., Hayashi, M., Shimada, H., Tanaka, N., Wakuri, S., Awogi, T., Yamamoto, K.I., Kodani, N.U., Nishi, Y., Nakadate, M., Sofuni, T.: Evaluation of the mouse lymphoma tk assay (microwell method) as an alternative to the *in vitro* chromosomal aberration test. Mutagenesis 14, 5-22 (1999)

7)　Chauvel-Lebret, D.J., Auroy, P., Tricot-Doleux, S., Bonnaure-Mallet, M.: Evaluation of the capacity of the SCGE assay to assess the genotoxicity of biomaterials. Biomaterials 22, 1795-1801 (2001)

8)　Kusakabe, H., Yamakage, K., Wakuri, S., Sasaki, K., Nakagawa, Y., Watanabe, M., Hayashi, M., Sofuni, T., Ono, H., Tanaka, N.: Relevance of chemical structure and cytotoxicity to the induction of chromosome aberrations based on the testing results of 98 high production volume industrial chemicals. Mutat. Res. 517, 187-198 (2002)

9)　Müller, B.P., Ensslen, S., Dott, W., Hollender, J.: Improved sample preparation of biomaterials for *in vitro* genotoxicity testing using reference materials. J. Biomed. Mater. Res. 61, 83-90 (2002)

10)　Kirsch-Volders, M., Sofuni, T., Ardema, M., Albertini, S., Eastmond, D., Fenech, M., Ishidate, M. Jr., Kirchner, S., Lorge, E., Morita, T., Norppa, H., Surralles, J., Vanhauwaert, A., Wakata, A.: Report from the *in vitro* micronucleus assay working group. Mutat. Res. 540, 153-163 (2003)

11)　Kirsch-Volders, M., Sofuni, T., Ardema, M., Albertini, S., Eastmond, D., Fenech, M., Ishidate, M. Jr., Kirchner, S., Lorge, E., Morita, T., Norppa, H., Surralles, J., Vanhauwaert, A., Wakata, A.: Corrigendum to "Report from the *in vitro* micronucleus assay working group" [Mutat. Res. 540 (2003) 153-163]. Mutat. Res. 564, 97-100 (2004)

12)　Muramatsu, K., Nakajima, M., Kikuchi, M., Shimada, S., Sasaki, K., Masuda, S., Yoshihara, Y.: *In vitro* cytocompatibility assessment of β-tricalcium phosphate/carboxymethyl-chitin composite. J. Biomed. Mater. Res. A. 71, 635-643 (2004)

13)　Matsuoka, A., Isama, K., Tsuchiya, T.: *In vitro* induction of polyploidy and chromatid exchanges by culture medium extracts of natural rubbers compounded with 2-mercaptobenzothiazole as a positive control candidate for genotoxicity tests. J. Biomed. Mater. Res. A. 75, 439-444 (2005)

14)　Matsuoka, A., Haishima, Y., Hasegawa, C., Matsuda, Y., Tsuchiya, T.: Organic-solvent extraction of model biomaterials for use in the *in vitro* chromosome aberration test. J.

6. References

1) Ishidate, M. (Ed.): "Data Book of Bacterial Reverse Mutation Assay" Life-science Information Center, Tokyo (1991)

2) The Japanese Tissue Culture Association (Ed.): "Toxicology Test Methods with Cells in Culture" Asakura Shoten, Tokyo (1991) in Japanese.

3) Hayashi, M.: "The Micronucleus Test-From experimental procedures to data evaluation-" Scientist Ltd., Tokyo (1999) in Japanese.

4) Sofuni, T. (Ed.): "Revised edition 1998 Data Book of Chromosomal Aberration Test *In vitro*" Life-science Information Center, Tokyo (1999)

5) Wever, D.J., Veldhuizen, A.G., Sanders, M.M., Schakenraad, J.M., van Horn J.R.: Cytotoxic, allergic and genotoxic activity of a nickel-titanium alloy. Biomaterials 18, 1115–1120 (1997)

6) Honma, M., Hayashi, M., Shimada, H., Tanaka, N., Wakuri, S., Awogi, T., Yamamoto, K.I., Kodani, N.U., Nishi, Y., Nakadate, M., Sofuni, T.: Evaluation of the mouse lymphoma tk assay (microwell method) as an alternative to the *in vitro* chromosomal aberration test. Mutagenesis 14, 5–22 (1999)

7) Chauvel-Lebret, D.J., Auroy, P., Tricot-Doleux, S., Bonnaure-Mallet, M.: Evaluation of the capacity of the SCGE assay to assess the genotoxicity of biomaterials. Biomaterials 22, 1795–1801 (2001)

8) Kusakabe, H., Yamakage, K., Wakuri, S., Sasaki, K., Nakagawa, Y., Watanabe, M., Hayashi, M., Sofuni, T., Ono, H., Tanaka, N.: Relevance of chemical structure and cytotoxicity to the induction of chromosome aberrations based on the testing results of 98 high production volume industrial chemicals. Mutat. Res. 517, 187–198 (2002)

9) Müller, B.P., Ensslen, S., Dott, W., Hollender, J.: Improved sample preparation of biomaterials for *in vitro* genotoxicity testing using reference materials. J. Biomed. Mater. Res. 61, 83–90 (2002)

10) Kirsch-Volders, M., Sofuni, T., Ardema, M., Albertini, S., Eastmond, D., Fenech, M., Ishidate, M. Jr., Kirchner, S., Lorge, E., Morita, T., Norppa, H., Surralles, J., Vanhauwaert, A., Wakata, A.: Report from the *in vitro* micronucleus assay working group. Mutat. Res. 540, 153–163 (2003)

11) Kirsch-Volders, M., Sofuni, T., Ardema, M., Albertini, S., Eastmond, D., Fenech, M., Ishidate, M. Jr., Kirchner, S., Lorge, E., Morita, T., Norppa, H., Surralles, J., Vanhauwaert, A., Wakata, A.: Corrigendum to "Report from the *in vitro* micronucleus assay working group" [Mutat. Res. 540 (2003) 153–163]. Mutat. Res. 564, 97–100 (2004)

12) Muramatsu, K., Nakajima, M., Kikuchi, M., Shimada, S., Sasaki, K., Masuda, S., Yoshihara, Y.: *In vitro* cytocompatibility assessment of β-tricalcium phosphate/carboxymethylchitin composite. J. Biomed. Mater. Res. A. 71, 635–643 (2004)

13) Matsuoka, A., Isama, K., Tsuchiya, T.: *In vitro* induction of polyploidy and chromatid exchanges by culture medium extracts of natural rubbers compounded with 2-mercaptobenzothiazole as a positive control candidate for genotoxicity tests. J. Biomed. Mater. Res. A. 75, 439–444 (2005)

14) Matsuoka, A., Haishima, Y., Hasegawa, C., Matsuda, Y., Tsuchiya, T.: Organic-solvent extraction of model biomaterials for use in the *in vitro* chromosome aberration test. J. Biomed. Mater. Res. A. 86, 13–22 (2008)

15) MHW Notification, YAKUKI No. 99, June 27, 1995 "Guideline on biological tests required for application for approval to manufacture (import) medical devices" (Note: abolition on February 13, 2003)

16) MHLW Memorandum, IRYOUKIKI-SHINSA No. 36, March 19, 2003 "Reference materials for basic principles of biological safety tests" (Note: abolition on March 1, 2012)

Biomed. Mater. Res. A. 86, 13-22（2008）

15)　薬機第99号：平成7年6月27日付け厚生省薬務局医療機器開発課長通知　薬機第99号「医療用具の製造（輸入）承認申請に必要な生物学的試験のガイドラインについて」（平成15年2月13日廃止）

16)　事務連絡医療機器審査 No. 36：平成15年3月19日付け厚生労働省医薬局審査管理課事務連絡　医療機器審査 No. 36「生物学的安全性試験の基本的考え方に関する参考資料について」（平成24年3月1日廃止）

第4部　埋植試験

1．適用範囲

　本試験は，埋植の評価を考慮すべき医療機器又は原材料の局所への影響を動物試験により評価するものである．埋植材料の材質，表面性状，又は分解過程などによって，周囲組織に引き起こされる組織反応の種類と程度を評価するもので，特に製品そのものを臨床模擬として埋植して評価する場合を除き，製品の設計仕様により引き起こされる影響を評価するためのものではない．また本試験により埋植試料の毒性病理学的異常だけではなく，新生骨の形成や組織再構築などの適合性を含め，生体適合性を総合的に評価することが可能である．

　試験に用いる埋植材料の形状による物理的刺激などの非特異的反応を引き起こさないよう注意すべきであり，またラット皮下への固形物の長期埋植による異物発がんなど，動物種，埋植期間によって特異的に引き起こされるが，ヒトでは想定されない傷害が発生する可能性のある試験設計をしてはならない．

　埋植初期から安定期にかけての組織反応の経時的変化を確認することは，ヒトでのインプラントの影響を予測する上で有用な情報を提供する．また吸収・分解性の医療機器では，吸収・分解過程で様々な分解物に局所がばく露されることから，どのような組織反応を惹起するかを確認することは極めて重要である．

　埋植試験の中で全身毒性を評価する場合の注意事項についても，本パートにおいて言及する．その場合は全身毒性の要求事項を満たすよう留意する．

　なお，脳内埋植試験においては，使用方法・使用条件を考慮した機能性（性能確認）試験が設定され，適切なリスク評価が実施されている場合には，改めて実施する必要はない．

2．引用規格

　ISO 10993-6: 2016, Biological evaluation of medical devices-Part 6: Tests for local effects after implantation

3．一般的注意事項

3.1　試験法

3.1.1　それぞれの埋植部位における試験法として，筋肉内，皮下，骨内及び脳内埋植試験法を例として後述する．

3.1.2　埋植試験による局所の炎症反応を考察するに際し，細胞毒性，感作性，刺激性などの試験データを参考にすることは重要である．

3.1.3　動物試験を実施する場合には，ISO 10993-2及び動物福祉に関する国内規制の要求事項に従わなければならない．

Part 4　Implantation Test

1.　Scope

This part specifies the test methods for the assessment of the local effects after implantation of medical devices or materials in animal studies. These tests are designed to evaluate the type and intensity of local effects caused in the surrounding tissues by their characteristics of materials, surface, degradation process of the implant specimen, and are not intended to evaluate the effect by the design specification except for the case when final products are implanted as clinical simulation. In addition to assessing toxicological impact of the implant specimen, these tests may also assess biocompatibility issues including new bone synthesis and tissue remodeling.

Non-specific tissue responses such as mechanical stress caused by the shape of test samples should be avoided. Inappropriate test protocol should not be designed such as the long-term implantation of solid materials in rat subcutaneous tissue which results in lesions due to a rodent-specific effect known as solid-state carcinogenesis.

Confirmation of the time-course effects of tissue response from the early (acute) to the steady-state stage may provide valuable information when predicting the implant device's effects on the human body. Moreover, since various degradation products generated in the absorption/decomposition process are exposed to local tissues, it is important to evaluate the tissue response due to the degradation product over the course of the study in the case of absorbable or degradable medical devices.

Notes in the case of systemic toxicity by implantation are referred in this part. Evaluation should be performed to satisfy the requirements for both the systemic toxicity test and the implantation test.

Another implantation tests into the brain is not required if functional tests (performance confirmation) have been performed in consideration of the method and condition of use, and an appropriate risk assessment has been performed.

2.　Normative reference

ISO 10993-6: 2016, Biological evaluation of medical devices-Part 6: Tests for local effects after implantation

3.　General aspects

3.1　Test methods

3.1.1　Implantation test methods for muscle, subcutaneous tissue, bone, and brain are described in latter parts.

3.1.2　It is important to consider other information such as, test data of cytotoxicity, sensitization, irritation, etc., when evaluating the local inflammatory reaction at the implantation site.

3.1.3　Animal testing must comply with the requirements of ISO 10993-2 and domestic regulations on animal welfare.

3.2　試験試料及び対照材料

3.2.1　最終製品を用いる場合は，最終製品そのもの又は最終製品の一部を切り出すなどして調製した試料を用いる．

3.2.2　埋植用試験試料を調製する場合には，その形状，断端の形状，大きさ，表面性状が組織反応に影響することを考慮し，物理的影響を最小限に抑えるために，できる限り平滑な形状とすることが求められる．また試験試料と同様の形状の対照材料を埋植することが評価を容易にする．なお，表面処理を施す場合は，最終製品と同じ表面性状に加工する．

3.2.3　滅菌は最終製品と同じ方法を用いる．試験試料を調製する場合は，無菌的に加工するか，滅菌前の製品を加工した後最終製品と同じ滅菌工程を経たものを用いることが望ましい．再滅菌する場合は，試料が変質などの影響を受けない方法を採用する．

3.2.4　評価は，臨床的許容性及び生体適合性が立証された同形状の材料に対する組織反応と比較する．具体的には，陰性対照材料としては，高密度ポリエチレンや純チタン，既承認 / 認証品として使用実績のある材料などを用いる．陽性対照材料は必須ではないが，試験法や動物の感度を比較したい場合などにおいて設定してもよい（8.4 項参照）．滅菌は，必ずしも試験試料と同じ方法にする必要はなく，材料が変質などの影響を受けない方法を採用する．

3.2.5　骨セメントや歯科材料など，生体内で硬化する医療機器を評価する場合は，臨床適用を摸擬して非硬化物を局所に埋植する．埋植が技術的に困難な材料に対しては，すでに硬化したものを整形して埋植する場合がある．後者の場合は，硬化中の生体反応について，別の生物学的安全性試験を実施することにより評価することが望ましい．

3.2.6　非固形（例：粉末）を評価する場合は，①ペレット化する，②粉末状態で臨床適用されるものであれば，臨床適用される形状で一定の面積，容積を埋植する，③シリコーンやポリプロピレン製などの刺激性の低いことが知られている開口チューブに充填して埋植するなどの設計とする．③の充填時にはコンタミネーションがないよう注意し，対照材料の一つとしてチューブのみを埋植する．

3.2.7　組織工学により製造される医療機器を試験する場合，生体由来材料は埋植する動物種に対して免疫反応を引き起こす可能性があることに留意する．

3.2.8　複数の部材からなる医療機器を埋植する場合，それぞれの部材による局所影響が明確に解析できる設計とする．最終製品そのものを埋植した時，それぞれの部材の組織反応が組織標本において特定できないと想定される場合は部材を単離して埋植する，表裏などが異なる材料ではそれが明確に区別できる方法で埋植するなどである．ただし，部材間の相互作用が予測される場合や，血管内埋植などにおいて臨床摸擬

3.2   Test sample and control material

3.2.1   For the final product, a representative portion of it (or a representative facsimile) is evaluated in the implantation study.

3.2.2   When preparing the implant specimen, the following factors can influence the tissue response: shape, size, shape of edge, and surface characteristics. The shape of the test sample shall be smooth, if possible, to reduce physical influences. The control material and test material should be of similar shape to minimize potential shape induced effects in the tissue response. The control material surface shall be the same as the test sample when surface processing.

3.2.3   Test sample shall be sterilized by the method intended for the final product. The test sample should be prepared for implantation aseptically or prepared for implantation after the unsterilized test sample is processed and then sterilized. If the test sample is re-sterilized, the re-sterilization must not change the test sample's properties.

3.2.4   The tissue response of the test sample should be evaluated by comparing to the material with same shape for which clinical acceptability and biocompatibility have been demonstrated. Specifically, high-density polyethylene, pure titanium, or approved medical devices are negative control candidates. Although the inclusion in the study of a positive control implant is optional, its inclusion in the study may be helpful for comparing the test method or sensitivity of test animals (refer to clause 8.4). It is not necessary to sterilize the controls using the same method as the test sample, but the sterilization method shall be selected not to change the control's properties.

3.2.5   When evaluating medical devices that harden in the body such as bone cement and dental materials, the pre-hardened form of the material is implanted into the animal to simulate the clinical use environment. If the pre-hardened form is technically difficult to implant, a hardened form of the material may be molded and implanted. In the latter case, it is desirable to use another biological safety test to evaluate the biological response during the hardening reaction.

3.2.6   When evaluating a non-solid material (such as powders), a) the non-solid may be pelleted, b) an adequate area or volume of non-solid material, which would be applied clinically, may be implanted, c) the non-solid material may be contained in open-ended cylindrical tubes made of low-irritating material such as silicone and polypropylene. In the last case, care should be taken to avoid contamination and empty tubes should serve as one of the controls.

3.2.7   When evaluating tissue-engineered medical devices, bioengineered material of human origin may cause an immune response in the implanted animals.

3.2.8   When evaluating medical device composed of two or more materials, the local biological effects of each material shall be determined. Each material may be separated and implanted, if the whole device is implanted and the tissue reaction caused by each material is unknown. If the material in the front and back of the test sample is different, the tissue response of each side shall be recorded. The final product may be implanted, when

試験として埋植試験を実施する場合は，最終製品そのものを埋植することにより評価する．

3.2.9　埋植試験により全身毒性を合わせて評価する場合，動物への埋植試料の総量とヒトの埋植量を比較して一定のばく露マージンを担保できる設計とすべきである．ただし，人工関節材料など，ヒトへの埋植量が大きいものについては，一定のばく露マージンを担保する設計は困難である．このような場合は，できる限りヒトの適用量を下回らない設計として，合わせて抽出液などによる全身毒性試験を検討する．また生体内分解材料の場合は，*in vitro* における分解動態が生体内と同程度であることが判明していない限り，抽出液を用いるべきではなく，埋植によって全身毒性を検索すべきである．

3.3　埋植部位

3.3.1　埋植部位は臨床適用部位に近い組織とする．本試験法では，例として筋肉内，皮下，骨内及び脳内埋植試験法について記載しているが，これ以外の組織・器官に臨床適用される場合は，その組織・器官の起原，構成組織，細胞種などを総合的に勘案して，例として挙げた組織のいずれか又は複数を選択する．また新たな組織への標準的な試験法が ISO 10993-6 などで明らかとなった場合は，それを示した上で，採用することができる．文献などで明らかとなった方法を採用する場合は，その妥当性を示した上で，十分なサンプル数（1 埋植期間について 10 箇所以上）の観察を行う設計とする．

3.3.2　吸収・分解性材料の場合は，消失した後に埋植部位を特定することが困難になるおそれがあるため，①埋植時に写真を撮影するなどして埋植位置を特定しておき，その位置に試験試料がない場合は吸収されたものとみなす，②陰性対照材料や局所への影響がないことが知られている物質をマーカーとして同時に埋植してその付近を観察する，③X 線撮影などを経時的に行って埋植部位を特定するなど，消失した後の取扱いを明確にしておく，あるいは消失した場合でも観察位置が特定できるよう工夫する．入墨又は試料の配置を示す模式図を利用してもよいが，短期の埋植期間のみとする．

3.3.3　埋植試験により全身毒性を合わせて評価する場合，あらかじめ試験計画立案の際に全身毒性を評価できるよう，血液学的，血液生化学的，病理組織学的検査などを計画する．対照材料と試験試料を同一の動物に埋植すると全身毒性の評価が困難となることから，試験試料埋植群と対照群は別々に設定する．また複数の材料を同一動物に埋植しても，全身毒性の評価は困難となる．ただし，複数の部材から構成される医療機器の埋植試験を設計する場合は，複数の部材を同一動物に埋植することで，臨床適用を摸擬することが可能となる．

3.4　埋植期間

3.4.1　埋植期間は，臨床適用期間を超える必要はないが，ヒトにおける埋植反応を予測し得る期間，若しくは，生体反応が安定した状態となるまでとする．

interaction between the material is predicted, or when the implantation test simulates clinical use conditions (e.g. implantation test in blood vessels).

3.2.9   When systemic toxicity is investigated in the implantation test, an adequate margin of exposure shall be considered in the test design by comparing total amount of implant for animals to that for human. However, for medical devices that are implanted in large quantities (such as artificial bone) it is difficult to include an adequate margin of exposure in the animal study. In such case, the implantation dose should not be less than the amount used in the clinical setting (if possible) and additional systemic toxicity test with extract should be considered. For biodegradable materials, systemic toxicity shall be investigated by implantation test, and biodegradable material extract shall not be used unless the decomposition kinetics *in vitro* are demonstrated to be the same as the *in vivo* situation.

3.3   Implantation site

3.3.1   Test sample shall be implanted into the tissue relevant to the intended clinical use of the medical device. In this part, detailed test methods for muscle, subcutaneous tissue, bone, and brain are given as examples. If the tissue intended clinical use is not those described, a more relevant tissue may be selected after a comprehensive evaluation is undertaken which consider the origin of the tissue and organ, tissue composition, and type of cells. Moreover, when the standard method for a new tissue becomes clear in ISO 10993-6, it can be available. When adopting a method described in literatures, justify the use of the test method and consider including sufficient number of test samples can be observed (ten or more test samples implanted per implantation period) in the test design.

3.3.2   For absorbable or degradable materials, mark the implantation site so that it can be identified after the test sample is absorbed or degraded; e.g., a) Take photographs during the implantation procedure, and the test sample must be considered to be absorbed if it is not found at the sites afterwards. b) Implant a negative control or an inert material as a reference point, and observe around the reference point. c) Take X-ray images of the implant site periodically to pinpoint the implantation sites. Tattoos or a schematic diagram showing the arrangement of samples may be used only for a short implantation period.

3.3.3   For combined test evaluating local implant effects and systemic toxicity, the protocol should include hematological, blood-biochemical, and histopathological examinations, etc. Since evaluation of systemic toxicity is confounded if the control and test samples are implanted into the same animal, the test and control articles should be implanted in separate animals. Implantation of two or more different materials in the same animal will confound evaluation of the systemic effects due to each individual material. However, the multiple material implantations for devices composed of two or more materials may better represent the clinical setting.

3.4   Implantation period

3.4.1   The implant study duration should be sufficient to predict the human response but the implantation duration does not have to be longer than the clinical use duration, or should be a period until the biological reaction becomes stable.

3.4.2　吸収・分解性材料でない場合

3.4.2.1　埋植初期の反応，埋植中期の埋植試料と生体界面の組織反応，そして安定化（すれば）した場合の反応を評価することが望ましい．複数の期間を観察して安定化することが明らかであった場合は，それ以上の期間の埋植群を省略することを検討する．ただし，試験計画を立案する際には，短中期の試験をあらかじめ行った上で長期埋植を計画するなど，動物愛護の観点から動物数を減らすことを検討する．

3.4.2.2　短期の埋植を1週から4週とし，長期埋植は12週を超える期間とする．またその間を中期埋植とする．生体適合性の高い材料の場合，短期において，埋植後2週間程度は埋植手術の影響が残るが，対照材料と比較することにより，試料に起因する炎症反応を区別して観察することができる．また器質化や新生骨の形成は埋植後2週間程度でも開始されており，生体適合性に関する情報が多く得られる．埋植後4週には，すでに安定化する場合が多い．中期では，周囲組織の多くは埋植前の状態に近づいており，界面や周囲はおおむね安定化し，その後の長期における反応を推測するための時期である．長期では，周囲組織は正常組織と同様となり，界面は非常に薄い被膜や新生骨で覆われ安定化する．

3.4.3　吸収・分解性材料の場合

3.4.3.1　吸収・分解過程で様々な物質が細粒化又は溶出するなどして，埋植局所は初期とは異なる環境となるため，分解過程を評価し得る埋植期間を設定する．具体的には，少なくとも以下の埋植期間を含むこと．

1)　短期（分解がない又は最低限の期間）：初期の組織反応を評価するため，通常1〜2週の埋植期間を設ける．

2)　中期（分解が進行中の期間）：崩壊/断片化などの組織学的変化が最も大きいと予測される時期を評価する．長期間の分解特性を有する場合には，予想される分解様式に応じた複数の埋植期間が必要な場合がある．異なる分解速度を有する複数の材料から構成される場合は，全ての材料の分解特性を評価可能な埋植期間を設定すべきである．

3)　長期（埋植試料がほぼ分解された期間）：埋植部位にごく少量しか残存していない時点の組織反応を評価する．なお，埋植試料が完全に吸収された後の評価が望ましいが，組織反応が安定化しており吸収性材料がごく少量しか残存していない場合でも，十分に局所への影響を評価し得ると思われる．可能な場合，試料の推定残存率を算出する．また加速分解した材料を埋植することにより，迅速に長期埋植の結果を確認することができるものの，実際の埋植期間のデータの代替にはならない．

3.4.2 Non-absorbable or non-degradable materials

3.4.2.1   The local tissue response around the implant should be evaluated at the acute and middle stage of the tissue response and when the tissue response has reached steady state. When the study results demonstrate that the tissue response has reached steady state for two or more implantation periods, one may end the study early and euthanize the animals that were planned to be followed further. Thus, to reduce animal usage, animals implanted for a longer duration may be added to the study after results are obtained from animals implanted with test samples for short and mid-duration.

3.4.2.2   Short-term tissue responses around the implant sites are assessed from 1 to 4 weeks following implantation and after 12 weeks for long-term tissue responses. Mid-term tissue responses are evaluated in the period between the two. Although the influences of the surgical procedure remain after 2 weeks, the local tissue response in animals implanted with a test sample can still be compared to the control material. Moreover, tissue reorganization and osteosynthesis begins about two weeks after implantation, and much biocompatibility information can be collected. At 4 weeks after implantation, most tissue response around the implant has reached steady state. In the middle stage, the appearances of the tissue surrounding the implant are similar in appearance to the tissue prior to implantation and the tissue response has generally reached steady state. At this stage it is suitable to speculate on the tissue response of animals that are being followed for longer durations. The surrounding tissue of animals implanted with the test sample long term is the same as the tissue prior to implantation, and the tissue-implant interface is covered with a very thin capsule or new bone and stabilized.

3.4.3 Absorbable and degradable materials

3.4.3.1   Implantation period shall be of sufficient duration and interval to fully capture the effects of the degradation or absorption process on the surrounding tissue since the rate that various substances and small fragments are released during the degradation process may change with time. Study intervals shall include the following time points as a minimum:

1) Early time frame (where there is no or minimal degradation): use usually a study interval of between 1 week and 2 weeks post-implantation to assess the early tissue response.

2) Mid time frame (when degradation is taking place): the period when the tissue response is expected to be most pronounced (e.g. substantial structural disruption and/or fragmentation of the device is most likely to occur). Implants with longer-term degradation profiles may require multiple assessment time points, with intervals targeted in accordance with the expected pattern of degradation. When a device with multiple materials with differing absorption rates is implanted, implant intervals reflecting the degradation profile of those components should be included.

3) Late time frame (when the implant is almost absorbed): this interval is targeted to observe when minimal amounts of the absorbable component remain at the implant site. Gross and microscopic evaluation after complete implant absorption is highly desirable. However, in the absence of complete absorption, the overall data collected should be sufficient to allow characterization of the local effects after implantation if the affected tissue's response have achieved an acceptable steady-state condition, and the absorbable material and/or its degradation products are in a state of limited visually-identifiable presence. If possible, calculate the estimated percentage of remaining absorbable materials. Although implantation of accelerated degraded material can be rapidly assessed the late stage events after implantation, these studies do not replace studies that characterize the real-time *in vivo* degradation profile of the absorbable devices.

3.4.3.2　埋植期間中に試料が完全に吸収されない場合，又は完全に分解されて試料が組織学的にも確認できない場合に備え，埋植期間を決めるためのサテライト群を設定することが有用な場合がある．また1年以上の分解期間が必要な場合では，サテライト群の動物を長期間にわたって観察することで有用な情報が得られることがある．

3.4.3.3　吸収・分解性材料の全身毒性を埋植試験により評価する場合，材料及びその分解物による毒性の両方を評価し得る適切な埋植期間を設定する．

3.5　試験動物

3.5.1　短中期の埋植試験には，げっ歯類，ウサギなどが一般的に用いられる．長期埋植では，げっ歯類，ウサギ，イヌ，ヒツジ，ヤギ，ブタなどが用いられる．ラットでは異物発がんが知られているため[1]，26週を超える皮下埋植試験に用いる場合は注意を要する．表1に長期埋植の際の動物種の選択を示した．

表1　長期埋植における動物種の選択

種	埋植期間（週）				
	13	26	52	78	(104)
マウス	○	○	○		
ラット	○	○	○		
モルモット	○	○	○		
ウサギ	○	○	○	○	○
イヌ	○	○	○	○	○
ヒツジ	○	○	○	○	○
ヤギ	○	○	○	○	○
ブタ	○	○	○	○	○

注：ISO 10993-6: 2016 Table 1 を引用した．医療機器の臨床適用に応じた試験期間とする．全ての期間を実施する必要はない．ラットの場合，26週を超える皮下埋植は異物発がんの可能性を考慮する．また104週は特定の場合のみに設計する．

3.5.2　吸収・分解性材料を試験する場合，げっ歯類を用いた事前のパイロット試験を行い，吸収・分解挙動について *in vitro* で得られた結果と比較しておくとよい．

3.5.3　局所への影響を確認する場合，動物の個体差の指標とするため，原則として対照材料と試験試料は同じ個体に埋植する．ただし，脳内埋植試験及び埋植試験により全身毒性を合わせて評価する場合，対照材料と試験試料を同じ個体に埋植することは適切ではない．

3.5.4　動物数は複数を用いることとするが，ISO 10993-6: 2016 に記載された動物数以上とする（4.2, 5.2, 6.2, 7.2 項参照）．

3.5.5　動物の性は，臨床適用の際にいずれかの性に特化される場合その性について設計

3.4.3.2 Satellite animals to determine the implantation period can be beneficial if the implants have not been completely absorbed within the implantation period, or completely degraded and cannot be observed microscopically. For materials which degrade or are absorbed for over a year, long-term observation of the satellite animals might give useful information.

3.4.3.3 When the systemic toxicity of the absorbable/degradable material is evaluated by an implantation test, implant an appropriate period when both the toxicity of the material and its degradation product can be evaluated.

3.5 Test animal

3.5.1 In general, rodents and rabbits are used for short and middle term implantation. For long-term implantation, rodents, rabbits, dogs, sheep, goats, and pigs is preferable. Tumors have been found in rats subcutaneously implanted with biocompatible material and followed for >26 weeks[1] and therefore, users should be aware of this phenomenon. Generally accepted observation periods are shown in Table 1.

Table 1 Selection of animal species for long-term implantation

Species	Implantation period (week)				
	13	26	52	78	(104)
Mice	◯	◯	◯		
Rats	◯	◯	◯		
Guinea pigs	◯	◯	◯		
Rabbits	◯	◯	◯	◯	◯
Dogs	◯	◯	◯	◯	◯
Sheep	◯	◯	◯	◯	◯
Goats	◯	◯	◯	◯	◯
Pigs	◯	◯	◯	◯	◯

Note: ISO 10993-6: 2016 Table 1 was referred. Depending on the intended use of the medical devices, not all implantation periods may be necessary. Oncogenesis caused by a foreign body should be considered when subcutaneously implanting the test sample in rats. An observation period of 104 weeks may be of interest in selected instances.

3.5.2 Before testing absorbable and degradable materials, it is preferable to compare the absorption and decomposition behavior *in vivo* with those *in vitro* by a pilot test using rodents.

3.5.3 In principle, both the test samples and control materials shall be implanted in the same animal to account for individual differences. However, the test samples and control materials shall not be implanted in the same animals when implantation test into the brain or the systemic toxicity test combined with the implantation test is conducted.

3.5.4 The number of animals shall be the same or greater than the number indicated in ISO 10993-6: 2016 (refer to clauses 4.2, 5.2, 6.2, and 7.2).

3.5.5 The selection of the animal's sex should depend on the specific sex of the intended pa-

し，性差が予測される場合は両性とし，それ以外はいずれかの性でよい．

3.5.6　各埋植期間終了後，動物を適切な方法で安楽死させる．

3.6　埋植方法

3.6.1　埋植手術は全身麻酔下で行う．全身麻酔には，一般的医薬品又は動物用医薬品を用い，動物に苦痛をもたらす薬品を用いてはならない．

3.6.2　術野は刈毛後，適切な消毒薬を用いて清拭する．熟練した術者により滅菌した清浄な器具を用いて切開し，出血は最小限になるよう埋植を行う．埋植後は，刺激性の低い縫合糸やステープラで切開創を閉じ，消毒する．また動物が縫合部位を舐めないよう，げっ歯類，ウサギやイヌの場合は埋植初期には首にカラーを装着するとよい．抗菌剤や抗生物質などの医薬品の投与は，知見や予備検討などにより当該医薬品が埋植部位の組織反応に影響しないことをあらかじめ確認する必要がある．例えば，ミノサイクリンなどの抗生物質は脳ミクログリア及びマクロファージの反応に影響を与えることが報告されている．

3.6.3　適当な対照材料がない場合や埋植術により手術の影響が残ることが予想される場合は，偽手術群を設定することを考慮する．偽手術群で著しい反応が見られた場合は，試験試料の反応がマスクされる可能性があるため，試験法に問題があると判断し，埋植法などを再検討する．

3.6.4　埋植期間中は，動物の一般状態を定期的に観察し，体重測定を行う．鎮痛剤を使用する場合には，ISO 10993-2 の規定に従う．

3.6.5　埋植期間中に動物の状態が悪化し，回復の見込みがない場合は，動物を安楽死させる．その場合，埋植局所の観察は通常どおり行い，全てのデータを記録する．この場合，状態の変化が試料の埋植に起因するか否かを十分検討する．評価の対象としない例としては，骨内埋植した直後に離断骨折し，治療を行わない限り苦痛を与え続けるなどの理由で安楽死させ，観察の結果埋植部位以外の骨折が原因であった場合など，原因が試料の埋植による影響ではないことが明らかな場合がある．

3.6.6　埋植部位の皮膚が哆開するなど，再手術の必要がある場合は，直ちに麻酔下で縫合するなどの処置を行う．化膿が見られる場合はできるだけ除去し，多量の生理食塩液や緩衝液を用いて洗浄する．抗菌剤や抗生物質を使用する際は，3.6.2 項を参考にして妥当性を確認しておく．これらの処置を行った場合は，全て記録する．

3.6.7　埋植期間終了後は，動物を全身麻酔下で安楽死させる．原則として放血処置を行

tient population, and on the predicted sex differences. In other cases, either sex may be used.

3.5.6   Animals are euthanized by an appropriate method after the end of implantation period.

3.6   Implantation method

3.6.1   Surgery shall be performed under general anesthesia. For general anesthesia, use common medicines or drugs for animals and the chemicals should not cause pain to the animals.

3.6.2   Remove the hair from surgical area, and disinfect the exposed area of the skin with an appropriate disinfectant. A person experienced in animal surgery should perform the implantation with aseptic clean instruments, and bleeding should be minimized. After implantation, close the wound using low−irritating sutures or surgical stapler, and disinfect the site. To prevent the animal from licking the closed site, a neck collar may be useful in rodents, dogs and rabbits during the early stages following implantation. Use medicine such as antibacterial drugs and antibiotics after it is confirmed by literature or preliminary examination that the medicine is unlikely to affect the tissue response around the implant site. For example, antibiotics such as minocycline have been reported to modulate the response of brain microglia and macrophages.

3.6.3   Sham−surgery control group should be considered if appropriate control materials are not available or if the surgical treatment effect may not be negligible. When remarkable responses are seen in sham−surgery control group, the test method is considered to be invalid since the reaction of the test sample may be masked by the surgical effect, and re-examination of the implantation method shall be considered.

3.6.4   Observe the general condition of the animals periodically and record their body weights during the implantation period. The use of analgesics shall be in line with the rules of ISO 10993−2.

3.6.5   If an animal's condition worsens and recover is unlikely, it should be humanely euthanized. The test samples from the euthanized animals should be sufficiently evaluated and recorded to determine if test sample implantation was a causative factor for the change in the animal's health. A euthanized animal may be excluded from the main test result evaluation if the implantation was not a causative factor for the change in the animal's health. An example where the animal may be excluded is an obvious bone fracture immediately after surgery and it is clear that the fracture is not due to the surgical procedure and not the test material.

3.6.6   If re−operation is needed such as opening of a closed wound, close the wound immediately while the animal in under anesthesia. If the wound has pus, remove as much pus as possible and wash the wound extensively with saline or buffered solution. Use of an antibacterial or antibiotic drug should be justified by referring to clause 3.6.2. All treatments shall be recorded.

3.6.7   After the end of implantation period, animals are euthanized under general anesthesia,

う.

3.7　観察
3.7.1　肉眼的観察
3.7.1.1　埋植試験試料周囲組織及び試料を肉眼又は拡大鏡を用いて,出血,浮腫,被包形成などの正常な構造からの変化について観察し,それらの範囲と合わせて記録する.なお,埋植周囲リンパ節[2]の腫脹なども観察する.試験動物に何らかの異常がある場合や全身毒性試験を兼ねる場合は,埋植部位以外の臓器を観察し,組織学的観察のための採材を行う.

3.7.1.2　埋植部位を破壊しないと観察できない場合は,組織観察標本用の組織を固定した後,埋植試料を引き抜く際などに埋植部位の肉眼観察を行い,組織観察用の標本と兼ねてもよい.この場合,あらかじめ試料が固定液により変色するか否かなどを確認しておく.

3.7.1.3　吸収性材料の場合,分解の程度,摘出時の状態を埋植部位ごとに記録する.

3.7.2　組織学的観察
3.7.2.1　埋植組織を,直ちに固定液に浸す.一般的には10％中性緩衝ホルマリン液で固定し,固定完了後,切り出し,パラフィン包埋,薄切を行う.ヘマトキシリン・エオジン染色を施して,光学顕微鏡下で観察する.必要に応じて,その他の固定法,包埋法及び染色方法を採用してもよい.埋植周囲リンパ節は,非吸収性材料の場合は肉眼的に異常が見られた場合,吸収性材料の場合は可能な限り採取して組織学的に観察する(分解材料のリンパ管内における移動を確認することができるため).

3.7.2.2　薄切片の作製に際し,ミクロトームによる薄切が可能な柔らかい試料の場合は,試料とともに薄切すると周囲組織を損傷せず,界面の観察が可能となる.

3.7.2.3　試料が硬い場合は,試料とともに薄切すると周囲組織を損傷するおそれがあるため,固定(脱灰)後に引き抜くか,適当な溶媒で溶解させるなど試料を除去し,組織損傷がないことを確認した後,薄切することを検討する.

3.7.2.4　試料が硬く有機溶媒などにも不溶である,多孔性であるなど,引き抜く際に界面の周囲組織を破壊してしまうおそれがある場合は,埋植部位全体を樹脂包埋し,研磨標本を作製する.一般的にギムザ染色やトルイジンブルー染色が用いられる.骨内埋植の場合,在来骨又は新生骨と試料の界面が重要な観察ポイントであり,研磨標本作製により,界面の保存が容易となる.またビラヌエバ染色を施した標本を蛍光顕微鏡で観察すると,石灰化骨と類骨の判別が容易になる.ただし,炎症性細胞の種類などを検索する際,標本が厚く細胞レベルの観察が困難である場合には,別

and bled in principle.

3.7 Observation
3.7.1 Macroscopic observation
3.7.1.1 Examine the implanted specimen and the surrounding tissue with the naked eye or a magnifying glass. Record any alterations of the normal structure such as hemorrhages, edema, and encapsulation with their area. Also observe the changes of the regional draining lymph nodes[2] such as swelling. If the animals show any abnormalities or systemic toxicity is also evaluated, other organs shall be observed and harvested for histological observation.

3.7.1.2 The test samples can be used for both macroscopic and microscopic observations. When the implantation site cannot be macroscopically observed unless the test sample is explanted, the macroscopic observation should be made when the test sample is explanted after tissue fixation. In this case, check the test sample for discoloration before tissue fixation.

3.7.1.3 For absorbable materials, record the degree of degradation and the shape of the residual samples at each implant site.

3.7.2 Histological observation
3.7.2.1 Immerse immediately implanted tissue in fixation solution. Generally, tissues are fixed in 10 % neutral buffered formalin solution, cut into blocks, embedded in paraffin, and processed for thin section. After hematoxylin and eosin staining, microscopic observation is made under a light microscopy. If needed, other fixation and staining methods may be appropriate. For non-absorbable materials, the regional draining lymph nodes should be observed histologically if gross abnormalities are noted. In the case of absorbable material, collect and observe the regional draining lymph nodes histologically as much as possible. This enables to evaluate the migration of the decomposed material via the lymph vessels.

3.7.2.2 If the test sample is soft enough to be cut by microtome, prepare thin sections without removing the test sample from the tissue to allow later observation of the undisturbed tissue-material interface.

3.7.2.3 If the test sample is hard, remove the test sample after fixation (decalcifying) or dissolve the test sample in the appropriate organic solvent, since the tissue interface may be destroyed if sectioned along with the test sample. After removal of the test sample, observe any tissue damage, and then prepare thin sections.

3.7.2.4 If tissue-device interactions may be affected when removing the test sample or if the test sample is difficult to dissolve in organic solvents, it may be useful to embed the whole implant and its surrounding tissue in resin and prepare ground section. In general, the ground section is stained with Giemsa or toluidine blue. In the bone implantation study, the native bone or new bone interface to the test sample is an important observation site. The undecalcified ground section makes assessment of the interface region easy. Additionally, if the specimen is stained with Villanueva stain and observed under fluorescence, calcified bone and osteoid are readily visible. However, if identification of the inflammato-

に骨組織を脱灰後，試料を引き抜くなどしてパラフィン包埋し，薄切標本を作製・観察する．

3.7.2.5　作製した標本は，顕微鏡下で観察する．埋植周囲に認められた炎症性細胞の種類や出現の程度及びその他の異常所見を記録する．例えば，被膜を構成する成分とその状態，線維芽細胞の増生，好中球（ウサギ及びモルモットの場合，偽好酸球），リンパ球，形質細胞，マクロファージ，巨細胞などの浸潤，変性・壊死，出血，脂肪化，新生骨形成などについて観察し，グレード分けして記録する．筋肉内埋植の場合，炎症性細胞の浸潤や炎症反応は筋線維間に延びる線維性結合組織の方向に拡大しやすく，また筋肉の収縮方向に長くなり，紡錘形となる傾向がある．観察に当たっては，そのようなことに留意して所見を記録する．

3.7.2.6　筋肉内埋植の場合は，炎症領域の幅を測定するなど，組織形態計測を行うことにより，局所への傷害を定量的に評価することが可能である．この際，標本中における試料の薄切面を一定にするなど，組織形態計測におけるばらつきを少なくすることに留意する．吸収・分解性の試料では貪食などにより形状が維持されないため，また多孔性や繊維状のものでは，内部に線維組織が侵入するため，炎症領域の幅を測定することはできない．また皮下や骨内埋植では，炎症領域の幅の計測が困難又は必ずしも炎症を定量化するための指標とはならないため，他に適切なパラメータがある場合はその根拠を示した上で組織形態計測を行ってもよい．

3.7.2.7　吸収性材料の場合，臓器のリモデリングを観察することが目的の一つであるため，埋植部位に正常な組織が形成されるかも考慮して評価する．

3.7.2.8　骨内埋植の場合，組織と埋植試料の界面は特に注意して観察する．埋植試料と骨が接触する程度，埋植試料近傍の骨組織の状況や非石灰化組織の介在，並びに骨吸収や骨新生の有無について記録する．

3.7.2.9　ヘマトキシリン・エオジン染色での病理組織学的評価で異常が認められた場合，評価方法を追加してもよい．

3.8　評価
3.8.1　各観察項目について，程度とともにその現象を観察する（評価基準を設けて観察し，表に示す）．表2に評価のために着目すべきポイントを示した．スコアリングの後，統計学的検定を行ってもよいが，その場合は観察項目ごとに比較する．全てのスコアの合計値を指標とする場合，それぞれの観察項目が評価において同等の重みとなるよう適切な係数を乗じるなどの処理を行うことを原則とする．なお，ISO 10993-6: 2016 Annex E などのスコア表を用いてもよい．

3.8.2　組織形態計測を行った場合は，その数値を表にして示す．

ry cells is difficult due to the thickness of the section, decalcify the bone tissue, pullout the test sample, embed the tissue in paraffin and cut thin sections for observation.

3.7.2.5 The histological sections are observed by microscopy. Inflammatory cell type, degree of inflammatory response, and abnormal appearances are recorded around the test sample. For example, components consisting of the capsule, proliferation of fibroblasts, neutrophils (pseudoeosinophils in rabbits and guinea pigs), lymphocytes, plasma cells, macrophages, and giant cells, tissue degeneration and/or necrosis, hemorrhages, fatty change, osteogenesis are observed and evaluated with grading. In the case of muscle implantation, infiltration of inflammatory cells and inflammatory response tend to expand in the direction of fibrous connective tissue which extend between muscle fibers, and becomes long in the muscular contraction direction, and the shape may be spindle. Careful attention should be taken in the observation.

3.7.2.6 In muscle implantation, morphometric analysis such as measuring the thickness of the inflammatory lesion may help to evaluate local effects quantitatively. Under the present procedures, it should be noted that the implanted site is kept constant when processing the section to minimize variation in morphometry measurement. Morphometric analysis is not applicable to absorbable or degradable test samples since the test sample shape is not uniform, and to porous or fibrous test samples since tissue can infiltrates into the porous material or vacancy of fibers. Moreover, since measurement of the inflammatory area is not always an indicator to quantify inflammation for subcutaneous and bone implantation tests, suitable parameter of morphometry may be used if the reliable reason can be shown.

3.7.2.7 For degradable/absorbable materials, restoration to normal structure at the implant site should also be observed to evaluate tissue remodeling.

3.7.2.8 For implants in bone, the interface between the tissue and the implant sample is of special interest. Evaluate the contact area between the implant and bone, the bone formation in the vicinity of the implant, the presence of non-calcified tissue, and the presence of bone resorption and osteogenesis.

3.7.2.9 When histopathological evaluation reveals abnormalities such as immune cell infiltration, additional methods other than hematoxylin/eosin staining are also recommended.

3.8 Evaluation

3.8.1 The appearance and the intensity for each observed histological characteristic is recorded (and the evaluation criteria should be defined and presented in a table). Histological characteristics evaluated for each implant site are described in Table 2. Statistical analysis may be applied to each graded histological characteristic to compare the tissue response to the control material. Comparisons between the test sample and control shall be made with individual response category. If the total sum of the score for individual animal is used, the score multiplied by suitable coefficient can be used for an indicator. Scoring systems given in ISO 10993-6: 2016 Annex E may also be used.

3.8.2 The morphometric analysis is presented in a table format.

3.8.3　ある観察期間において，試験試料の反応が陰性対照材料と比較して有意（8.7 項参照）に強い場合，陽性反応を認めたと判定する．

3.8.4　肉眼的観察では，反応の広がりを全体として捉えることが可能であり，組織学的観察では肉眼的観察で見られた反応がどのような細胞が主体になって起きているのかがわかる．反応が微弱であれば，組織学的観察でのみ見られるにとどまり，局所的反応は肉眼的観察においてしか見られない可能性もある．したがって，組織学的観察を評価するに当たっても，肉眼的観察結果も考慮すべきである．

3.8.5　まれに動物個体の感受性が異常に高い（陰性対照でも細胞浸潤などの反応が見られる）場合があり，評価が困難となることがある．このような場合には，その動物を評価の対象から外し，新たに動物を追加，補充する．ただし，評価の対象外とした動物のデータも試験の報告に含めるべきである．

表2　埋植局所の組織学的観察ポイント

埋植組織	観察ポイント
筋肉内	線維性被膜の状態（被膜，被包の成熟度合いと線維芽細胞の増生程度）及びその厚み，細胞浸潤（マクロファージ，巨細胞，好中球（偽好酸球），リンパ球，形質細胞，好酸球など），変性・壊死，出血，血管新生，脂肪化など
皮下	筋肉内と同様
骨内	組織と埋植試料の界面の状態（軟組織又は骨の介在の程度），新生骨の形成（埋植試料周囲の骨新生の程度と石灰化骨/類骨の割合など），細胞浸潤（マクロファージ，巨細胞，好中球（偽好酸球），リンパ球，形質細胞，好酸球など），変性・壊死，出血など
脳内	筋肉内の観察ポイント及び神経病理学的評価．上衣層及びくも膜顆粒についても調査する．

注：吸収・分解性の試料の場合は，残存した試料の形状や残存の程度などについて評価する．

3.9　試験報告書

試験報告書には，少なくとも以下の事項を記載する．

1) 試験実施機関及び試験責任者
2) 試験実施期間
3) 試験試料（最終製品又は原材料）を特定する情報
    （例：医療機器の名称，製造販売業者名，製造番号，原材料名など）
4) 対照材料
    （例：対照材料名，入手先，入手年月日，製造番号など）
5) 試験試料及び対照材料の調製方法
    （例：切断，滅菌，サイズなど）
6) 試験動物（種，系統，性，週齢，体重，入手元．動物の収容方法及び飼育方法）
7) 試験方法（麻酔方法及び術後処置を含む試料の埋植方法，回収方法，病理組織標本

3.8.3 For certain implantation period, if the local effects of the test sample are severer compared to the negative control (refer to clause 8.7), the tissue response to the test sample is concluded positive.

3.8.4 Macroscopic observation enables to understand the extent of the biological response as a whole, while the microscopic observation provides one with an understanding of the number and type of cells that make up the biological response observed at the macroscopic level. If the biological reaction is weak, it will mainly be detected by histological observation, and a local reaction may be only observed macroscopically. Therefore, in histological evaluation, the macroscopic results should also be taken into consideration.

3.8.5 With some animals, a significant biological response is seen even with the negative control implant. Therefore, it may become difficult to differentiate between the animal's response to the test sample and its response to the procedure. In such a case, replace the animal showing the unusual response with a new animal that has been prepared similarly. However, the data of all animal, including the one that was removed, shall be documented in the final report and a justification provided explaining the protocol deviation.

Table 2   Histological observation points of local implantation sites

Implanted tissue	Observation point
Muscle	Extent of fibrosis (degree of membrane or capsule formation, and fibroblast increase), its thickness, cellular infiltrates (macrophages, giant cells, neutrophils (pseudeosinophils), lymphocytes, plasma cells, eosinophils etc.), tissue degeneration and necrosis, hemorrhage, neovascularization, fatty change etc.
Subcutis	Same as muscle implantation.
Bone	Extent of tissue–material interface (degree of intervention of soft tissue and bone), new bone formation (degree of osteogenesis surrounding the test sample and calcified bone/osteoid ratio etc.), cellular infiltrates (macrophages, giant cells, neutrophils (pseudeosinophils), lymphocytes, plasma cells, eosinophils etc.), tissue degeneration and necrosis, hemorrhage, and neovascularization etc.
Brain	Observation point of muscle implantation and neuropathological evaluation. Changes in the ependymal layer and the arachnoid granulations should also be investigated.

Note: Shape and amount of the residual test sample are evaluated for absorbable/degradable materials.

3.9   Test Report

In the test report, the following items are included at least.
1) Information of the test facility and the study director
2) Test period
3) Information of the test sample (final product or raw material)
   (Example: name of the medical device, manufacturer name, serial number, name of raw materials)
4) Information of the control material
   (Example: name of the control materials, origin, date of arrival, serial number)
5) Preparation of the test sample and control
   (Example: cutting, sterilization, size)
6) Test animals
   (Species, strain, sex, age, body weight, vendor, husbandry, animal care)
7) Test methods

の作製方法）

8)　試験結果

試料，試料周囲組織及び埋植周囲リンパ節の肉眼的観察結果

試料周囲組織（加えて，吸収性材料の場合は採取できた埋植周囲リンパ節）の組織学的観察結果（組織形態計測結果を含む）

統計学的検定結果（実施した場合）

9)　結果の評価と考察

10)　参考文献

4．筋肉内埋植試験法

4.1　試験試料の大きさ

4.1.1　埋植する動物によって適切な大きさを設定する．なお，ウサギの場合は，幅（又は直径）1〜3 mm，長さ約10 mmの棒状とし，断端の角をできるだけ滑らかにする．より大きい試料は筋肉を切開して埋植するが，15ゲージ程度の穿刺針を用いて埋植する方が，動物の全身状態と周囲組織へのダメージが少ない．

4.1.2　製品の材質や形状，サイズなどにより，試験試料が整形不可能な場合，あるいは最終製品が試験試料の規定サイズよりも細かい若しくは薄い場合で，それらを規定サイズに整形した場合に，臨床適用の場合とはかけ離れた組織反応が生じると推定される場合は，その旨を示した上で規定サイズとは異なるサイズの試験試料を埋植しても差し支えない．その場合は，できる限り陰性対照材料も同じ形状に整形する．

4.2　試験動物と埋植部位

4.2.1　ウサギの脊柱傍筋肉内への埋植が推奨される．ウサギであれば左右の脊柱傍筋肉内へ各4箇所程度の埋植が可能である．試験試料が小さい場合，ラット臀部及びウサギ大腿部筋肉へも埋植可能である．

4.2.2　一つの埋植期間につき，3匹以上の動物を用い，試験試料及び対照材料ともに，10箇所以上の埋植部位を観察する．なお，肉眼的観察用と組織学的観察用は，兼ねることができる．

4.2.3　既承認/認証品などの対照材料を用いる場合で，ある程度の組織反応を呈することが予測されるときは，動物の感受性の確認のため陰性対照材料を埋植する．

4.2.4　全ての埋植期間において非吸収性の陰性対照材料を埋植，観察すべきであるが，やむを得ず1埋植期間のみにしか設定しなかった場合には，その妥当性を記録する．

(Anesthesia, implantation procedures including post-operative care, retrieval of the test sample, histopathological procedure)

8) Test results

Macroscopic appearances of the test sample, surrounding tissue, and draining lymph nodes

Microscopic observation of the surrounding tissue (including morphometric analysis), as well as those of the draining lymph nodes for absorbable materials

Statistical analysis when applied

9) Assessment of results and discussion

10) References

4. Test method for implantation in muscle

4.1 Size of the implants

4.1.1 Implant size is dependent on animal species. For rabbits, implants with rounded edges of 1 mm to 3 mm width (diameter) and approximately 10 mm length are recommended. Implantation of the test sample into the muscle with approximately 15-gauge needle reduces trauma to the test animal and implant sites. Larger specimens are implanted by the surgical techniques.

4.1.2 When the test sample cannot be remodeled due to its material property, shape, and size of the final product, or the size of the final product is smaller or thinner than the recommended implant size and the tissue response in the implant study differ from the clinical use situation, it may be reasonable to use test samples in the implant study that are different from the recommended sizes. The use of test samples different from the standard shape and size should be documented and justified. The negative control should be prepared in the similar shape to the test sample as much as possible.

4.2 Test animals and implantation sites

4.2.1 The rabbit paraventricular muscles are recommended for muscle implantation. In rabbits, approximately 4 implants can be implanted into either side of the paraventricular muscles. Small test samples can also be implanted into the gluteal muscles in rats and the thigh muscles in rabbits.

4.2.2 Use at least 3 animals, and sufficient implants to yield a total 10 test and 10 control specimens for each implantation period. One implant site can be observed both macroscopically and histologically.

4.2.3 When a control material (such as an approved medical device) is included in the study and the control material is expected to elicit a significant tissue reaction, a negative control material should be included in the study to confirm the animal's response to the negative control.

4.2.4 Non-absorbable negative control material shall be implanted and evaluated at all implantation periods. When a study is designed with only one implantation period for negative control material, record their validity.

4.3　埋植方法

4.3.1　埋植時は全身麻酔下で，皮膚を切開し，埋植は 15 ゲージ程度の穿刺針か，トロッカーを用いて埋植する．

4.3.2　穿刺針などに試料が装填できない場合は，筋肉を外科的に切開して埋植する．この場合は，陰性対照材料などの対照材料も同様の方法で埋植する．

4.3.3　筋線維方向に並行するよう各試料を埋植する．

4.3.4　埋植箇所は 25 mm 程度の間隔を開ける．

4.3.5　必要に応じて，切開部位を非刺激性の縫合糸，若しくはステープラで閉じる．

4.4　埋植期間
埋植箇所の反応が安定期を迎えるまでの期間を 3.4 項に従って設定する．

4.5　評価方法
3.8 項参照．

4.6　試験報告書
3.9 項参照．

5．皮下埋植試験法

5.1　試験試料の大きさ

5.1.1　シート状の場合は，厚み 0.3〜1.0 mm，直径約 10〜12 mm の円板状とする．

5.1.2　直径約 1.5〜2 mm，長さ約 5〜10 mm の棒状として，断端を丸く加工したものでもよい．

5.1.3　非固形試料の場合は，直径約 1.5 mm，長さ約 5 mm のチューブに充填する．
チューブに充填した量を記録すること．可能な場合，非固形試料を直接埋植してもよいが，吸収される場合には埋植位置を特定する工夫を施す．

5.1.4　試験試料を規定以外のサイズに調製する場合は，4.1.2 項を参照する．

5.2　試験動物と埋植部位

5.2.1　成熟したマウス，ラット，モルモット，ウサギのうち 1 種を用いる．

5.2.2　埋植期間につき，少なくとも 3 匹の動物を用いて，試験試料及び対照材料ともにそれぞれ合計 10 箇所以上の埋植部位を観察する．

4.3   Implantation procedure

4.3.1   Under general anesthesia, the implant is introduced with a 15-gauge hypodermic needle or trocar. An incision in the skin may be made before implantation to avoid contaminating the implant site with epithelial tissue.

4.3.2   Implantation by surgical technique is available when the test samples cannot be inserted into a needle/trocar. Controls, such as the negative control, should also be implanted in the same manner as the test sample.

4.3.3   Each specimen is implanted so that it is parallel in the muscle fibers.

4.3.4   Specimens are implanted at intervals of about 25 mm.

4.3.5   The incision site is closed with non-irritating suture or staples, if needed.

4.4   Implantation period

The implantation period shall be of sufficient duration until tissue reactions at the implantation sites has reached steady state according to clause 3.4.

4.5   Evaluation

Refer to clause 3.8.

4.6   Test report

Refer to clause 3.9.

5.   Test method for implantation in subcutaneous tissue

5.1   Size of the implants

5.1.1   If the test sample is a sheet, implant it as a disk of 0.3 mm to 1.0 mm in thickness and approximately 10 mm to 12 mm in diameter.

5.1.2   Implant of approximately 1.5 mm to 2 mm in diameter and 5 mm to 10 mm length with rounded ends may be used.

5.1.3   Non-solid specimen shall be filled in tubes of approximately 1.5 mm diameter and 5 mm length. The mass of the filled specimen shall be recorded. Non-solid specimen may be directly implanted if feasible. Mark the implantation site for the absorbable materials.

5.1.4   When the test sample is not prepared in the standard size, refer to clause 4.1.2.

5.2   Test animals and implantation sites

5.2.1   Select one species among mature mice, rats, guinea pigs or rabbits.

5.2.2   Use at least 3 animals, and sufficient implants to yield a total 10 test and 10 control specimens for each implantation period.

5.2.3　既承認 / 認証品などの対照材料を用いる場合である程度の組織反応を呈することが予測されるときは，動物の感受性の確認のため，陰性対照材料を埋植する．

5.2.4　全ての埋植期間において非吸収性の陰性対照材料を埋植，観察すべきであるが，やむを得ず 1 埋植期間のみにしか設定しなかった場合には，その妥当性を記録する．

5.3　埋植方法
5.3.1　背部皮下に埋植する場合
5.3.1.1　全身麻酔下で，皮膚を切開して切開部位から約 1 cm 以上の深さで鈍性剥離して皮下ポケットを作製し，1 個の試料を埋植する．複数の試料を埋植する場合は，それぞれを 1 cm 程度離す．

5.3.1.2　穿刺針などを用いて埋植してもよい．

5.3.1.3　切開部位を非刺激性の縫合糸，若しくはステープラで閉じる．

5.3.2　頚部皮下に埋植する場合
5.3.2.1　マウスを用いる場合は，全身麻酔下で腰部を切開して，頚部までゾンデなどを用いて皮下を鈍性分離して皮下トンネルを作製し，1 個の試料を頚部皮下に埋植する．

5.3.2.2　ラットの場合は，全身麻酔下で両側の頚部に皮下トンネルを作製して埋植する．体幹，後肢に埋植してもよい．

5.3.2.3　切開部位を非刺激性の縫合糸で縫合するとともに，皮下トンネルを通して試料が移動しないよう，縫合しておく．

5.4　埋植期間
埋植箇所の反応が安定期を迎えるまでの期間を 3.4 項に従って設定する．

5.5　評価方法
3.8 項参照．

5.6　試験報告書
3.9 項参照．

6．骨内埋植試験法
6.1　試験試料の大きさ
6.1.1　円柱状に加工したものとする．スクリュー状に加工したものの方が骨への初期密着性に優れるが，標本作製時は試料の長軸に沿って切断しないと骨と試料の界面の観

5.2.3   When a control material (such as an approved medical device) is included in the study and the control material is expected to elicit a significant tissue reaction, a negative control material should be included in the study to confirm the animal's response to the negative control is appropriate.

5.2.4   Non-absorbable negative control shall be implanted and evaluated at all implantation periods. When a study is designed with only one implantation period for negative control material, record their validity.

5.3   Implantation procedure
5.3.1   Implantation in the back
5.3.1.1   Under general anesthesia, make incisions of the skin and create subcutaneous pockets at approximately 1 cm apart from incision sites by blunt dissection, and then place one implant in each pocket. In the case of multiple specimens, each implant site is separated at approximately 1 cm.

5.3.1.2   The implants may be delivered by a trocar.

5.3.1.3   An incision site is closed with non-irritating suture or a stapler if needed.

5.3.2   Implantation in the neck
5.3.2.1   In mice, under general anesthesia, make an incision on the hip and prepare a subcutaneous tunnel by blunt dissection towards the neck. One implant is placed in the subcutaneous tissue.

5.3.2.2   In the case of rats, both sides of the neck are available. Alternatively, both flanks and/or hind legs may be used.

5.3.2.3   An incision site is closed with non-irritating suture and make some stitches to prevent the implant moving through the subcutaneous tunnel.

5.4   Implantation period
The implantation period shall be of sufficient duration until tissue reactions at the implantation sites has reached steady state according to clause 3.4.

5.5   Evaluation
Refer to clause 3.8.

5.6   Test report
Refer to clause 3.9.

6.   Test method for implantation in bone
6.1   Size of the implants
6.1.1   Rod-shaped specimen is preferably used. Although a screw-shaped test sample provides better initial adherence to the bone, the bone-test sample interface is difficult to evaluate as far as the implant site is cut along the long axis of the test sample in tissue

察がしづらい.

6.1.2　ペースト状のものは, そのまま骨に充填するが, あらかじめ骨に埋植腔を作製して充填する. 埋植前後の容器込み重量を差し引きするなどして埋植量を記録しておく.

6.1.3　ラットなどの小動物の場合は, 直径約1mm, 長さ約5mmの円柱状とする.

6.1.4　ウサギなどの中型動物の場合は, 直径約2mm, 長さ約6mmの円柱状とする.

6.1.5　イヌ, ヒツジ, ヤギなどの大型動物の場合は, 直径約4mm, 長さ約12mmの円柱状とする.

6.1.6　スクリュータイプのインプラントをウサギ, イヌ, ヒツジ, ヤギ, ブタに埋植する場合は, 2〜4.5mmの径とする.

6.1.7　試験試料を規定以外のサイズに調製する場合は, 4.1.2項を参照する.

6.2　試験動物と埋植部位

6.2.1　成熟したげっ歯類, ウサギ, イヌ, ブタ, ヒツジ, ヤギのうち1種を用いる. 若齢の動物を用いる場合, 骨端及び骨が未熟な部位は避ける.

6.2.2　埋植部位はできるだけ臨床適用部位に近い部位とする. 大腿骨や脛骨が用いられることが多いが, いずれにおいても, 骨体部の緻密骨に埋植する場合と, 骨端部の海綿骨部に埋植する場合では, 組織反応は異なるため, 注意を要する.

6.2.3　埋植期間につき, 少なくとも3匹の動物を用い, 試験試料及び対照材料ともにそれぞれ合計10箇所以上の埋植部位を観察する.

6.2.4　既承認/認証品などの対照材料を用いる場合である程度の組織反応を呈することが予測されるときは, 動物の感受性の確認のため, 陰性対照材料を埋植する.

6.2.5　1個体に複数の試料を埋植してもよいが, ウサギでは骨が比較的薄く, 骨折する場合があるため, 左右の大腿骨と脛骨にそれぞれ1箇所ずつ, 計4箇所の埋植が現実的である.

6.2.6　全ての埋植期間において非吸収性の陰性対照材料を埋植, 観察すべきであるが, やむを得ず1埋植期間のみにしか設定しなかった場合には, その妥当性を記録する.

preparation.

6.1.2 Paste-like material is filled into implantation hole as it is. The amount of paste-like material should be recorded by subtracting the total container weight before and after the implantation procedures.

6.1.3 For small animals, like rats, cylinder-shaped implants with approximate dimensions of 1 mm diameter and 5 mm length may be used.

6.1.4 For middle-sized animals, like rabbits, cylinder-shaped implants with approximate dimension of 2 mm diameter and 6 mm length may be used.

6.1.5 For larger animals like dogs, sheep, and goats, cylinder-shaped implants with approximate dimensions of 4 mm diameter and 12 mm length may be used.

6.1.6 Screw-type implants with approximate diameter from 2 to 4.5 mm may be implanted in rabbits, dogs, sheep, goats, and pigs.

6.1.7 When the test sample is not prepared in the standard size, refer to clause 4.1.2.

6.2 Test animals and implantation sites
6.2.1 Select one species among mature rodents, rabbits, dogs, pigs, sheep, or goats. For younger animals, avoid the epiphyseal area and other immature bones as implant sites.

6.2.2 Implantation sites shall be equivalent to intended clinical use. Femurs or tibiae are used in many cases. It is cautioned that the biological responses of cortical and cancellous bones are different.

6.2.3 Use at least 3 animals and sufficient implants to yield a total 10 test and 10 control specimens for each implantation period.

6.2.4 When a control material (such as an approved medical device) is included in the study and the control material is expected to elicit a significant tissue reaction, a negative control material should be included in the study to confirm the animal's response to the negative control is appropriate.

6.2.5 Two or more implants may be implanted per animal. To minimize fracture of the rabbit bones, a proposed implantation scenario is to implant one test sample in each femur and tibia (4 total implants per animal).

6.2.6 Non-absorbable negative control shall be implanted and evaluated at all implantation periods. When a study is designed with only one implantation period for negative control material, record their validity.

6.3　埋植方法

6.3.1　全身麻酔下で，埋植局所の皮膚を切開し，骨を露出した後，リーマを用いて孔を開ける．この際，熱による局所の組織ダメージを最小にするよう，また切削した組織片が周囲に付着しないように生理食塩水などを注水して洗浄する．

6.3.2　埋植孔は，試料のサイズにできるだけ一致するものとし，ギャップをできる限り少なくする．

6.3.3　切開部位を非刺激性の縫合糸，若しくはステープラで閉じる．

6.4　埋植期間

埋植箇所の反応が安定期を迎えるまでの期間を 3.4 項に従って設定する．

6.5　評価方法

3.8 項参照．

6.6　試験報告書

3.9 項参照．

7．脳内埋植試験法

7.1　試験試料の大きさ

7.1.1　埋植する動物によって適切な大きさを設定する．

7.1.2　ラット及びウサギの脳実質内に埋植する場合，幅 1 mm × 1 mm 又は直径 1 mm 以下，長さ 2 ～ 6 mm の棒又は楔状とする．

7.1.3　主に脳実質表面に接するよう意図された医療機器の場合，脳表面に埋植する．ラット及びウサギの脳表面に埋植する場合，直径 8 mm 以下のディスク状とし，その厚さは医療機器の用途に応じて決定する．

7.1.4　陰性対照材料は全ての埋植期間において埋植，観察すべきであるが，やむを得ず 1 埋植期間のみにしか設定しなかった場合には，その妥当性を記録する．

7.2　試験動物と埋植部位

7.2.1　ラット又はウサギを用いた試験法を示したが，医療機器の特性を考慮して他の動物種を使用する場合，試験法を変更してもよい．

7.2.2　性差が報告されているため，雌雄動物を同数使用する．片性のみを用いる十分な正当性がある場合はこの限りではない．

6.3 Implantation procedure

6.3.1 Under general anesthesia, make an incision on the implantation sites and expose bone, bore a hole in the bone with a reamer. To minimize local tissue damages from the heat generated by drilling and to minimize adherence of bone fragments to the circumference, wash and cool the hole with physiological saline.

6.3.2 Implant the test sample into the hole. The hole should be sized to minimize the gap between the test sample and the bone.

6.3.3 Close the incision with non-irritative suture or staple.

6.4 Implantation period

The implantation period shall be of sufficient duration until tissue reactions at the implantation sites has reached steady state according to clause 3.4.

6.5 Evaluation

Refer to clause 3.8.

6.6 Test report

Refer to clause 3.9.

7. Test method for implantation in brain tissue

7.1 Size of the implants

7.1.1 Implant size is dependent on animal species.

7.1.2 For the brain parenchyma of rats and rabbits, rods or wedges with $1 \text{ mm} \times 1 \text{ mm}$ or less in width (diameter) and 2 mm to 6 mm length are used.

7.1.3 For medical devices intended to contact the surface of the brain, implant them on the parenchymal surface. For the brain surface of rats and rabbits, a disk with 8 mm or less in diameter is used. The thickness should be justified according to the use of the material.

7.1.4 Negative control material shall be implanted and evaluated at all implantation periods. When a study is designed with only one implantation period for negative control material, record their validity.

7.2 Test animals and implantation sites

7.2.1 This protocol is for studies using rats or rabbits. If other animal species are used based on device considerations, the protocol may be modified.

7.2.2 Equal numbers of males and females are used due to sex differences. If sufficient justification is provided, a single sex may be applicable.

7.2.3　健康で過去に実験に用いられていない動物を用いる．動物種及び週齢は神経生理学
及び生物学的反応において重要な要素であるため十分に考慮する．

7.2.4　試験試料及び陰性対照材料ともに，各埋植期間で 8 箇所以上（両性を用いる場合は，
各性 4 箇所以上）に埋植する．試験試料及び対照材料ともに，解剖学的に同等な部
位に埋植する．機械的外傷を最小限にするために，埋植部位及び外科的処置法は慎
重に選択する．

7.2.5　1 個体につき片側の脳半球にのみ埋植し，1 個体につき試験試料又は対照材料の 1
種類のみを埋植する．その理由は，筋肉内，皮下及び骨内埋植試験と異なり，神経
系器官の埋植試料に対する反応は必ずしも局所的ではなく，他側の脳半球まで広範
囲に波及し得るためである．ラットの場合は脳半球に 1 箇所，ウサギの場合は 2 箇
所埋植可能である．

7.3　埋植方法

7.3.1　全ての試験動物に対し，埋植前及び埋植後（定期的）に体重を測定する．適切な鎮
痛及び麻酔処置を埋植時及び埋植後の適切な期間行う．

7.3.2　手術中に動物が動かないよう適切に固定する．頭部固定装置を用いると試料を正確
に配置でき，物理的損傷を最小限とすることができる．動物の固定に関しては，他
の方法を考慮してもよい．

7.3.3　無菌的に頭蓋骨を露出させ，そこに埋植試料を挿入するのに十分な大きさの孔を開
ける．さらに，硬膜に小さな穴を開け，埋植試料を脳の適切な部分に慎重に挿入す
る．

7.4　埋植期間

7.4.1　細胞死は埋植後数日で起こり，神経変性過程は迅速で一過性となり得るため，1 週
間の埋植期間が必要である．加えて，埋植箇所の反応が安定期を迎えるまでの期間
を 3.4 項に従って設定する．

7.4.2　長期の埋植期間は，医療機器の臨床適用を考慮して設定する．

7.5　埋植期間中の観察方法

7.5.1　神経系組織の損傷は異常行動を引き起こすため，埋植試料の評価には一般状態観察
結果を加味する．

7.5.2　埋植後初期には，試験動物を個別収容して 1 日 2 回観察することで埋植部位が適切
に治癒しているか，飲食行動が正常に回復しているか，外科的処置による異常な臨
床症状が認められるかなどを確認する．

7.2.3   Animals that are healthy and have not been subjected to previous experiments shall be used. It is noted that animal species and age are important factors in neurophysiology and biological response.

7.2.4   At least 8 test samples and 8 negative control materials (at least 4 materials to both males and females when using both sexes) should be implanted for each implantation period. Anatomically equivalent site shall be used for both the test samples and negative control materials. The implant site and surgical procedure is also critical to minimize the risk of mechanical trauma.

7.2.5   Only one type of implant, either test or control is implanted in only one hemisphere per animal. The tissue responses to implants of neural tissues is not always localized and may spread widely across the contralateral hemisphere of the brain unlike those of the muscle, subcutis and bone. Implantation can be performed at one site per hemisphere in rats, and at two sites per hemisphere in rabbits.

7.3 Implantation procedure
7.3.1   Each animal should be weighed prior to implantation and periodically thereafter. Appropriate analgesia and anesthesia shall be maintained during surgical procedures and for an identified period after implantation.

7.3.2   Animals should be appropriately restrained during the operation procedure. Stereotactic methods may allow accurate placement of the implants and minimize physical damage to the puncture location. The animal may be restrained in alternative methods.

7.3.3   Aseptically expose the skull and make a hole in the skull of sufficient diameter to insert the implant sample. In addition, a small hole is made in the dura and the implant is gently inserted into the appropriate site of the brain.

7.4 Implantation period
7.4.1   A one-week implantation period is required, since neurodegenerative processes can be rapid and transient, and cell death can occur within the first few days following implantation. Other appropriate periods shall be also determined according to clause 3.4 to ensure a steady-state conditions of biological tissue response.

7.4.2   Long-term implantation periods shall be considered in view of the clinical applications of the medical device.

7.5 Post-implantation observation
7.5.1   As damage to neural tissue can result in abnormal behavior, clinical observations should be included in the evaluation of the effects of brain implants.

7.5.2   Animals should be initially housed individually and observed twice daily. This ensures proper healing of the implant sites, return to normal eating and drinking behavior, and any abnormal clinical signs due to the surgical procedure.

7.5.3　毎週，各動物に対して詳細な観察を行う．観察項目には，埋植試料に起因する全ての異常な臨床兆候，異常行動又は全身性 / 中枢神経性の臨床兆候を含める．臨床兆候には，皮膚，被毛，眼，粘膜，分泌物，排泄物の変化又は他の自律神経活動の存在（流涙，立毛，瞳孔の大きさ，異常な呼吸パターン）が含まれるが，これらに限定されるものではない．加えて，歩様，姿勢及びハンドリングに対する応答の変化，並びに間代性又は強直性痙攣の存在，常同行動（過度のグルーミング，旋回行動），異常行動（自傷行動，後ろ向き歩行）について記録する．

7.5.4　中枢神経系の障害を評価する際に，functional observation battery（FOB）又は modified Irwin test を用いることができる．

7.5.5　行動学的及び神経学的兆候については，いつ最初に観察されたか，その後，いつ進行度合いが変化又は解消したかを記録する．異常行動，神経学的兆候，歩行，姿勢，又は反射の所見を発見した場合，関連する兆候を毎日観察することとする．

7.5.6　脳内埋植試験法は処置後に重度のストレスや痛みを伴う可能性があるため，試験動物をできる限り早期に除外するためのエンドポイントを試験に先立って設定しておき，重篤な臨床作用を認めた場合，動物愛護の観点から動物を安楽死処置する．安楽死動物のデータの採否は 3.6.5 項を参照する．

7.6　評価方法

7.6.1　3.7 項及び 3.8 項参照．脳内埋植に固有の注意点を以下に記載する．

7.6.2　浸漬固定でアーティファクトを生じる可能性がある場合，還流固定を用いる．

7.6.3　適切な組織学的染色，傷害の生化学的指標又はそれら両者を用いて，神経病理学的評価を実施する（表 3）．使用した特殊染色 / 傷害指標は，それら手法について記述された参考文献を明示する．評価項目には神経変性（変性ニューロン及び神経突起の切断），グリオーシス，アストロサイトーシス，ミクログリア活性化が含まれる．アストロサイト及びミクログリアに関しては，その形態学的反応の特徴を同定する．

7.5.3   A detailed physical examination shall be performed on each animal weekly. The observations include all abnormal clinical signs, abnormal behaviors, or systemic or central nervous system manifestations caused by the implant. Clinical signs could include, but are not limited to, changes in skin, fur, eyes or mucous membranes, occurrence of secretions and excretions, or other evidence of autonomic activity (e.g. lacrimation, piloerection, pupil size, unusual respiratory pattern). Additionally, changes in gait, posture, and response to handling, as well as the presence of clonic or tonic seizures, stereotypes (e.g. excessive grooming, repetitive circling) or bizarre behavior (e.g. self–mutilating, walking backwards) shall be recorded.

7.5.4   To help with assessment of central nervous system disorder, a functional observation battery (FOB) or modified Irwin's test can be used.

7.5.5   For the behavior and neurological signs, time of first observation and subsequent progression or resolution should be recorded. If any abnormal behavior, neurological signs, ambulation, posture, or reflexes are found, the relevant signs should be observed daily.

7.5.6   Since implantation in the brain can induce severe stress and pain after the procedure, endpoints for early removal of an animal from the test should be set prior to the test. Once severe clinical effects have been identified, test animals should be removed from the test and euthanized. Refer to clause 3.6.5 to determine whether to include data from euthanized animals.

7.6   Evaluation

7.6.1   Refer to clauses 3.7 and 3.8. The precautions specific to implantation in the brain tissue are described below.

7.6.2   Perfusion fixation should be used if immersion fixation might produce artefacts in the tissue.

7.6.3   The neuropathological evaluation should be performed using appropriate histological stains, biochemical indicators of damage, or both (Table 3). The use of specific stain/damage indicator should be stated along with appropriate references describing those techniques for the neuropathological evaluation. Parameters include neurodegeneration (degenerative neurons and disruption in the neuronal processes), gliosis, astrocytosis, microglia activation. The characteristics of morphological response of astrocytes and microglia should be identified.

表 3　脳組織のバイオマーカー及び染色法の例

染色法及びバイオマーカー	細胞種及び細胞構成成分
ヘマトキシリン・エオジン	全ての中枢神経系及びリンパ節
Fluoro-Jade	変性ニューロン
自家蛍光	神経変性
抗 Glial Fibrillary Acidic Protein（GFAP）抗体	アストロサイトマーカー
抗 Ionized calcium binding adaptor molecule 1（Iba-1）抗体	ミクログリアなどのマーカー
Luxol fast blue	ミエリン
Amino Cupric Silver Stain	変性ニューロン

注：特異的抗体は全ての動物種とは交差しない可能性がある.

7.6.4　試料周囲組織に加え，埋植部位近傍（〜 3 mm，同側の脳半球）及びさらに離れた部位の評価が有用な場合がある. 埋植部位近傍を評価する際は，炎症細胞／浸潤細胞，出血，壊死，グリオーシス（灰白質及び白質）などを観察し，さらに離れた部位を評価する際は，これらに加えて他の非局所的影響も含める.

7.7　評価方法

　3.9 項参照. ただし，一般状態観察結果も加味して埋植試料の評価を行う.

8.　参考情報
8.1　試験法の選択

　埋植試験法としては，ISO 10993-6: 2016, Biological evaluation of medical devices-Part 6: Tests for local effects after implantation があり，インプラントの原材料を試験する際には，ISO 規格に従うことで基本的には十分である. 一方，Nakamura らの報告[3, 4]にあるように，筋肉内埋植試験では炎症領域の幅が細胞毒性などとの相関性がよいことも事実であるため，組織学的評価のみならず，炎症領域の幅のような定量的指標を利用することが望ましい. また骨内埋植試験では，標準仕様書[5]において新生骨形成におけるいくつかの形態計測パラメータが示されており，これを利用することで生体適合性評価の一助となる.

8.2　滅菌法

　高圧蒸気滅菌，乾熱滅菌，煮沸滅菌などの加熱による滅菌の場合には，熱による試験試料の変質，変形に注意する必要がある（例：純ニッケルなどは，酸化被膜の形成により毒性発現に影響があるため，乾熱滅菌などの高温環境を避ける）. エチレンオキサイドガスなどを用いてガス滅菌を行う場合には，ガスの残留のないよう注意しなくてはならない. またアルコールに長時間浸漬して消毒する場合には，試料中に含まれる化合物がアルコール中に溶出しやすく，真の毒性を検出し得ないおそれがあるため，本試験の滅菌法としては不適切である[6]. また他に γ 線滅菌や電子線，紫外線滅菌などがあるが，照射によって試料の変質や劣化が起こる場合があるので注意しなくてはならない. いずれにしても，採用した滅菌法によって，試験試料とする原材料の変質や変形，及びガスや化合物の残留・吸着などによって実際に生体に適用する最終製品と異なった組織反応

Table 3   Examples brain biomarkers and stains

Stain and biomarker	Cell type or cellular component evaluated
Hematoxylin and eosin (H&E)	All CNS and lymph node tissue
Fluoro–jade	Degenerating neurons
Autofluorescence	Neurodegeneration
Anti–Glial fibrillary acidic protein (GFAP) antibody	Astrocyte marker
Anti–Ionized calcium binding adaptor molecule 1 (Iba–1) antibody	Markers for microglia etc.
Luxol fast blue	Myelin
Amino cupric silver stain	Degenerating neurons

Note: Specific antibodies are not available for all animal species.

7.6.4   It can be useful to examine the brain adjacent to implant track (3 mm or less, ipsilateral) and away from the implant track. Parameters for the brain adjacent to the implant track includes inflammatory cell/infiltrates, hemorrhage, necrosis, gliosis in both grey matter and white matter, and others. In addition to these, parameters for the brain away from the implant track include other non–local effects.

7.7   Evaluation

Refer to clause 3.9. It is noted that the clinical observations should be included in the evaluation of the effects of brain implants.

8.   Reference information

8.1   Selection of test methods

Basically, the testing standard, ISO 10993–6: 2016, Biological evaluation of medical devices–Part 6: Tests for local effects after implantation, is available for evaluating raw materials of implant devices. Additionally, it is recommended that quantitative parameter such as width of inflammation as well as histological evaluation be used, since the width of inflammation correlates well with cytotoxicity determined in Nakamura *et al.*[3, 4]. For the bone implantation test, the use of morphometric parameters in new bone formation, as described in JIS[5], should aid the biocompatibility evaluation.

8.2   Sterilization method

Deterioration and deformation of the test samples by heat should be noted in cases of autoclave, dry–heat sterilization, and boiling sterilization (e.g., for pure nickel, high–temperature condition should be avoided so that toxicity is affected by formation of oxidation layer). For ethylene oxide gas sterilization, remain of the gas should be negligible. Disinfection by a long duration exposure to alcohol is not appropriate since toxicity cannot be detected due to elution of toxic compounds of the test sample[6]. If gamma ray, electron beam, and ultraviolet sterilization are used, care should be taken not to cause deterioration or degradation of the test sample by the irradiation. Anyway, the test and control specimens shall not induce tissue responses that never cause in the case of the final product applying in human body, due to deterioration or deformation of the test sample and residue or adhesion of gas or compounds to the test sample. A suitable sterilization method shall be selected after

を起こすような変化が試験試料及び対照材料に生じてはならず，原材料の性質や臨床適用時の滅菌法などを十分に考慮した上で適切な滅菌法を選択すべきである．

8.3　動物数

ISO 10993-6: 2016 においては，肉眼観察用の動物と組織学的観察用の動物の区別について言及されていない．一方で，過去の国内試験法においては，短期筋肉内埋植試験で双方を別に設定するよう規定されてきた．本ガイダンスにおいては，筋肉内埋植試験法においても ISO 10993-6: 2016 に調和させる目的で肉眼観察用と組織学的観察用の動物を兼ねることができるよう変更した．

8.4　陽性対照材料

陽性対照材料としては，天然ゴム製品の毒性原因物質の一つであるジエチルジチオカルバミン酸亜鉛（ZDEC）を種々の濃度で含有させたポリウレタンシート / ロッドが代表的である．これは，ZDEC の含有量と，ウサギ筋肉内埋植試験における「炎症領域の幅」及び *in vitro* 細胞毒性試験との相関性を調べた結果をもとに設定されたものである[7]．陰性対照材料（検定済み高密度ポリエチレンシート / ロッド）とともに，陽性対照材料も一般財団法人食品薬品安全センター秦野研究所（第 1 部細胞毒性試験 4.6 項参照）から入手可能である．

また骨内埋植試験の場合は，純ニッケルを用いることができる．

8.5　埋植期間による組織像の変化

陽性対照材料などを用いたウサギ筋肉内埋植における組織反応の経時的検索では，「炎症領域の幅」が最大となるピークは偽好酸球などの炎症細胞浸潤のピーク時期とほぼ一致しており，その後，肉芽形成，瘢痕化による線維性被膜の形成へと組織反応の進行に伴って徐々に幅は狭くなっていくようである．この炎症性細胞浸潤のピークの時期は，試料中に含まれる毒性物質の絶対量，溶出速度，毒性強度などによって異なるものと考えられる．したがって，幅の計測部位の名称を便宜上「炎症領域の幅」としているものの，組織傷害性が低い物質であれば，埋植から 1 週間後では，マクロファージや線維芽細胞を主体とする細胞浸潤から肉芽形成に至るステージ， 4 週間後では線維性被膜が形成されるステージにあると考えられ，主として線維性被膜の幅を測定することとなる．

8.6　埋植周囲リンパ節の変化

局所に炎症がある場合，その支配領域下のリンパ節にリンパ管を経由して異物あるいは抗原物質などが達すると，炎症が起きてリンパ節が腫脹することがある．組織学的には，充血，リンパ組織の増生，胚中心細胞の増生が認められる[8]．埋植試験では埋植局所の生体組織に及ぼす影響を検索することが目的であるが，支配領域のリンパ節を確認することにより，局所に生じた炎症の種類や程度を把握する一助となる．また吸収性材料の場合は分解材料のリンパ管内における移動を確認する一助となる．なお，ラットなどでは安楽死操作に起因して，アーティファクトとしてリンパ洞や皮質に赤血球が見られることがある[9]．

taking into consideration the raw material characteristics and sterilization method used in the clinical setting.

8.3　Number of animals

Unlike ISO 10993-6: 2016, previous domestic test guidelines of implantation test have stipulated that different animals should be allocated for macroscopic and histological observation in short-term muscle implantation tests. This guidance has been revised so that the same animals can be used both for macroscopic and histological observations in the intramuscular implantation test, for the purpose of harmonization to ISO 10993-6: 2016.

8.4　Positive control material

The representative positive control material is the polyurethane sheet/rod that incorporates various concentrations of zinc diethyldithiocarbamate (ZDEC), a causative toxic compound found in natural rubber products. This control material was selected followed by investigation of correlation with thickness of inflammation region in the rabbit muscle implantation test and *in vitro* cytotoxicity[7]. The negative control material (authorized high-density polyethylene sheet/rod) and positive control material is obtained from Hatano Research Institute, Food and Drug Safety Center (refer to part I cytotoxicity test, clause 4.6). For bone implantation tests, pure nickel is available.

8.5　Histological alteration during the implantation period

Histological findings in rabbit muscle implanted with positive control material showed that the time maximal "thickness of inflammation lesion" corresponds with maximal inflammatory cells infiltration such as pseudoeosinophils, and the thickness of the inflammation lesion shrinks gradually along with the progress of tissue reactions such as formation of granulation tissue and fibrous membrane by scarring. The peak time of inflammatory cell infiltration depends on the absolute content of the toxic substances in the test sample, elution rate, toxic intensity, etc. For weakly toxic substance that cause tissue injury, the period from the implantation day to 1 week after implantation is thought to be the stage of cellular infiltration of mainly macrophages and fibroblasts, and formation of granulation tissue, and after 4 weeks is the stage of fibrous membrane formation. In these cases, although measurement of thickness is called "thickness of inflammation lesion" for convenience, it means that thickness of fibrous membrane is measured.

8.6　Alteration of lymph nodes draining the implantation site

Local inflammation may cause enlargement of regional draining lymph nodes when the foreign body or antigen reaches via lymphatic vessel. Histologically, congestion, proliferation of lymph tissue and germinal center cells are found[8]. Evaluation of the regional draining lymph nodes may help to clarify the type and degree of local inflammation, since the objective of the implantation test is to determine effects on local tissue. The evaluation of lymph nodes also helps to confirm the migration of absorbed degradable material via the lymph vessels. In rats, red blood cells may be seen in lymphatic sinus and cortex as an artifact in euthanasia[9].

8.7　組織反応について

　「有意に強い組織反応」とは，単に統計学的手法を用いた判定のみを意味するものではなく，対照材料の観察結果と比較して，試験試料の炎症性あるいは組織傷害性が強く認められた場合や質的に異なる反応が生じる場合を指すと考える．ただし，組織形態計測を実施した場合は，対照材料と試験試料との微妙な差の判定根拠について苦慮することが想定され，判定に客観性を持たせる方法として統計学的手法を用いることも一つの対応策と思われる．なお，炎症とは，静的な反応ではなく，時間の経過とともに循環障害や浸潤細胞の種類と，反応の強さが変化する動的な反応であるため，組織像の評価に際しては炎症反応の時間的経過を十分に考慮しておく必要がある．複数の観察期間を設けているのは，このような動的な反応の変化を検索するためであり，いずれかの埋植期間の情報が重要というわけではなく，全ての情報から総合的に組織反応を評価すべきである．

8.8　脳内埋植試験について

　適用を検討する医療機器としては，脳の電極や水頭症のドレインとなるシャントなど，脳組織に埋植されるものが対象となる．脳血管に留置されるような血管内壁と接触する医療機器は，神経組織に直接ばく露されないため，脳内埋植試験は適用されない．

8.9　肉眼及び組織の代表例の写真について

　試験報告書に記載すべき事項から肉眼及び組織の代表例の写真を除外した．その目的は ISO 10993-6: 2016 に調和させることであり，写真の撮影，試験への使用及び試験報告書への掲載を妨げるものではない．

8.10　安楽死処置について

　実験動物医学専門医（qualified laboratory animal veterinarian）や選任獣医師（attending veterinarian）が設置されている施設では，安楽死の要否などについてこれらの専門家に相談できる．なお，前者については，国際実験動物医学専門医協会（IACLAM: International Association of Colleges of Laboratory Animal Medicine）のもとで認定される専門医制度があり，国内では日本実験動物医学専門医協会のもとに実験動物医学専門医制度がある．

9．薬食機発 0301 第 20 号からの変更点

1)　吸収分解性材料を試験する際の注意事項を追記した．
2)　脳内埋植試験法を追加した．
3)　その他 ISO 10993-6: 2016 で改訂された詳細な事項を反映した．

10．引用文献

1)　Maekawa, A., Ogiu, T., Onodera, H., Furuta, K., Matsuoka, C., Ohno, Y., Tanigawa, H., Salmo, G.S., Matsuyama, M., Hayashi, Y.: Malignant fibrous histiocytomas induced in rats by polymers. J. Cancer Res. Clin. Oncol. 108, 364–365（1984）
2)　Tilney, N.: Patterns of lymphatic drainage in the adult laboratory rat. J. Anat. 109, 369–

8.7　Tissue reactions

Statistical significance is not the only factor for determining a "significant tissue reactions". Strong reactions such as inflammation and tissue injury at the test sample site and qualitatively different reactions compared to those observed in the control sites are also factors for "significant tissue reactions" factors. When morphometrical analysis is performed, the use of statistical technique can be considered to increase the evaluation's objectivity since clarification of slight differences between control and test samples may be difficult. Inflammation is not static, but dynamic response whereby circulatory failure (such as hyperemia, congestion, edema, bleeding, etc.), type of infiltrating cells, and strength of the reaction changes with time, and therefore changes of inflammatory reactions over time shall be considered when evaluating histological data. Multiple observation periods in the study are recommended in order to investigate the full spectrum of the host tissue response to the test sample. Information from a specific time point is not sufficient.

8.8　Medical devices to which implantation test in brain tissue is applied

Medical devices directly contact with or implanted in neural tissue shall be considered for the evaluation by the implantation test in brain tissue, e.g. an electrode implanted into the brain, shunts for hydrocephalus correction, drains. For the material for a neuro-interventional device which contact with the inner wall of blood vessels, the brain implant test is not applied since they are not directly exposed to neural tissue.

8.9　Typical photos of macroscopic and histological examination

Typical photos of macroscopic and histological examination have been removed from the items to be included in the test report. Its purpose is the harmonization with ISO 10993-6: 2016, and does not preclude capture of the images, use in testing and inclusion in the test report.

8.10　Euthanasia of animals

Study director can consult for the necessity of euthanasia and other veterinary care with an attending veterinarian or a Diplomate of the Japanese College of Laboratory Animal Medicine, the latter is certified by Japanese College of Laboratory Animal Medicine (JCLAM), a member of International Association of Colleges of Laboratory Animal Medicine (IACLAM).

9.　Points changed from MHLW Notification, YAKUSHOKUKI-HATSU 0301 No. 20

1) Precautions for testing absorbable and degradable materials were described.
2) Tests methods for implantation in brain tissue was indicated.
3) The other details revised in ISO 10993-6: 2016 were included.

10.　References cited

1) Maekawa, A., Ogiu, T., Onodera, H., Furuta, K., Matsuoka, C., Ohno, Y., Tanigawa, H., Salmo, G.S., Matsuyama, M., Hayashi, Y.: Malignant fibrous histiocytomas induced in rats by polymers. J. Cancer Res. Clin. Oncol. 108, 364–365 (1984)
2) Tilney, N.: Patterns of lymphatic drainage in the adult laboratory rat. J. Anat. 109, 369–

383（1971）

3）　Nakamura, A., Ikarashi, Y., Tsuchiya, T., Kaniwa, M.A., Sato, M., Toyoda, K., Takahashi, M., Ohsawa, N., Uchima, T.: Correlation among chemical constituents, cytotoxicities and tissue: in the case of natural rubber latex materials. Biomaterials 11, 92–94（1990）

4）　Ikarashi, Y., Toyoda, K., Ohsawa, N., Uchima, T., Tsuchiya, T., Kaniwa, M.-A., Sato, M., Takahashi, M., Nakamura, A.: Comparative studies by cell culture and implantation test on the toxicity of natural rubber latex materials. J. Biomed. Mater. Res. 26, 339–356（1992）

5）　TS T 0011: 2008 骨組織の薄切標本の作製方法

6）　Bouet, T., Toyoda, K., Ikarashi, Y., Uchima, T., Nakamura, A., Tsuchiya, T., Takahashi, M., Eloy, R.: Evaluation of biocompatibility, based on quantitative determination of the vascular response induced by material implantation. J. Biomed. Mater. Res. 25, 1507–1521（1991）

7）　Tsuchiya, T., Ikarashi, Y., Hata, H., Toyoda, K., Takahashi, M., Uchima, T., Tanaka, N., Sasaki, T., Nakamura, A.: Comparative studies of the toxicity of standard reference materials in various cytotoxicity tests and *in vivo* implantation tests. J. Appl. Biomat. 4, 153–156（1993）

8）　菊池浩吉，吉木敬編：新病理学各論，pp.109–113，南山堂（1992）

9）　Stefanski, S.A., Elwell, M.R., Strongberg, P.C.: Spleen, lymph nodes, and thymus. *In:* Pathology of the Fischer Rat. Boorman, G.A., Eustis, S.L., Elwell, M.R., Montogomery, C.A., MacKenzie, W.F.（eds.）pp.369–393, Acad. Press, San Diego（1990）

11.　参考文献

1）　IARC Monographs on the Evaluation of Carcinogenic Risks to Humans, Vol. 74 Surgical Implants and Other Foreign Bodies. IARC, Lyon（1999）

383 (1971)

3) Nakamura, A., Ikarashi, Y., Tsuchiya, T., Kaniwa, M.A., Sato, M., Toyoda, K., Takahashi, M., Ohsawa, N., Uchima, T.: Correlation among chemical constituents, cytotoxicities and tissue: in the case of natural rubber latex materials. Biomaterials 11, 92-94 (1990)

4) Ikarashi, Y., Toyoda, K., Ohsawa, N., Uchima, T., Tsuchiya, T., Kaniwa, M.-A., Sato, M., Takahashi, M., Nakamura, A.: Comparative studies by cell culture and implantation test on the toxicity of natural rubber latex materials. J. Biomed. Mater. Res. 26, 339-356 (1992)

5) TS T 0011: 2008 Making method for the thin bone tissue samples for observation with optical microscope

6) Bouet, T., Toyoda, K., Ikarashi, Y., Uchima, T., Nakamura, A., Tsuchiya, T., Takahashi, M., Eloy, R.: Evaluation of biocompatibility, based on quantitative determination of the vascular response induced by material implantation. J. Biomed. Mater. Res. 25, 1507-1521 (1991)

7) Tsuchiya, T., Ikarashi, Y., Hata, H., Toyoda, K., Takahashi, M., Uchima, T., Tanaka, N., Sasaki, T., Nakamura, A.: Comparative studies of the toxicity of standard reference materials in various cytotoxicity tests and *in vivo* implantation tests. J. Appl. Biomat. 4, 153-156 (1993)

8) Kikuchi, H., Yoshiki, K.: New Pathology-Detailed Discussion, pp.109-113, Nanzando (1992)

9) Stefanski, S.A., Elwell, M.R., Strongberg, P.C.: Spleen, lymph nodes, and thymus. *In*: Pathology of the Fischer Rat, Boorman, G.A., Eustis, S.L., Elwell, M.R., Montogomery, C.A., MacKenzie, W.F. (eds.) pp.369-393, Acad. Press, San Diego (1990)

11. Reference

1) IARC Monographs on the Evaluation of Carcinogenic Risks to Humans, Vol. 74 Surgical Implants and Other Foreign Bodies. IARC, Lyon (1999)

第5部　刺激性試験

1．適用範囲

　本試験は，試験試料（最終製品又は原材料）の抽出液による，刺激性を評価するものである．ここでは，皮膚刺激性試験，皮内反応試験及び眼刺激試験の標準的な方法を記載した．刺激性試験の項目は，当該医療機器の臨床適用部位に応じて選択する．なお，ISO 10993-10 には，口腔粘膜刺激試験や膣粘膜刺激試験などの記載もあることから，これらを利用してもよい．また試験試料の臨床適用方法あるいは性状により，動物への投与物質は必ずしも抽出液でなく，最終製品など，より適切なリスク評価ができるものを用いるべきである．近年，医療機器の抽出物の皮膚刺激性評価のための in vitro 皮膚刺激性試験の有用性が実証されたことから，本ガイダンスにも in vitro 皮膚刺激性試験法の概要を記載した．

　なお，引用規格などに挙げた試験基準で既に実施された試験結果がある場合には，本試験を改めて実施する必要はない．

2．引用規格

2.1　ISO 10993-10: 2010, Biological evaluation of medical devices-Part10: Tests for irritation and skin sensitization

2.2　ASTM Standard F 719-81 (2012): Standard Practice for Testing Biomaterials in Rabbits for Primary Skin Irritation

2.3　ASTM Standard F 749-13: Standard Practice for Evaluating Material Extracts by Intracutaneous Injection in the Rabbit

2.4　USP General Chapters: ⟨88⟩ Biological Reactivity Tests, *In vivo*-Intracutaneous Test

3．皮膚刺激性試験

3.1　*in vitro* 皮膚刺激性試験（再構築ヒト表皮試験法）（6.1 項参照）

3.1.1　目的

　本試験は試験試料（最終製品又は原材料）から抽出した抽出液（以下「試験液」とする．）中に，皮膚刺激性を有する物質が存在するかどうかを確認する *in vitro* 試験である．

3.1.2　試験の要約

　試験試料から生理食塩液及び植物油を用いて抽出した試験液を，正常ヒト由来表皮角化細胞からなる再構築ヒト表皮モデル（以下「RhE モデル」とする．）に添加して，細胞生存率を指標として，炎症カスケードの起因現象である細胞の損傷を測定することで，刺激性の有無を判定する．

Part 5   Irritation Test

1.   Scope
This test is to evaluate irritancy of extracts of the test sample (final products or materials). Standard methods for skin irritation, intracutaneous response and eye irritation studies are described in this guidance. Select an appropriate irritation test based on the expected clinical application site of the medical device. Oral mucosa irritation or vaginal mucosa irritation test can be selected as they are also included in ISO 10993-10. Additionally, more suitable test sample for risk assessment such as a final product should be selected for animal administration rather than extract, depending on clinical use or chemical characterization of test sample. In recent years, the usefulness of the *in vitro* skin irritation test has been demonstrated for the evaluation of skin irritation of extracts from a medical device. For this reason, an overview of *in vitro* skin irritation test methods is described in this guidance.

It is not necessary to conduct an irritation test in a case there are test results from studies conducted in accordance with test standards.

2.   Normative references
2.1   ISO 10993-10: 2010, Biological evaluation of medical devices-Part 10: Tests for irritation and skin sensitization

2.2   ASTM Standard F 719-81 (2012): Standard Practice for Testing Biomaterials in Rabbits for Primary Skin Irritation

2.3   ASTM Standard F 749-13: Standard Practice for Evaluating Material Extracts by Intracutaneous Injection in the Rabbit

2.4   USP General Chapters: ⟨88⟩ Biological Reactivity Tests, *In vivo*-Intracutaneous Test

3.   Skin irritation test
3.1   ***In vitro* skin irritation test (reconstructed human epidermis test method) (refer to Section 6.1)**

3.1.1   Purpose
The test is an *in vitro* test designed to confirm existence of a potential substance that exhibits skin irritation in the extracts (referred to below as "test solutions") that are prepared by extraction from test samples (final products or their raw materials).

3.1.2   Summary of the test
Test solutions extracted from test samples using physiological saline or vegetable oil are applied on a reconstructed human epidermis model composed of normal human-derived epidermal keratinocytes (hereinafter referred to as "RhE model"). Irritation is determined by measuring cellular damage triggering inflammatory cascade using cell viability as an indicator.

3.1.3　試験液の調製
3.1.3.1　抽出溶媒
　　抽出には，生理食塩液（日局又は同等品），植物油（綿実油又はゴマ油，日局又は同等品）を用いる．

3.1.3.2　抽出溶媒と試験試料量の比
　　原則として，付録 1 の規定に従うものとする．

3.1.3.3　抽出条件
　　原則として，付録 2 の規定に従うものとする．

3.1.3.4　操作方法
　　抽出後，直ちに室温（25℃以下にならないよう）に冷却する．次いで，容器の内容液を別の乾燥した滅菌容器に集め，付録 3 に従い，25℃前後で保存し，これを試験液として 24 時間以内に試験を実施する．滅菌品に関しては一連の操作を無菌的に行うこと．

3.1.3.5　対照液の調製
　　陰性対照液は Phosphate Buffered Saline（PBS）とする．陽性対照液は生理食塩液で 1 ％に調製したラウリル硫酸ナトリウム（SDS）とする．溶媒対照液は抽出溶媒単独（試験試料を加えない）で，試験液調製と同条件で操作を行ったものとする．陽性対照材料としては Y-4 が推奨される．Y-4 の抽出条件は 37℃若しくは 50℃で 72±2 時間抽出とする（6.4 項参照）．

3.1.4　試験法
3.1.4.1　三次元 RhE モデル
　　適切に評価された RhE モデルを使用する．1 試料ごとに 3 ウェル使用する（6.3 項参照）．

3.1.4.2　試験操作
　　RhE モデルを使用した試験法の概要を下記に示すが，各段階の操作の詳細は，使用する RhE モデルの手順書に従って行うこと．
1) 　RhE モデルは適切な培養条件下で，37℃の 5 ％炭酸ガス培養器内にいれて，静置して前培養する．
2) 　試験液，対照液，溶媒対照液をそれぞれ RhE モデルに添加する．
3) 　37℃の 5 ％炭酸ガス培養器内に静置して，一晩培養する．
4) 　PBS を用いて洗浄する．
5) 　MTT 溶液をウェルに添加し，37℃の 5 ％炭酸ガス培養器内で約 3 時間浸漬させる．
6) 　RhE モデルを適切な量のイソプロパノールに室温で約 2 時間若しくは一晩（容器の周りをシールする）浸漬して，ブルーホルマザンを抽出する．
7) 　イソプロパノール抽出溶液を 96 ウェルプレートへ移して適切な OD を測定し（例：図 1，6.5 項参照），生存率（％）を算出する（6.6 項参照）．

3.1.3　Preparation of test solution
3.1.3.1　Extraction solvent
Use physiological saline (Japanese Pharmacopoeia (JP) or equivalent products) and vegetable oil (cotton seed oil or sesame oil, JP or equivalent products) for extraction.

3.1.3.2　Extraction solvent/test sample ratio
Basically follow standards shown in Attachment 1.

3.1.3.3　Extraction condition
Basically follow standards listed in Attachment 2.

3.1.3.4　Handling of test solution
Cool the extract to ambient temperature (not below 25 ℃) immediately after extraction. Then, aseptically transfer the liquid into a separate, dry and sterile container, store it at around 25 ℃ in accordance with Annex 3, and perform the irritation test within 24 hours using it as the test solution. For sterile products, perform the series of procedures under aseptic conditions.

3.1.3.5　Preparation of control solution
Use phosphate buffered saline (PBS) as a negative control solution. Use 1 % Sodium Lauryl Sulfate (SDS) prepared with physiological saline as a positive control solution. Use the solution prepared from the extraction solvent alone (without addition of the test sample) as a vehicle control under the same conditions as the test solution preparation. Y‑4 is a recommended as a positive reference material. Extraction conditions for Y‑4 should be 72 ± 2 hours at 37 ℃ or 50 ℃ (refer to Section 6.4).

3.1.4　Test method
3.1.4.1　Three‑dimensional RhE model
Use an adequately evaluated RhE model. Use 3 wells per one test sample (refer to Section 6.3).

3.1.4.2　Test procedure
An overview of a test method using the RhE model is shown below. Details of procedures for each step should follow the procedures specified for the RhE model to be employed.
1) Preculture the RhE model in a 5 % carbon dioxide incubator maintained at 37 ℃ under appropriate culture conditions and leave it.
2) Add the test, control and solvent control solutions to each RhE model.
3) Incubate each RhE model in a 5 % carbon dioxide incubator maintained at 37 ℃ overnight.
4) Rinse each RhE model with PBS.
5) Add an MTT solution to each well, which is then placed in a 5 % carbon dioxide incubator maintained at 37 ℃ for about 3 hours to soak MTT into the cells.
6) Soak each RhE model in an appropriate amount of isopropanol at room temperature for about 2 hours or overnight (tightly seal around the container) to extract blue formazan.
7) Transfer the isopropanol extract solution to a 96‑well plate in order to measure a suitable optical density (OD) (refer to Figure 1 and Section 6.5) and calculate cell viability (%) (refer to Section 6.6).

	1	2	3	4	5	6	7	8	9	10	11	12
A	ブランク	ブランク	ブランク	ブランク	ブランク	ブランク						
B	陰性対照1	陽性対照1-1	溶媒対照1-1	溶媒対照2-1	試験液1-1	試験液2-1						
C	陰性対照1	陽性対照1-1	溶媒対照1-1	溶媒対照2-1	試験液1-1	試験液2-1						
D	陰性対照2	陽性対照1-2	溶媒対照1-2	溶媒対照2-2	試験液1-2	試験液2-2						
E	陰性対照2	陽性対照1-2	溶媒対照1-2	溶媒対照2-2	試験液1-2	試験液2-2						
F	陰性対照3	陽性対照1-3	溶媒対照1-3	溶媒対照2-3	試験液1-3	試験液2-3						
G	陰性対照3	陽性対照1-3	溶媒対照1-3	溶媒対照2-3	試験液1-3	試験液2-3						
H												

図 1　96 ウェルプレートへの配置例

3.1.4.3　試験成立条件

　下記 3 条件を全て満たした場合に試験成立とみなす.

1) 　陰性対照の平均 OD 測定値の範囲は, 使用する各 RhE モデルの手順書に記載されている範囲に従う.

2) 　陰性対照液の生存率に対する陽性対照液平均生存率の範囲は, 生存率が<40 % である.

3) 　全ての対照液及び全ての試験液において, 生存率の標準偏差 (N = 3) SD が≦20 % である.

3.1.4.4　評価

　陰性対照液に対する生存率が≦50 %の場合を刺激性, 陰性対照に対する生存率が>50 %の場合を非刺激性と判定する.

3.1.5　試験報告書

　試験報告書には, 少なくとも以下の事項を記載する.

1) 　試験実施機関及び試験責任者

2) 　試験実施期間

3) 　試験試料を特定する要素
　　（例：医療機器の名称, 製造販売業者名, 製造番号, 原材料名など）

4) 　対照液を特定する要素
　　（例：対照液名, 入手先, 製造番号など）

5) 　試験試料の試験への適用方法（滅菌した場合は, その方法を含む）
　　（例：採取重量又は面積, 細切の方法, 滅菌方法など）

6) 　試験液の調製方法
　　（例：抽出方法など）

7) 　使用した RhE モデル

8) 　試験方法

9) 　試験結果

	1	2	3	4	5	6	7	8	9	10	11	12
A	Blank	Blank	Blank	Blank	Blank	Blank						
B	Negative control 1	Positive control 1-1	Vehicle control 1-1	Vehicle control 2-1	Test sample 1-1	Test sample 2-1						
C	Negative control 1	Positive control 1-1	Vehicle control 1-1	Vehicle control 2-1	Test sample 1-1	Test sample 2-1						
D	Negative control 2	Positive control 1-2	Vehicle control 1-2	Vehicle control 2-2	Test sample 1-2	Test sample 2-2						
E	Negative control 2	Positive control 1-2	Vehicle control 1-2	Vehicle control 2-2	Test sample 1-2	Test sample 2-2						
F	Negative control 3	Positive control 1-3	Vehicle control 1-3	Vehicle control 2-3	Test sample 1-3	Test sample 2-3						
G	Negative control 3	Positive control 1-3	Vehicle control 1-3	Vehicle control 2-3	Test sample 1-3	Test sample 2-3						
H												

Figure 1   Examples of arrangement in a 96-well plate

3.1.4.3   Test acceptance criteria

A test is considered valid when all three criteria mentioned below are met:

1) Mean OD value of the negative control (NC) is within the range specified in the procedures for individual RhE models used.
2) The range of mean viability in the positive control solution compared to that of the NC solution is $<40\ \%$.
3) The standard deviation (SD) of viability (N = 3) is $\leq 20\ \%$ for all control and test solutions.

3.1.4.4   Evaluation

The test solution is considered to be irritant when viability compared to the NC solution is $\leq 50\ \%$. The test solution is considered a non-irritant when the viability is $>50\ \%$.

3.1.5   Test report

The test report shall include the following items at the minimum:

1) Name of the testing agency and study director
2) Test period
3) Factors to identify the test sample
   (e.g., name of the medical device, manufacturer's name, serial number, and names of raw materials, etc.)
4) Factors to identify the control solution
   (e.g. name of the control solution, supplier, serial number, etc.)
5) Method of application of the test sample to the test (including sterilization process if practiced)
   (e.g. sampling weight or area, cut and sterilization processes, etc.)
6) Preparation method for test solution
   (e.g., extraction method, etc.)
7) RhE model used
8) Test method
9) Test results
10) Evaluation of the results and discussion

10)　結果の評価と考察

11)　参考文献

3.2　*in vivo* 皮膚一次刺激性試験

3.2.1　目的

本試験は試験液中に，皮膚刺激性を有する物質が存在するかどうかを確認する *in vivo* 試験である．

3.2.2　試験の要約

試験試料から生理食塩液及び植物油を用いて抽出した試験液を，1 溶媒当たりウサギ 3 匹を用い，背部の無傷皮膚区画に塗布し，刺激性を観察する（6.2 項参照）．なお，3 匹の動物を用いた試験の反応が疑わしい場合は，さらに 3 匹を追加して試験を実施する．

3.2.3　試験液の調製

3.1.3 項に従う．ただし，対照液の調製については，抽出溶媒単独（試験試料を加えない）で，試験液調製と同条件で操作を行ったものを対照液とする．

3.2.4　試験法

3.2.4.1　試験動物

健康で体重が 2 kg 以上のウサギ計 6 匹（1 群 3 匹，2 溶媒）を使用する．週齢及び性は特に規定しないが，試験の評価が可能な皮膚を有する動物を用いる（6.7 項参照）．使用前 1 週間以上，馴化する．

投与前までに背部の毛を刈り（又は剃り），投与及び皮膚観察が容易な状態にする（6.8 項参照）．

3.2.4.2　投与液量

試験液及び対照液の投与液量は，原則として 1 投与区画当たり 0.5 mL とする．

3.2.4.3　投与経路及び投与期間

塗布による投与を 1 回行う．

3.2.4.4　投与部位

背部を上下，左右計 4 区画に分け試験液及び対照液をそれぞれ 2 区画に投与する（例：図 2 参照）．投与液量は 1 区画につき 0.5 mL とし，これを 1 枚の不織布（リント布）など（2.5 cm 角）にしみ込ませてテープで貼りつける．その上をポリエチレンフィルムなどで覆い，固定する．

11)　References

3.2　*In vivo* primary skin irritation test

3.2.1　Purpose

The test is an *in vivo* test designed to confirm the presence of potential substances that exhibit skin irritation in the test solution.

3.2.2　Summary of the test

Test solutions extracted from test samples using physiological saline or vegetable oil are applied on intact dorsal regions of three rabbits for each vehicle to observe irritancy (refer to Section 6.5). If the response in the test using three animals is equivocal, further testing using another three animals should be considered.

3.2.3　Preparation of test solution

Follow the procedure described in 3.1.3. For the preparation of the control solution, use the solution prepared from the extraction solvent alone (without addition of the test sample) as a solvent control under the same conditions as the test solution preparation.

3.2.4　Test method

3.2.4.1　Test animal

Use six healthy rabbits of each weighing 2 kg or more (three animals per group, two solvents). Age by weeks and sex are not specified, but the skin condition at testing site should be good for evaluation of the results (refer to Section 6.7). Animals should be acclimatized and cared for under specific laboratory conditions for one week or longer before use.

Clip (or shave) hair from a dorsal region before topical application to have the skin condition better to apply or observe at the site (refer to Section 6.8).

3.2.4.2　Dose level

Apply 0.5 mL of the test and control solution at each treatment site.

3.2.4.3　Administration route and period

Apply topically to dorsal regions once.

3.2.4.4　Administration site

Divide a dorsal region into four regions, top and bottom and right and left portions, and administer the test and control solutions in two regions each (refer to Figure 2). Apply one non-woven fabric (such as lint, a 2.5 cm square) impregnated with the test or control solution (0.5 mL each) on each area and fix each area with tape. Then fix the dorsal area by covering with a polyethylene film.

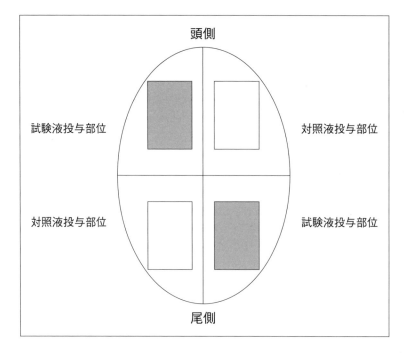

図 2　皮膚一次刺激性試験（例）ウサギ背部図

表 1　皮膚（皮内）反応の評点付けシステム（ISO 10993-10, 6 *In Vivo* irritation tests）

	評点
紅斑及び痂皮の形成	
紅斑なし	0
非常に軽度な紅斑（認識下限レベル）	1
軽度な紅斑	2
中程度の紅斑	3
高度な紅斑（ビート赤），紅斑の評点付けを妨げる痂皮の形成	4
	［最高点 4 点］
浮腫の形成	
浮腫なし	0
非常に軽度な浮腫（認識下限レベル）	1
軽度な浮腫（膨隆により縁が明確に識別可能なレベル）	2
中程度の浮腫（約 1 mm の膨隆）	3
高度な浮腫（1 mm 以上の膨隆とばく露範囲を超えた広がり）	4
	［最高点 4 点］
	［紅斑・痂皮及び浮腫の合計点数の最高点 8 点］

投与部位に見られた他の有害作用も記録及び報告すること．

3.2.4.5　観察

　投与直前に皮膚の状態を観察する．投与後 24 時間目に不織布を除去し，丁寧に塗布面を拭き取る（6.9 項参照）．不織布除去 1 ±0.1 時間後，24 ± 2 時間後，48 ± 2 時間後及び 72 ± 2 時間後に皮膚の状態を観察し，表 1 に従って観察・記録する．不織布除去 72 時間後に持続性の病変が認められた場合，病変が可逆性か非可逆性かを評価するた

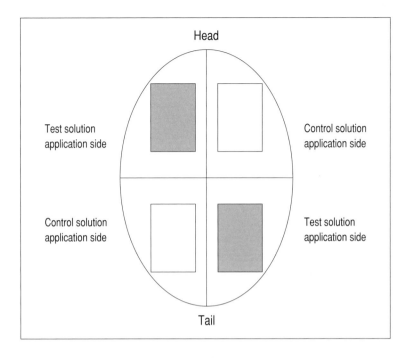

Figure 2   Rabbit dorsal region for primary skin irritation test (example)

Table 1   Grading system for intracutaneous (intradermal) reactions (ISO 10993-10, 6 *In Vivo* irritation tests)

Reaction	Irritation score
Erythema and eschar formation	
No erythema	0
Very slight erythema (barely perceptible)	1
Well-defined erythema	2
Moderate erythema	3
Severe erythema (beet-redness) to eschar formation preventing grading of erythema	4
	[Maximal possible score 4]
Oedema formation	
No oedema	0
Very slight oedema (barely perceptible)	1
Well-defined oedema	2
Moderate oedema (raised approximately 1 mm)	3
Severe oedema (raised more than 1 mm and extending beyond exposure area)	4
	[Maximal possible score 4]
	[Maximal possible score for irritation 8]

Other adverse changes at the skin sites shall be recorded and reported

3.2.4.5 Observation

Observe skin conditions of all animals immediately before administration. Remove non-woven fabrics 24 hours after administration and wipe the application area carefully (refer to Section 6.9). Observe and record skin conditions 1 ± 0.1, 24 ± 2, 48 ± 2 and 72 ± 2 hours after removal of them in accordance with Table 1. Extended observation is necessary if there are persistent lesions 72 hours after removal of non-woven fabrics, in order to evaluate

めに，必要に応じて14日を超えない範囲で観察期間を延長する．

体重は，投与日及び観察終了日に測定し，記録する．

3.2.4.6　評価

観察結果より刺激性を評価する．例えば，個々の動物において試験液及び対照液ごとに，24±2，48±2及び72±2時間の2投与部位の評点スコアを合計し，各合計を6（3時点×2試験液又は対照液投与部位）で除して，個別の平均一次刺激点数を求める．各試験液群及び対照液群の平均一次刺激点数を求めるため，各群3匹の動物の点数を合計し，3で除す．試験液群の平均一次刺激点数から対照液群の平均一次刺激点数を差し引いて一次刺激指数（PII）を求める．一次刺激指数を表2に規定する一次刺激指数カテゴリと比較し，適切な反応カテゴリを報告書に記載する．

表2　一次刺激指数カテゴリ

平均点数	反応カテゴリ
0〜0.4	無視できる程度
0.5〜1.9	多少
2.0〜4.9	中程度
5.0〜8.0	激しい

3.2.5　試験報告書

試験報告書には，少なくとも以下の事項を記載する．

1) 試験実施機関及び試験責任者
2) 試験実施期間
3) 試験試料を特定する要素
　　（例：医療機器の名称，製造販売業者名，製造番号，原材料名など）
4) 対照液を特定する要素
　　（例：対照液名，入手先，製造番号など）
5) 試験液の調製方法
6) 試験動物の種と系統，数，週齢，性別，個別体重
7) 試験方法
8) 試験結果（6.10参照）
　　表：個々の動物の皮膚反応結果（評点スコア）
9) 結果の評価と考察
10) 参考文献

4．皮内反応試験

4.1　目的

本試験は試験液を皮内投与し，刺激性の有無を確認するための*in vivo*試験である．

the reversibility or irreversibility of the lesions over a period of time not exceeding 14 days.

Weigh and record the body weights of all animals at the administration day and the last day of the observation.

3.2.4.6 Evaluation

Evaluate irritancy from observation results. For example, all erythema grades plus oedema grades from two application sites at 24 ± 2 hours, 48 ± 2 hours and 72 ± 2 hours are summed separately for each test and control solution for each animal. The primary irritation score for each animal is calculated by dividing the sum of all the scores by 6 (three time points × two test sites or two control sites). To obtain the primary irritation score for each test and control group, add all the primary irritation scores of the three individual animals and divide by three. To obtain the primary irritation index (PII), subtract the primary irritation score for the test group from that for the control group. The PII is compared with the categories of irritation response given in Table 2 and the appropriate response category is recorded for the report.

Table 2   Primary irritation index category

Mean score	Reaction category
0–0.4	Negligible
0.5–1.9	Slight
2.0–4.9	Moderate
5.0–8.0	Severe

3.2.5 Test report

The test report shall include the following items at the minimum:
1) Name of the testing agency and study director
2) Test period
3) Factors to identify the test sample
   (e.g., name of the medical device, manufacturer's name, serial number, and names of raw materials, etc.)
4) Factors to identify the control solution
   (e.g. name of the control solution, supplier, serial number, etc.)
5) Preparation method for test solution
6) Species, strain, number, age and sex of animals
7) Test method
8) Test results
   Table: Skin response results of individual animal (score points)
9) Evaluation of the results and discussion
10) References

4.   Intracutaneous reactivity test
4.1   Purpose

This test is designed to confirm irritancy of the test solution by intracutaneous administration.

4.2　試験の要約

　試験試料から生理食塩液及び植物油を用いて抽出した試験液を，3匹のウサギの背部に皮内投与し，投与部位を投与後72±2時間まで観察して，刺激性の有無を評価する（6.2項参照）．なお，3匹の動物を用いた試験の反応が疑わしい場合は，さらに3匹を追加して試験を実施する．

4.3　試験液の調製

　3.1.3項に従う．ただし，対照液の調製については，抽出溶媒単独（試験試料を加えない）で，試験液調製と同条件で操作を行ったものを対照液とする．

4.4　試験法
4.4.1　試験動物

　栄養状態のよい健康で体重が2kg以上のウサギ3匹を使用する．週齢及び性は特に規定しないが，試験の評価が可能な皮膚を有する動物を用いる（6.7項参照）．使用前1週間以上，馴化する．

　投与前までに背部の毛を刈り（又は剃り），投与及び皮膚観察が容易な状態にする（6.8項参照）．

4.4.2　投与液量

　試験液及び対照液の投与液量は，原則として1ヶ所当たり0.2mLとする．

4.4.3　投与経路及び投与期間

　背部皮内投与を1回行う．

4.4.4　投与部位

　脊柱をはさみ，両側20ヶ所（片側10ヶ所）に2種類の溶媒で得られた各試験液及び各対照液を各5ヶ所ずつ投与する（例：図3参照）．

4.4.5　観察

　全例について投与直前に皮膚の状態を観察する．全例について投与直後並びに投与後約24±2，48±2及び72±2時間に，投与部位の皮内反応状態を，表2に従って観察・記録する．体重は，投与日及び観察終了日に測定し，記録する．

　備考：オイルの皮内注射は炎症を誘発することがある．

4.4.6　評価

　観察結果より刺激性を評価する．例えば，個々の動物において試験液及び対照液ごとに，24±2，48±2及び72±2時間の5投与部位の評点スコアを合計し，各合計を15（3時点×5試験液又は対照液投与部位）で除して，個別動物の点数を求める．各試験液群及び対照液群の平均点を求めるため，各群3匹の動物の点数を合計し，3で除す．試験液の最終評価点は，試験液群の平均評価点から対照液群の平均評価点を差し引いて求める．試験液の最終評価点が1.0以下であれば試験の要求事項が満たされた（刺激性

4.2   Summary of the test

Test solutions extracted from test samples using physiological saline or vegetable oil as a vehicle will be administered intracutaneously to dorsal regions of three rabbits to evaluate irritancy by observation of administration sites until 72 ± 2 hours of administration (refer to Section 6.2). If the response in the test using three animals is equivocal, further testing using another three animals should be conducted.

4.3   Preparation of test solution

Follow the procedure described in 3.1.3. For the preparation of the control solution, use the solution prepared from the extraction solvent alone (without addition of the test sample) as a solvent control under the same conditions as the test solution preparation.

4.4   Test method
4.4.1   Test animal

Use three healthy rabbits of each weighing 2 kg or more in good nutrition. Age by weeks and sex are not specified, but the skin condition at testing site should be good for evaluation of the results (refer to Section 6.7). Animals should be acclimatized and cared for under specific laboratory conditions for 1 week or longer before use.

Clip (or shave) hair from a dorsal region before topical application to have the skin condition better to apply or observe at the site (refer to Section 6.8).

4.4.2   Dose level

Administer 0.2 mL of the test and control solution at each administration site.

4.4.3   Administration route and period

Administer intracutaneously to dorsal regions once.

4.4.4   Administration site

Administer the test and the control solutions (two vehicles, five injections for each solution, total 20 injections) on both sides of the spinal column (10 injections on each side) (refer to figure 3).

4.4.5   Observation

Observe skin conditions of all animals just before administration. Observe and record skin conditions of the injection sites of all animals approximately 24 ± 2, 48 ± 2 and 72 ± 2 hours after administration in accordance with Table 2. Weigh and record the body weights of all animals on the administration day and the last day of the observation.

Remark: Intradermal injection of oil frequently elicits an inflammatory response.

4.4.6   Evaluation

Evaluate irritancy from observation results. For example, all erythema grades plus oedema grades at 24 ± 2 hours, 48 ± 2 hours and 72 ± 2 hours are summed separately for each test and control solution for each animal. The irritation score for each animal is calculated by dividing the sum of all the scores by 15 (three time points $\times$ five test sites or five control sites). To determine the overall mean irritation score for each test and control group, add the scores for the three individual animals and divide by three. The final test sample score is obtained by subtracting the score of the control from the test sample score. The require-

陰性）とする.

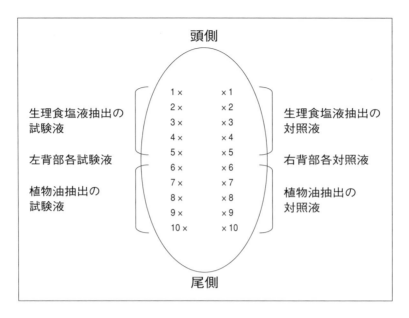

図3　皮内反応試験（例）投与部位

4.5　試験報告書

3.2.5 項参照すること.

5．眼刺激試験
5.1　目的

本試験は，ウサギの眼に試験液を点眼することによって眼組織に及ぼす影響を評価するためのものである.

5.2　試験の要約

試験試料から生理食塩液及び植物油を用いて抽出した試験液を，それぞれ3匹のウサギに点眼し，前眼部を点眼後72±2時間まで観察して，眼組織への影響を評価する（6.2 項参照）. 点眼72±2時間後に持続性の病変が認められた場合，病変が可逆性か非可逆性かを評価するために，必要に応じて21日を超えない範囲で観察期間を延長する（6.11, 6.12 項参照）.

5.3　試験液の調製

3.1.3 項に従う. ただし，対照液の調製については，抽出溶媒単独（試験試料を加えない）で，試験液調製と同条件で操作を行ったものを対照液とする.

5.4　試験法
5.4.1　試験動物

1)　健康で，前眼部に異常がなく体重が2～3kgのウサギ計6匹（1群3匹，2溶媒）

ments of the test are met if the final test sample score is 1.0 or less (non-irritant).

Figure 3   Arrangements of the injection sites (example)

4.5   Test report
Refer to Section 3.2.5.

5.   Ocular irritation test
5.1   Purpose
This test is designed to confirm effects of test samples (final products or materials) on ocular tissues by instillation of the extract of the test sample to rabbit eyes.

5.2   Summary of the test
Test solutions extracted from test samples using physiological saline or vegetable oil as a vehicle is applied to one eye (three rabbits for each vehicle) to evaluate eye irritancy for 72 ±2 hours after instillation (refer to Section 6.2). Extended observation may be necessary if there are persistent lesions observed at 72 ±2 hours after instillation, in order to evaluate the reversibility or irreversibility of the lesions over a period of time not exceeding 21 days (refer to Section 6.11, 6.12).

5.3   Preparation of test solution
Follow the procedure described in 3.1.3. For the preparation of the control solution, use the solution prepared from the extraction solvent alone (without addition of the test sample) as a solvent control under the same conditions as the test solution preparation.

5.4   Test method
5.4.1   Test animal
1)   Use six healthy rabbits, each weighing 2 to 3 kg, without any abnormalities in the anterior chamber of the eyes (three animals/group, two vehicles). Age and sex are not speci-

を使用する．週齢及び性は特に規定しないが，試験の評価が可能な眼を有する動物を用いる．

2)　使用前1週間以上，馴化する．角膜をスリットランプで観察する場合，瞬膜を切除した方が容易に観察できるため，瞬膜の切除は適宜とする．切除する場合は，試験に使用する2週間以上前に行う．

3)　投与前にウサギの前眼部を観察し，結膜充血，角膜混濁などの異常がないことを確認する．さらに，角膜については，フルオレセインナトリウム溶液又は試験紙などを用いて観察し，染色のないことを確認する（6.13項参照）．

5.4.2　試験方法

1)　ウサギの片目の下眼瞼を引っ張り，袋状にし，その中に生理食塩液抽出の試験液を0.1 mL点眼し，眼を閉じて約30秒間そのままの状態にする．

2)　他眼には，生理食塩液抽出の対照液を同様に点眼する．

3)　1)から2)の操作を3匹のウサギに実施する．

4)　同様に，植物油抽出の試験液を残り3匹のウサギの片目に点眼し，他眼には，植物油抽出の対照液を点眼する．

5)　点眼1 ±0.1, 24± 2, 48± 2及び72± 2時間後に，スリットランプを用いて両眼を観察し，ISO 10993-10の眼病変の評点付けシステム（付表1）又はMcDonald-Shadduckの評価基準（付表2）に従い評価し，記録する．点眼72± 2時間後に持続性の病変が認められた場合，病変が可逆性か非可逆性かを評価するために，必要に応じて21日を超えない範囲で観察期間を延長する（6.11, 6.12項参照）．

5.5　試験報告書

試験報告書には，少なくとも以下の事項を記載する．

1)　試験実施機関及び試験責任者

2)　試験実施期間

3)　試験試料を特定する要素

（例：医療機器の名称，製造販売業者名，製造番号，原材料名など）

4)　対照液を用いた場合は，それを特定する要素

（例：対照液名，入手先，製造番号など）

5)　試験液の調製方法

6)　試験動物の種と系統，数，週齢，性別，個別体重

7)　試験方法

8)　試験結果（6.10参照）

表：個々の動物の眼反応結果（評点のスコア）

個々の動物の結果は，表3の様な表形式にした全データを添付することが望ましい．

9)　結果の評価と考察

10)　参考文献

fied, but the eye condition at testing sites should be good for evaluation of the results.

2) Animals should be acclimatized and cared for under specific conditions for one week or longer before use. To make corneal observation with slit lamp easier, the nictitating membranes may be excised as appropriate. If used, perform the excision at least two weeks before initiation of a test.

3) Observe anterior portions of eyes before administration to confirm the absence of abnormalities such as conjunctivae hyperemia or corneal opacity. Additionally, observe corneas after instillation of fluorescein sodium solution or using a test paper to confirm absence of stained area (refer to Section 6.13).

5.4.2 Test procedure

1) Open a lower eyelid of the one side of eyes, instill 0.1 mL of the test solution extracted with physiological saline into the conjunctival sac, and then close the eye for 30 seconds.

2) Instill a control solution prepared with physiological saline into the other eye in the same manner as the test solution.

3) Treat the rest rabbits in a same manner as the procedures 1) and 2)

4) Similarly, instill a test solution extracted with vegetable oil to one eye of the other three rabbits and a control solution prepared with vegetable oil into the other eye

5) Observe both eyes using a slit lamp 1 ± 0.1, 24 ± 2, 48 ± 2 and 72 ± 2 hours after instillation, evaluate in accordance with Attachment 1 (Systems for grading ocular lesions) or McDonald−Shadduck's standard (Attachment 2) and record scores. Extended observation can be necessary if there are persistent lesions 72 ± 2 hours after instillation, in order to evaluate the reversibility or irreversibility of the lesions over a period of time not exceeding 21 days (refer to Section 6.11, 6.12).

5.5 Test report

The test report shall include the following items at the minimum:

1) Name of the testing agency and study director

2) Test period

3) Factors to identify the test sample
(e.g., name of the medical device, manufacturer's name, serial number, and names of raw materials, etc.)

4) Factors to identify the control solution
(e.g. name of the control solution, supplier, serial number, etc.)

5) Preparation method for test solution

6) Species, strain, number, age and sex of animals

7) Test method

8) Test results (refer to Section 6.10)
Table: Ocular response results of individual animals (score points)
It is desirable to attach individual data from all animals as a table like Table 3.

9) Evaluation of the results and discussion

10) References

6．参考情報

6.1　刺激性試験実施の基本的な考え方

　医療機器の刺激性評価を行う場合，まずは被験物質の毒性情報などを収集し，試験実施の必要性について検討する．刺激性を判定できる十分な情報がなく，試験以外の方法で刺激性の有無を評価できない場合は，動物福祉の観点から，まず *in vitro* 試験の実施を考える方が望ましい．*in vitro* 試験の実施や評価が難しい場合，初めてウサギなどの動物での試験実施を考える．

　ISO 10993-10 では 2019 年現在，刺激性試験と感作性試験を分離し，刺激性試験全般を ISO 10993-23 として改訂する作業が進められている．さらに皮膚刺激性試験では，*in vitro* 皮膚刺激性試験のラウンドロビン試験が ISO/TC 194/WG8 主導で実施され，その有用性が実証されたことから[1]，新たな評価法として改訂版への採用に向けた検討がなされている．

　ただし，現時点では RhE モデルを用いた *in vitro* 皮膚刺激性試験では刺激性の有無のみが判定され，ウサギを用いた *in vivo* 試験のように刺激性の強弱の判定まではできない．一方，5 つの刺激性物質（乳酸，ヘプタン酸，Y-4，Genapol X-80，SDS）の刺激性能を *in vivo* 試験であるウサギを用いた皮膚一次刺激性試験及び皮内反応試験，ヒトパッチテスト及び RhE モデルを用いた *in vitro* 皮膚刺激性試験で検証された報告があり，各試験とも同一被験物質濃度条件で実施された結果，RhE モデルを用いた *in vitro* 皮膚刺激性試験が他の試験法よりも低濃度の刺激性物質も陽性と判定できることが示されている[2]．この結果から，RhE モデルを用いた *in vitro* 皮膚刺激性試験で陰性と判定された検体については，動物試験を新たに実施する必要はないと考えられる．一方，RhE モデルを用いた *in vitro* 皮膚刺激性試験で陽性と判定された検体については，*in vivo* 試験を実施し，刺激性の強弱の情報を入手することも有用と考えられる．

6.2　試験液の調製

　in vivo 試験を実施する場合，試験液の pH が強酸性又は強アルカリ性（pH ≦ 2 又は ≧ 11.5）を示す場合は試験を実施しない．必要に応じて生理食塩液抽出液（極性液）については，調製後に pH を確認して記録する．

　被験物質細切時の破片などが不溶性異物として抽出液に含まれる場合がある．このような抽出液の性状観察（色調変化や微粒子の有無）は投与前の確認として重要である．不溶性異物の物理的刺激により皮内に炎症を生じる可能性が予期される場合，不溶性異物ができる限り入り込まないような調製方法が推奨される．

6.3　RhE モデル

　OECD No. 439 で化学物質の刺激性評価について検証された RhE モデルとして，Epi-Derm™ SIT（EPI-200），SkinEthic™RHE，LabCyte EPI-MODEL 24 SIT，EpiSkin™（SM），epiCS® 及び Skin + ® が記載されている．このうち，EpiDerm™SIT と SkinEthic™RHE は ISO TC194 WG8 で行われたラウンドロビンテストによって，医療機器の抽出液の刺激性評価への有用性が示されている．その他の RhE モデルについては，医療機器の抽出液の刺激性評価についての適切な検証がなされた後に使用することを推奨する．

6. Reference information

6.1 Basic principles for conducting irritation test

In order to evaluate the irritancy of medical devices, first, collect toxicological information of the test substance and then consider whether further testing is necessary. When there is not enough information to determine the irritancy of a medical device, and the irritancy of a medical device can only be evaluated by conducting an irritation test, it is preferable to consider conducting an *in vitro* test first from the viewpoint of animal welfare. If it is difficult to conduct an *in vitro* test and evaluate irritancy of a medical device, consider conducting a test with animals such as rabbits.

As of 2019, revision of ISO 10993-10 is in progress to separate the irritation test and sensitization test, and standardize the irritation test including both *in vitro* and *in vivo* testing as ISO 10993-23. The usefulness of the *in vitro* skin irritation test has been demonstrated in the ISO/TC 194/WG8-conducted Round Robin Study[1], so that adoption of this new evaluation method is being considered to the revised version.

However, the current *in vitro* skin test with the RhE model estimates only the presence or absence of irritation, unlike *in vivo* rabbit test, where the grade of irritation can be determined. On the other hand, the irritation potency of five irritants (lactic acid, heptanoic acid, Y-4, Genapol-X80 and SDS) has been evaluated in both primary skin irritation test and intracutaneous reactivity test using rabbits, the human patch test, and the *in vitro* skin irritation test using the RhE model. The results of these tests with same test sample concentration demonstrate that the *in vitro* test with the RhE model can judge irritancy of a test sample at a lower concentration than other test methods[2]. These results suggest that samples, which have been judged negative in the *in vitro* skin irritation test using the RhE model do not require further *in vivo* test. In contrast, it may be useful to perform an *in vivo* test to obtain the degree of irritancy for samples that have been judged positive in the *in vitro* skin irritation test using the RhE model.

6.2 Preparation of test solution

When the pH of test solution indicates strong acidity or strong alkaline (pH≤2 or ≥15), *in vivo* test should not be performed. If necessary, pH of test solutions extracted using physiological saline (polar solution) would be measured and recorded at the time of dose preparation.

When the test sample is cut into small pieces to prepare a test solution, the solution may contain insoluble foreign substances such as small fragments derived from the sample. It is important to observe and evaluate the properties of the test solution (color change and presence of particles) prior to application of it to the test. If it can be expected that a physical stimulation by the substances causes inflammation in the skin, an appropriate preparation method, which prevents contamination of the substances as much as possible, is recommended.

6.3 RhE models

EpiDerm™ SIT (EPI-200), SkinEthic™ RHE, LabCyte EPI-MODEL 24 SIT, EpiSkin™ (SM), epiCS® and Skin + ® are listed in the OECD Test Guideline 439 as RhE models validated for evaluating the irritancy of chemicals. The Round Robin Study conducted by the ISO/TC 194/WG8 revealed the usefulness of only EpiDerm™ SIT and SkinEthic™ RHE models for evaluating the irritancy of medical device extracts. For the other RhE models, it is recommended to use it once appropriate confirmation regarding irritancy evaluation for extractables of medical devices is performed.

6.4　陽性対照材料

　　陽性対照材料としては，Y-4（Genapol X-080 を 10 パーツ含有する PVC ペレット）がある．Y-4 の刺激性試験用陽性対照材料としての性能は，海外研究施設と共同で実施した予備検討において実証され，その再現性・頑健性も ISO/TC 194/WG8 で行われたラウンドロビン試験により検証されている．一般財団法人食品薬品安全センター秦野研究所（第 1 部細胞毒性試験 4.6 項参照）から入手可能である．

　　当該ラウンドロビン試験において，Y-4 の極性及び非極性抽出液はほとんどの RhE モデルにおいて明瞭な陽性反応を呈した．ただし，その他のモデルと比較してバリアー機能が高いと考えられる EpiDerm™SIT（EPI-200）を用いた試験では，付録に提示した抽出条件（0.2 g/mL，37℃，72 時間）により非極性溶媒抽出液を調製すると生存率が 40 ％を越える施設が散見された．この状況に鑑みて，Y-4 の非極性溶媒抽出液を用いた試験を行う場合は各 RhE モデルの特性を考慮して，各試験施設で適切な条件を設定し，その刺激性を確認した上で試験に供することを推奨する．

6.5　OD 測定例

　　イソプロパノール抽出液 200 μl を 96 ウェルプレートの各ウェルに入れる．1 検体につき測定するウェル数は，各 RhE モデルのマニュアルに従うこと．ブランクとしてイソプロパノールを 200 μl 入れる（配置例：図 1 参照）．570 nm でホルマザンの OD を測定する．必要に応じて波長基準を測定して差し引く場合もある．

6.6　生存率の算出法例

　　ブランク値として 6 ウェルのブランクの平均値を求める．検体の吸光度値からブランク値を引いたものを各検体の測定値とする．陰性対照の生存率は 3 ウェルの陰性対照の測定値の合計を 3 で除し，陰性対照の測定値平均を求め，これを生存率 100 ％とする．各検体の生存率は（各検体の測定値平均*/ 陰性対照の測定値平均）× 100 の式で算出できる．*N＝3 の試験から算出した平均値

6.7　動物種

　　試験に使用するウサギとしては，日本白色種，ニュージーランド白色種などが汎用される．皮内反応試験及び皮膚刺激性試験は，いずれも背部皮膚を用いるので，皮膚の状態が試験結果の評価に大きな影響を与える．すなわち，ウサギには皮膚の生理的現象としてヘアサイクルがあり，いわゆるアイランドスキンと呼ばれる皮膚が部分的に肥厚した状態の動物は試験動物としては適さない．試験には，ヘアサイクルができるだけ休止期（スムーススキン）にある動物を選択する必要がある．

6.8　動物の毛刈り

　　ISO 10993-10 では，投与の 18〜4 時間前に毛刈りするよう規定されているが，これは投与時に毛刈りの影響が残っていないこと，毛の伸びが観察に影響しないこと，あるいは動物福祉の観点から動物を必要以上に毛のない状態にしないことなどを目的としたものと考えられる．したがって，上記目的が達せられることが明らかな場合には，毛刈りの時期を変更することも可能である．なお，刺激性の無いことが確認できている場合

6.4 Positive control material

Y-4 (PVC pellet containing 10 parts of Genapol X-080) is available as a positive control material. The Performance of Y-4 as a positive control material for irritation tests has been verified in a preliminary study conducted in collaboration with overseas research laboratories, and its reproducibility and robustness have also been verified by the Round Robin Study conducted by the ISO/TC 194/WG8. Y-4 is available from Hatano Research Institute, Food and Drug Safety Center (refer to Section 4.6 Part 1, Test for cytotoxicity).

In the Round Robin Study, polar and non-polar extracts of Y-4 showed a clear positive reaction in most of the RhE models. However, in the test using EpiDerm™ SIT (EPI-200), which is considered to have a higher barrier function than other models, with non-polar solvent extract prepared under the extraction conditions (0.2 g/mL, 37 ℃, 72 hours) presented in the Appendix, survival rates were above 40 % in some laboratories. Therefore, it is recommended to check the irritancy before performing a test using Y-4 non-polar solvent extract, considering the properties of each RhE model and extraction conditions be set at each test facility.

6.5 Example for absorbance measurements

Transfer 200 μL isopropanol extract from each test sample into each well of 96-well plate. According to the manual for each RhE model, determine the number of wells to be measured per sample. Add 200 μL of isopropanol as a blank (refer to Figure 1 for example of arrangement). Read the OD of formazan at 570 nm. In some cases, the wavelength reference may be measured and subtracted from the value at 570 nm.

6.6 Example of viability calculation

Calculate the mean OD from the six blank wells as a blank value. The measured value for each test sample is the value for subtracting the absorbance of the blank to that of each test sample. To calculate the viability of the negative control, divide the sum of the measurements of the 3-well negative control by 3 and then determine the mean of the negative controls, that is converted into 100 % viability. The viability of each test sample can be calculated by the formula of (mean measured value of each test sample[*]/mean measured value of negative control). [*]A mean value calculated from the test results (N = 3).

6.7 Animal species

Japanese white or New Zealand white rabbits are commonly used in studies. Both intracutaneous response test and skin irritation test use dorsal skin, and the skin condition heavily influences the evaluation of test results. The hair cycle is a physical event in rabbit skin, which commonly results in the condition called island skin (that is the condition a part of skin with thick hair), which is not suitable for the testing. Therefore, it is necessary to select animals whose hair cycle is at rest time (smooth skin).

6.8 Clipping hair

In ISO 10993-10 it is specified that animals should have their hair clipped 18 to 4 hours before administration. The rationale for this period is to decrease the potential for residual irritancy as a result of clipping, avoid hair re-growth and minimize the time of the animals maintained without a normal hair in accordance with animal welfare. Therefore, if it is clear to achieve the purpose for hair clipping, changing the time schedule for hair clipping is available. A hair-removing cream may be used when it is confirmed that the cream does

には，脱毛クリームを使用してもよい.

6.9   試験液の接触時間

　　ここでは，皮膚における一次刺激性を評価する方法を示した. そのため，試験液の接触時間は標準的に 24 時間としたが，当該医療機器の接触期間により変更することも可能である（ISO 10993-10 参照）. また当該医療機器が臨床において反復使用される場合には，皮膚刺激性試験においても，反復投与による影響を評価する必要がある.

6.10   動物の投与日及び観察終了日の個別体重及び試験液投与部位の写真

　　試験報告書に記載すべき事項から投与日及び観察終了日の個別体重や試験液投与部位の写真を除外した. その目的は ISO-10993-10: 2010 に調和させることであり，投与日及び観察終了日の個別体重の測定，試験液投与部位の写真撮影及び試験報告書への掲載を妨げるものではない.

6.11   眼刺激の評価基準

　　ISO 10993-10 の眼病変の評価システム（付表 1）でアスタリスクが付された所見は，刺激性陽性反応と考えられている.

6.12   試験動物の福祉

　　ISO 10993-10 には，非常に強い眼の損傷，出血性又は化膿性の分泌物，あるいは著しい角膜潰瘍が見られる動物は，直ちに安楽死させるように記載されている. さらに，点眼後 24 時間以内に回復の徴候が見られない対光反射消失又は角膜混濁，あるいは点眼後 48 時間以内に回復の徴候の見られない結膜炎症が見られる動物も安楽死させるよう記載されている. 眼刺激試験においては，必要に応じて局所麻酔及び鎮痛剤を使用してもよい.

6.13   フルオレセインナトリウム溶液の点眼

　　フルオレセインナトリウム（日局）溶液をウサギ眼に直接点眼し，染色をすることは避けることが望ましい. 1 ～ 2 ％フルオレセインナトリウム溶液を涙液の分泌の少ないウサギ眼に直接点眼するとフルオレセインナトリウムの蛍光が強く，染色された組織を識別することが困難である. フルオレセインナトリウム溶液でウサギ眼を染色する場合，まずウサギ眼に生理食塩液を点眼しフルオレセインナトリウム溶液を眼科用の硝子棒に採り，上又は下眼瞼を引っ張り投与する. 両眼瞼を指で軽く閉じ，角膜などを染色する. 直接フルオレセインナトリウム溶液を点眼し染色する場合は 2 ％フルオレセインナトリウム溶液を生理食塩液で 5 ～10 倍に希釈使用するとよい. なお，この場合，希釈したフルオレセインナトリウム溶液は防腐性を失うため，調製後長期間保存しないこと.

　　フルオレセインナトリウム溶液又は試験紙などを用いて観察すると，ひっかき傷や毛が眼に入ったための傷によると思われる染色がよく観察される. このような場合は試験に使用しても構わない. ただし，記録を残すこと.

not possess irritancy.

6.9 Contact duration of test solution

This guidance includes the method to evaluate the primary irritation on skin. Therefore, the contact duration of a test solution was set at 24 hours in accordance with the standard; however, it is possible to change the duration based on the actual contact duration of the medical device (refer to ISO 01993-10). In case where the medical device is used repeatedly in the clinical practice, it is necessary to evaluate the effect of the test sample after repeated administration in skin irritation test.

6.10 Individual animal weights and photograph of the test solution administration sites on the administration day and the last day of observation

Individual animal weights and photograph of the test solution administration sites at initiation and completion of test have been excluded from the list of items to be included in the test report in order to harmonize with ISO-10993-10: 2010. This does not prevent measurement of individual animal weights at initiation and completion of test and taking photographs of the test solution administration sites and describing them in the test report.

6.11 Evaluation of eye irritation

If the treated eye shows findings (footnoted grades, with an asterisk given Attachment 1), the response is evaluated as positive.

6.12 Animal welfare

In ISO 10993-10, described as following considerations:
Immediately withdraw an animal from the study and humanely euthanized it if, at any time, it shows: very severe ocular damage, blood-stained or purulent discharge, or significant corneal ulceration. Additionally, it is described that the animal should be euthanized if it shows absence of a light reflex or corneal opacity without evidence of recovery within 24 hours after instillation or maximum conjunctival inflammation without evidence of recovery within 48 hours after instillation. In an ocular irritation test, if necessary, local anesthetic and analgesic agents can be used.

6.13 Instillation of fluorescein sodium solution

Because 1-2 % solution of fluorescein sodium (Japanese Pharmacopoeia) is a high concentration, it is difficult to distinguish specific stained tissue of rabbit eyes that secrete only a small amount of lacrimal fluid. Therefore, when staining rabbit eyes with 1-2 % fluorescein sodium solution, first instill physiological saline and then administer 1-2 % fluorescein sodium solution with a glass bar while pulling an upper or lower eyelid. Close both eyelids gently with fingers in order to stain corneas, etc. If staining of corneas by direct instillation of fluorescein sodium solution is desirable, it is recommended to dilute 1-2 % fluorescein sodium solution 5 to 10-fold with physiological saline. In this case do not store the diluted fluorescein sodium solution for a long period, as it loses the antiseptic properties.

In observations using fluorescein sodium solution or a test paper, scratches or scars likely to be caused by a hair gotten in the eye may be stained and frequently observed. In such cases the animals may be used in the test, but findings should be recorded.

6.14　コンタクトレンズの眼装用試験

コンタクトレンズの生物学的安全性試験として，ウサギを用いる眼装用試験が要求される．眼装用試験は，通常"ISO 9394: 2012, Ophthalmic optics-Contact lenses and contact lens care products-Determination of biocompatibility by ocular study with rabbit eyes"に従って実施され，眼組織への影響を，肉眼的及び病理組織学的観察結果をもとに評価されることから，対象試験試料がコンタクトレンズで，眼装用試験が実施されている場合には，抽出液による眼刺激試験を実施する必要はない．

7．薬食機発0301第20号からの変更点

1) 3.2.4.6 評価及び 4.4.6 評価について参考情報を参照となっていたが，現在ほぼ ISO 10993-10 の判定方法に従って評価されていることから，具体的な判定方法を記載し，現状と合わせた．
2) 再構築ヒト皮膚モデルを使用した医療機器の *in vitro* 皮膚刺激性試験を採用した．
3) *in vivo* 皮膚一次刺激性試験，皮内反応試験及び眼刺激試験で使用するウサギの体重を規定した．
4) *in vivo* 皮膚一次刺激性試験において，ISO 10993-10 では健常皮膚だけ試験するため，擦過傷処理部分を削除した．
5) 試験報告書に記載すべき事項から投与日及び観察終了日の個別体重や試験液投与部位の写真を除外した．
6) 参考情報に，刺激性試験実施の基本的な考え方を追加した．
7) 全体の構成について整合をとった．

8．引用文献

1) De Jong W.H, Hoffmann S, Lee M, Kandárovád H, Pellevoisine C, Haishima Y, Rollins B, Zdawzcyk A, Willoughby J, Bachelorj M, Schatzk T, Skoog S, Parker S, Sawyer A, Pescioo P, Fant K, Kim K-M, Kwon J.S, Gehrke H, Hofma-Hutherr H, Meloni M, Julius C, Briotet D, Letasiova S, Kato R, Miyajima A, Fonteyne L. De L, Videau C, Tornier C, Turley A, Christiano N, Coleman K.P.: Toxicology *In Vitro* 50, 439-449 (2018)
2) Kabdarova H, Bendovoa H, Letasiova S, Coleman K.P, De Jong W.H.: Toxicology *In Vitro* 50, 433-438 (2018)

9．参考文献

1) OECD No. 439: OECD Guidelines for the Testing of Chemicals. *In vitro* Skin Irritation: Reconstructed Human Epidermis Test Method 439 (2019)
2) Nomura Y, Lee M, Fukui C, Watanabe K, Olsen D, Turley A, Morishita Y, Kawakami T, Yuba T, Fujimaki H, Inoue K, Yoshida M, Ogawa K, Haishima Y.: J Biomed Mater Res B Appl Biomater 106(8), 2807-2814 (2018)
3) Francis, N., Marzulli, H.L. edited: Dermatoxicology, 4th ed., Eye irritation (Robert B. Hackett, T. O. McDonald), pp.749-815, Hemisphere Publishing (1991)
4) McDonald, T.O., Shadduck, J.A.: Dermatoxicology and Pharmacology, pp.139, John Wiley & Sons, New York (1977)

6.14 Ocular simulation study with rabbit eyes for contact lenses

As a biocompatibility test of contact lenses, ocular simulation study with rabbit eyes are recommended. Generally, the test will be conducted in accordance with "ISO 9394: 1998, Ophthalmic optics-Contact lenses and contact lens care products-Determination of biocompatibility by ocular study using rabbit eyes" and the degree of irritation to the ocular tissue produced by the device under test be assessed by macroscopic findings and histopathological findings. Accordingly, it is not necessary to perform an eye irritation test using extracts when the device is a contact lens and the ocular simulation study has been performed.

7. Points changed from MHLW Notification, YAKUSHOKUKI-HATSU 0301 No. 20

1) At present, *in vivo* test evaluation is generally performed according to the ISO 10993-10, so detailed judgment methods have been described (Section 3.2.4.6 and section 4.4.6).

2) The *in vitro* skin irritation test of a medical device using a reconstructed human skin model has been adopted.

3) The body weight of rabbits used in the *in vivo* primary skin irritation test, intradermal reaction test and eye irritation test has been defined.

4) In the *in vivo* primary skin irritation test, ISO 10993-10 tests only healthy skin, so the abraded area has been deleted.

5) Individual animal weights and photograph of the test solution administration sites at initiation and completion of test have been exclude from list of Items to be included in the test report.

6) Basic principles for conducing irritation test have been added to the reference information.

7) Consistency has been assured for overall composition of the Guideline.

8. References cited

1) De Jong W.H, Hoffmann S, Lee M, Kandárovád H, Pellevoisine C, Haishima Y, Rollins B, Zdawzcyk A, Willoughby J, Bachelorj M, Schatzk T, Skoog S, Parker S, Sawyer A, Pescioo P, Fant K, Kim K-M, Kwon J.S, Gehrke H, Hofma-Hutherr H, Meloni M, Julius C, Briotet D, Letasiova S, Kato R, Miyajima A, Fonteyne L. De L, Videau C, Tornier C, Turley A, Christiano N, Coleman K.P.: Toxicology *In Vitro* 50, 439-449 (2018)

2) Kandárovád H, Bendovoa H, Letasiova S, Coleman K.P, De Jong W.H. Jirouá D.: Toxicology *In Vitro* 50, 433-438 (2018)

9. References

1) OECD No. 439: OECD Guidelines for the Testing of Chemicals. *In vitro* Skin Irritation: Reconstructed Human Epidermis Test Method 439 (2019)

2) Nomura Y, Lee M, Fukui C, Watanabe K, Olsen D, Turley A, Morishita Y, Kawakami T, Yuba T, Fujimaki H, Inoue K, Yoshida M, Ogawa K, Haishima Y.: J Biomed Mater Res B Appl Biomater 106(8), 2807-2814 (2018)

3) Francis, N., Marzulli, H.L. edited: Dermatoxicology, 4th ed., Eye irritation (Robert B. Hackett, T. O. McDonald), pp.749-815, Hemisphere Publishing (1991)

4) McDonald, T.O., Shadduck, J.A.: Dermatoxicology and Pharmacology, pp.139, John Wiley & Sons, New York (1977)

表 3 眼の刺激性反応結果の記載例

		試験液を点眼した眼（右眼）			対照液を点眼した眼（左眼）		
動物番号		2481	2482	2483	2481	2482	2483
開始時体重（kg）		2.96	3.31	2.99			
終了時体重（kg）		3.05	3.34	3.02			
点眼前	角膜混濁	0×0	0×0	0×0	0×0	0×0	0×0
	角膜新生血管	0	0	0	0	0	0
	角膜染色	0	0	0	0	0	0
	前房	0	0	0	0	0	0
	虹彩	0	0	0	0	0	0
	結膜充血	0	0	0	0	0	0
	結膜浮腫	0	0	0	0	0	0
	分泌物	0	0	0	0	0	0
点眼1時間後	角膜混濁	0×0	0×0	0×0	0×0	0×0	0×0
	角膜新生血管	0	0	0	0	0	0
	角膜染色	0	0	0	0	0	0
	前房	0	0	0	0	0	0
	虹彩	0	0	0	0	0	0
	結膜充血	0	0	0	0	0	0
	結膜浮腫	0	0	0	0	0	0
	分泌物	0	0	0	0	0	0
点眼24時間後	角膜混濁	0×0	0×0	0×0	0×0	0×0	0×0
	角膜新生血管	0	0	0	0	0	0
	角膜染色	0	0	0	0	0	0
	前房	0	0	0	0	0	0
	虹彩	0	0	0	0	0	0
	結膜充血	0	0	0	0	0	0
	結膜浮腫	0	0	0	0	0	0
	分泌物	0	0	0	0	0	0

Table 3 Results of eye irritation test (Example)

		Eyes instilled with a test solution (right eye)			Eyes instilled with a control solution (left eye)		
Animal No.		2481	2482	2483	2481	2482	2483
Body weight at initiation of the test (kg)		2.96	3.31	2.99			
Body weight at completion of the test (kg)		3.05	3.34	3.02			
Before instillation	Corneal opacity	0 × 0	0 × 0	0 × 0	0 × 0	0 × 0	0 × 0
	Corneal neovascularity	0	0	0	0	0	0
	Corneal staining	0	0	0	0	0	0
	Anterior chamber	0	0	0	0	0	0
	Iris	0	0	0	0	0	0
	Conjunctival hyperemia	0	0	0	0	0	0
	Chemosis	0	0	0	0	0	0
	Discharge	0	0	0	0	0	0
1 hour after instillation	Corneal opacity	0 × 0	0 × 0	0 × 0	0 × 0	0 × 0	0 × 0
	Corneal neovascularity	0	0	0	0	0	0
	Corneal staining	0	0	0	0	0	0
	Anterior chamber	0	0	0	0	0	0
	Iris	0	0	0	0	0	0
	Conjunctival hyperemia	0	0	0	0	0	0
	Chemosis	0	0	0	0	0	0
	Discharge	0	0	0	0	0	0
24 hour after instillation	Corneal opacity	0 × 0	0 × 0	0 × 0	0 × 0	0 × 0	0 × 0
	Corneal neovascularity	0	0	0	0	0	0
	Corneal staining	0	0	0	0	0	0
	Anterior chamber	0	0	0	0	0	0
	Iris	0	0	0	0	0	0
	Conjunctival hyperemia	0	0	0	0	0	0
	Chemosis	0	0	0	0	0	0
	Discharge	0	0	0	0	0	0

付表 1　ISO 10993-10 の眼病変の評点付けシステム

Ⅰ　角膜

不透明度：混濁の程度（最も混濁した領域を読み取る）

不透明度なし	0
虹彩を明視できる程度の散在からび慢性の不透明化	1*
容易に識別できる半透明，虹彩の細部がわずかにぼやけて見える	2*
真珠様，虹彩の細部が観察できないが，瞳孔の大きさはかろうじて識別できる	3*
不透明，虹彩が透視できない	4*

角膜損傷域

1/4 未満，0 ではない	0
1/4 以上，1/2 未満	1
1/2 以上，3/4 未満	2
3/4 以上，全域に及ぶまで	3

Ⅱ　虹彩

正常	0
皺襞形成亢進，充血，腫脹，角膜周囲の充血（いずれか 1 つ，あるいは全て，若しくは組合せ）が見られるが，対光反射は認められる（緩徐反応陽性）	1*
対光反射消失，出血，広範囲の破壊（いずれか 1 つ，あるいは全て）が見られる	2*

Ⅲ　結膜

A　発赤（角膜及び虹彩を除く眼瞼，眼球結膜）

正常	0
充血亢進	1
広範囲かつ深紅色となり，血管の識別困難	2*
全域の深紅色化	3*

B　結膜浮腫

正常	0
腫脹亢進（瞬膜を含む）	1
眼瞼の部分的外反を伴う明らかな腫脹	2*
1／2 程度の眼瞼閉鎖を伴う腫脹	3*
1／2 以上の眼瞼閉鎖を伴う腫脹	4*

C　分泌物

正常	0
常量以上の分泌物（正常な動物の内眥に見られる少量は含まない）	1
眼瞼及び眼瞼に接する被毛を湿潤	2
眼瞼及び眼の周囲を相当範囲湿潤	3

＊：刺激性陽性反応

Attachment 1   System for grading ocular lesions (ISO 10993-10)

1. Cornea

    Degree of opacity (most dense area)

No opacity	0
Scattered or diffuse area, details of iris clearly visible	1[*]
Easily discernible translucent areas, details of the iris slightly obscured	2[*]
Opalescent areas, no details of iris visible, size of pupil barely discernible	3[*]
Opaque, detail of iris not visible	4[*]

    Area of cornea involved

One-quarter (or less), not zero	0
Greater than one-quarter, but less than half	1
Greater than half, but less than three-quarters	2
Greater than three-quarters, up to whole area	3

2. Iris

Normal	0
Folds above normal, congestion swelling, circumcorneal injection (any or all or combination of these), iris still reacting to light (sluggish reaction is positive)	1[*]
No reaction to light, hemorrhage, gross destruction (any one or all of these)	2[*]

3. Conjunctiva

    Redness (refers to palpebral and bulbar conjunctiva excluding cornea and iris)

Vessels normal	0
Vessels definitely injected above normal	1
More diffuse, deeper crimson red, individual vessels not easily discernible	2[*]
Diffuse beefy red	3[*]

    Chemosis

No swelling	0
Any swelling above normal (includes nictitating membrane)	1
Obvious swelling with partial eversion of lids	2[*]
Swelling with lids about half-closed	3[*]
Swelling with lids about half-closed to completely closed	4[*]

    Discharge

No discharge	0
Any amount different from normal (dose not include small amounts observed in inner canthus of normal animals)	1
Discharge with moistening of the lids and hairs just adjacent to lids	2
Discharge with moistening of the lids and hairs, and considerable area around the eye	3

[*]Positive result.

付表2　Scale for Scoring Ocular Lesions-Slit Lamp（McDonald-Shadduck）

角膜
　　0 ＝正常．スリットランプでは，上皮及び内皮表面は明るいグレイに，実質は大理石様のグレイにみえる．
　　1 ＝わずかに透明性を失う．実質の前1/2程度が損傷している．下部構造は，わずかな曇りがあるが，散乱光ではっきりと見える．
　　2 ＝中程度に透明性を失う．曇りが内皮まで広がる．実質は均一な白色となる．下部構造は，散乱光ではっきりと見える．
　　3 ＝実質は全体が損傷しているが，内皮表面は見える．散乱光により，下部構造はわずかに見える．
　　4 ＝実質は全体が損傷し，内皮表面は見えない．散乱光でも，下部構造も見えない．

角膜不透明度
　　0 ＝混濁のない正常な角膜．
　　1 ＝ 1〜25 ％の実質混濁．
　　2 ＝ 26〜50 ％の実質混濁．
　　3 ＝ 51〜75 ％の実質混濁．
　　4 ＝ 76〜100 ％の実質混濁．

角膜血管新生
　　0 ＝血管新生なし．
　　1 ＝血管新生は存在するが，血管は角膜周辺部以内に侵入せず，侵入部位は限られている．
　　2 ＝血管が2 mm 又はそれ以上にあらゆる方向から角膜内に侵入する．

角膜染色
　　0 ＝フルオレセイン染色なし．
　　1 ＝わずかな範囲に限られたかすかなフルオレセイン染色．散乱光による下部構造の観察は容易である．
　　2 ＝わずかな範囲に限られた中程度のフルオレセイン染色．散乱光による下部構造の観察では，細部がはっきりと判らない．
　　3 ＝著しいフルオレセイン染色．染色が角膜の広い範囲に及ぶ．散乱光による下部構造の観察は，全く見えないことはないが困難である．
　　4 ＝著しいフルオレセイン染色．散乱光による下部構造の観察は，不可能．

前房
　　0 ＝前房内に光の乱反射を認めない．
　　1 ＝チンダル現象をわずかに認める．前房内の光は，水晶体を通過した光より弱い．
　　2 ＝チンダル現象を明らかに認める．前房内の光は，水晶体を通過した光と同程度である．
　　3 ＝チンダル現象を明らかに認める．前房内の光は，水晶体を通過した光より強い．

虹彩
　　0 ＝充血のない正常な虹彩．時々，12時から1時及び6時から7時方向の瞳孔縁に直径1〜3 mm のかすかに充血した部位が存在する．
　　1 ＝ 2次血管がわずかに充血しているが，3次血管は充血していない．
　　2 ＝ 2次血管が中程度に充血し，3次血管がわずかに充血している．
　　3 ＝虹彩実質のわずかな腫脹を伴う，2次及び3次血管の中程度の充血．
　　4 ＝虹彩実質の著しい腫脹を伴う，2次及び3次血管の著しい充血．

結膜充血
　　0 ＝正常．
　　1 ＝ 4〜7時及び11〜1時の部分に限られたリンバス周辺部の充血を伴う眼瞼結膜の紅赤色．
　　2 ＝ 75 ％程度のリンバス周辺部の充血を伴う眼瞼結膜の赤色．
　　3 ＝明白なリンバス周辺部の充血と，結膜の点状出血を伴った暗赤色の眼瞼，眼球結膜充血．

結膜浮腫
　　0 ＝正常．
　　1 ＝眼瞼の外反のない腫脹．
　　2 ＝上眼瞼の部分的外反を伴った腫脹．
　　3 ＝上下眼瞼の同程度の部分的外反を伴った腫脹．
　　4 ＝下眼瞼の部分的外反と上眼瞼の著しい外反を伴った腫脹．

分泌物
　　0 ＝正常．
　　1 ＝常量より多く眼内に存在するが，眼瞼や被毛には存在しない．
　　2 ＝豊富で容易に見られ，眼瞼や眼瞼周囲の被毛に付着する．
　　3 ＝眼瞼周囲の被毛を十分に湿らし，眼瞼より流出する．

Attachment 2   Scale for Scoring Ocular Lesions–Slit Lamp (McDonald–Shadduck)

Cornea
    0 = Normal, the epithelial or endothelial surfaces looks light–gray lamp and the parenchyma marble gray
    1 = Lose clarity slightly, Anterior 1/2 portion of the parenchyma injured, substructure slightly cloudy, but clearly visible with scattering light
    2 = Lose clarity slightly, Anterior 1/2 portion of the parenchyma injured, substructure slightly cloudy, but clearly visible with scattering light
    3 = The parenchyma overall injured but the endothelium visible, substructure slightly visible with scattering light
    4 = The parenchyma overall injured and the endothelium not visible, substructure invisible with scattering light

Corneal opacity
    0 = Normal cornea with no opacity
    1 = 1 to 25 % cloudiness of the parenchyma
    2 = 26 to 50 % cloudiness of the parenchyma
    3 = 51 to 75 % cloudiness of the parenchyma
    4 = 76 to 100 % cloudiness of the parenchyma

Corneal angiogenesis
    0 = No angiogenesis
    1 = Angiogenesis exists but vessels not invading within circumcorneal region and invaded area light
    2 = Vessels invading into cornea from various directions 2 mm or over

Corneal staining
    0 = No fluorescein staining
    1 = Slight fluorescein staining in limited area, easy to observe substructure with scattering light
    2 = Moderate fluorescein staining in limited area, details of substructure not clear scattering light
    3 = Marked fluorescein staining substructure is barely visible, but difficult to observe
    4 = Marked fluorescein stain, impossible to observe substructure with scattering light

Anterior chamber
    0 = No diffusion of light noted in the anterior chamber
    1 = Tyndall phenomenon slightly noted, light within an anterior chamber is weaker than that the transmitted light through a crystalline lens
    2 = Tyndall phenomenon clearly noted, light within an anterior chamber is equivalent to the transmitted light through a crystalline lens
    3 = Tyndall phenomenon clearly noted, light within an anterior chamber is stronger than the light transmitted through a crystalline lens

Iris
    0 = Iris with no congestion, occasionally mydriasis noted at the direction of 12:00 to 01:00 and 06:00 to 07:00, 1 to 3 mm diameter slight congestion noted at the margin
    1 = Secondary vessels slightly congested but tertiary vessels not congested
    2 = Secondary vessels moderately congested and tertiary vessels slightly congested
    3 = Moderate congestion of secondary and tertiary vessels with slight swelling of the iris parenchyma
    4 = Marked congestion of secondary and tertiary vessels with marked swelling of the iris parenchyma

Conjunctival congestion
    0 = Normal
    1 = Reddening of eyelids and conjunctiva with limited congestion around limbus in the direction of 04:00 to 07:00 and 11:00 to 01:00
    2 = Reddening of eyelids and conjunctiva with approximately 75 % of congestion around limbus
    3 = Dark–red eyelids accompanied by clear congestion around limbus and petechial hemorrhage of congestion, congestion of bulbar conjunctiva

Chamosis
    0 = Normal
    1 = Swelling with no palpebral valgus
    2 = Swelling with partial valgus of upper eyelid
    3 = Swelling with partial valgus of lower and upper eyelids int the same level
    4 = Swelling with partial valgus of lower eyelid and marked valgus of upper eyelid

Discharge
    0 = Normal
    1 = Amount of discharge is more than normal in the eye but none on eyelids and eyelashes
    2 = Abundant amount of discharge attaching to the eyelids and eyelashes
    3 = Moisturizing the eyelids and eyelashes and flows from the eyelids

第6部　全身毒性試験

1．適用範囲

　本ガイダンスは，医療機器又は原材料の全身毒性を評価するためのものである．実施に当たっては動物福祉への配慮が必要である．試験液の刺激性，腐食性が強いことが推定され，投与により試験動物に著しい苦痛を与える可能性が考えられる場合などには，その旨を報告し，試験条件の変更あるいは全身毒性試験に代わる方法がないかを検討すべきである．また著しい苦痛に耐えている兆候が試験動物に確認された場合，直ちに安楽死を検討する必要がある．

2．引用規格

　ISO 10993-11: 2017, Biological evaluation of medical devices-Part 11: Tests for systemic toxicity

3．用語及び定義

　引用規格に記載されている以下の定義を用いる．

3.1　急性全身毒性

　試験検体の単回，又は継続的ばく露後24時間以内に生じる毒性作用．

3.2　亜急性全身毒性

　試験検体の反復又は継続的ばく露後24時間以降，28日間までの時期に生じる毒性作用．

　　注：この毒性の評価のために行われる反復投与による全身毒性試験の投与期間は，最も一般的な国際的ガイドラインでは14日～28日間とされている．一方，静脈内投与による亜急性全身毒性試験の投与期間は，一般的に24時間より長く14日間より短いとされている．

3.3　亜慢性全身毒性

　寿命の一部の期間，試験検体を反復又は継続的にばく露することにより生じる毒性作用．

　　注：亜慢性全身毒性試験は，通常，げっ歯類では90日間，他の動物種では寿命の10％を超えない期間で行われる．一方，静脈内投与による亜慢性全身毒性試験の投与期間は，14日間から28日間とされている．

3.4　慢性全身毒性

　寿命の過半の期間（通常，寿命の10％を超える期間）にわたり，試験検体を反復又は継続的にばく露することにより生じる毒性作用．

　　注：慢性全身毒性試験は，通常，6～12ヶ月間の期間で実施される．

Part 6   Tests for systemic toxicity

1.   Scope

These test methods are intended to evaluate systemic toxicity of medical devices or raw materials. Procedures should be designed to avoid animal welfare problems. If the test solution is strongly irritating or corrosive and administration causes marked pain in test animals, report as such and consider modifying test conditions or an alternative to systemic toxicity testing. In addition, if a test animal shows any sign that it is in severe pain, euthanasia needs to be considered without delay.

2.   Normative reference

ISO 10993-11: 2017, Biological evaluation of medical devices-Part 11: Tests for systemic toxicity

3.   Terms and definitions

The terms and definitions given in the normative reference apply.

3.1   Acute systemic toxicity

Adverse effects occurring at any time within 24 hours after single or continual administration of a test sample.

3.2   Subacute systemic toxicity

Adverse effects occurring after multiple or continual administration of a test sample between 24 hours and 28 days.

> Note: The selection of time intervals of between 14 days and 28 days for the multiple exposure in this subacute systemic study is consistent with most international regulatory guidelines. Subacute intravenous studies are generally defined as treatment durations of more than 24 hours but not more than 14 days.

3.3   Subchronic systemic toxicity

Adverse effects occurring after the repeated or continual administration of a test sample for a part of the lifespan.

> Note: Subchronic toxicity studies are usually 90 days in rodents but not exceeding 10 % of the lifespan of other species. Subchronic intravenous studies are generally defined as treatment durations of 14 days to 28 days for rodents or non-rodents.

3.4   Chronic systemic toxicity

Adverse effects occurring after the repeated or continual administration of a test sample for a major part of the life span (period exceeding 10 % of the lifespan in general).

> Note: Chronic toxicity studies usually have a duration of 6 months to 12 months.

4．急性全身毒性試験

4.1　目的

　本試験は，試験試料（最終製品又は原材料）から抽出した抽出液（以下「試験液」とする．）中に，急性全身毒性を有する物質が存在しないことを確認するための試験である．

4.2　試験の要約

　本ガイダンスに示す試験法は，基本的に引用規格に基づくものである．試験試料から生理食塩液又は植物油を用いて抽出した試験液を，1群5匹のマウスに対し，それぞれ静脈内投与（生理食塩液抽出液）又は腹腔内投与（植物油抽出液）する．投与72時間経過後まで観察し（6.2項参照），対照液投与群と比較して，急性全身毒性の有無を評価する．本試験法は，米国薬局方[1]などで医薬品容器の毒性試験として古くから用いられてきた，いわゆる pharmacopoeia-type の試験である．

4.3　試験液の調製

4.3.1　抽出溶媒

　抽出には，生理食塩液（日局又は同等品），植物油（綿実油，ゴマ油など，日局又は同等品）を用いる．対象となる医療機器の臨床適用条件がこれらの溶媒の性質と大きく異なるなど，リスク評価のためにより適切な溶媒を選定する必要がある場合には ISO 10993-12 を参考にするとよい．

4.3.2　抽出溶媒と試験試料量の比

　原則として，付録の1項又は ISO 10993-12 の規定に従うものとする．

4.3.3　抽出条件

　原則として，付録の2項又は ISO 10993-12 の規定に従うものとする．

4.3.4　操作方法

　抽出後，直ちに室温（25℃前後を下回らないよう）まで冷却し，振とうする．ISO 10993-12 に従い，抽出中に攪拌又は循環を実施した場合には，抽出後の振とう操作は行わなくてもよい．次いで容器の内容液を無菌的に別の乾燥した滅菌容器に回収し，25℃前後で保存し，24時間以内に試験に用いる．

4.3.5　対照液の調製

　対照液は，抽出溶媒単独（試験試料を加えない）で，試験液調製と同一の条件で加熱処理し調製する．

4.4　試験法

4.4.1　試験動物

　体重17〜25gの健康なマウスで，1週間程度馴化後，体重の減少をみなかったものを試験動物として使用する．雌雄どちらを用いてもよいが，試験液投与群と対照液投与

4.   Acute systemic toxicity

4.1   Objectives

This test method is intended to confirm absence of a substance exhibiting acute systemic toxicity in the extract from the test sample (final products or raw materials) (hereinafter referred to as "test solutions").

4.2   Summary of the test

The test method described in this Part is based on the normative reference. The test solutions prepared with physiological saline or vegetable oil are administered intravenously (physiological saline extract) or intraperitoneally (vegetable oil extract) in 5 mice per group. The animals are observed up to 72 hours after administration (see Section 6.2) and acute systemic toxicity is evaluated by comparison with the control group. This test method is a so-called pharmacopoeia-type test that has been conducted for long time as a toxicity test for containers of pharmaceutical products in US Pharmacopoeia[1], etc.

4.3   Preparation of test solutions

4.3.1   Extraction solvents

Use physiological saline (JP or equivalent) and vegetable oils (cotton seed oil, sesame oil, etc. [JP or equivalent]) for extraction. If a more suitable solvent is needed for risk assessment in a case where clinical application conditions of the medical device in question are greatly different from the properties of these solvents, ISO 10993-12 may be used as a reference.

4.3.2   Proportion of extraction solvent and test sample

In principle, follow the rules in Section 1 of the Attachment of this guidance or ISO 10993-12.

4.3.3   Extracting conditions

In principle, follow the rules in Section 2 of the Attachment of this guidance or ISO 10993-12.

4.3.4   Operating procedures

After extraction, cool the solution immediately to room temperature (not below about 25 ℃) and shake. When it is agitated or circulated during extraction in accordance with ISO 10993-12, the resultant extract does not need to be shaken. Then, collect the extraction solution in the container aseptically into another dry sterilized container. Obtained test solution is stored at around 25 ℃ and use in the test within 24 hours.

4.3.5   Preparation of control solutions

Use the solutions prepared from the extraction solvent alone (without addition of the test sample) by heating under the same conditions as in the preparation of the test solutions as the control solution.

4.4   Test methods

4.4.1   Test animals

Use healthy mice, each weighing 17 to 25 g, which have not lost body weight during the acclimatization period of about one week. Either male or female animals are used as long

群を構成する動物の性は同一とする．想定される医療機器が，いずれかの性に用いられるものである場合，試験動物の性別はその性を選択することが望ましい．雌動物を使用する場合は妊娠していない未経産の動物を用いる．

4.4.2　投与液量

試験液の投与液量は，原則として，体重1kg当たり50mLとする（6.3項参照）．

4.4.3　投与経路

生理食塩液抽出液及び生理食塩液対照液は静脈内投与とし，植物油抽出液及び植物油対照液は腹腔内投与とする．

4.4.4　観察及び測定項目

一般状態観察：全例について投与直後，4時間後，その後は投与から24時間，48時間，72時間経過後に行う．一般状態は，引用規格のAnnex Cの指標などを参考に観察し記録する．死亡例が認められた場合，直ちに剖検する．毒性兆候が発現した場合に，この消長を確かめるため観察期間を延長したり，観察頻度を増やすことが推奨される．

体重測定：全例について投与前，投与から24時間，同48時間，同72時間経過後に測定する（6.4項参照）．

病理解剖：観察期間終了後，全例について，投与部位，心臓，肺，消化管，肝臓，脾臓，腎臓，及び生殖器を含む主要臓器を肉眼的に観察する．

血液検査・尿検査・病理組織学的検査：血液学並びに血液生化学検査，病理組織学的検査は臓器・組織における毒性作用の内容，強さを精査するために実施される（6.6項参照）．病理解剖によって異常所見が認められた場合には，これらの検査の実施を考慮するとよい．また尿検査は，影響が予測される場合に実施を考慮するとよい（表2参照）．

4.4.5　判定方法

観察期間を通して，試験液投与群の全例に，対照液投与群の動物と比較して強い生物学的反応が認められない場合に急性全身毒性はないと判定する．

試験液投与群の動物が2匹以上死亡した場合，あるいは2匹以上の動物で痙攣や衰弱など著しい毒性症状を示した場合や，体重減少が認められ，最終体重が投与時体重の10％を超える減少動物が3匹以上の場合は急性全身毒性ありと判定する．

試験液投与群のいずれかの動物が，対照液投与群の動物と比較してわずかな生物学的反応を示した場合，あるいは1匹の動物だけが強い生物学的反応又は死亡が認められた場合には，試験液投与群及び対照液投与群の例数を各々10匹にして再試験を実施する．

再試験を実施した結果，試験液投与群の動物が対照液投与群と比較し，全観察期間を通して，科学的に有意な生物学的反応を示さなかった場合，急性全身毒性はないと判定

as the animals in the test group and control group are the same sex. When the concerned medical device is intended for use in only one sex, it is preferred to perform the test for that sex. If female animals are used, they shall be nulliparous and non-pregnant.

4.4.2 Dosing volume
Generally, the dosing volume of the test solution is 50 mL per kg body weight (see Section 6.3).

4.4.3 Route of administration
Use the physiological saline extract and the physiological saline control for intravenous administration and the vegetable oil extract and the vegetable oil control for intraperitoneal administration.

4.4.4 Observation and parameters
Observation of general conditions:
Observe all animals immediately after administration, and 4, 24, 48 and 72 hours after administration. Observe and record general conditions by referring to the indices in Annex C of the normative reference. Perform autopsy immediately for dead animals, if any. When signs of toxicity are found, it is recommended to extend the observation period or increase the frequency of observation to confirm appearing and disappearing of observations trend

Body weight measurement:
Measure the body weight of all animals before administration and 24, 48 and 72 hours after administration (see Section 6.4).

Pathological dissection:
After completion of the observation period, observe major organs of all animals macroscopically including the administration site, heart, lungs, gastrointestinal tract, liver, spleen, kidneys and reproductive organs.

Haematology and clinical chemistry, urinalysis and histopathology:
If needed, perform haematology and clinical chemistry and histopathological examination to investigate details and intensity of toxic effects in the organs and tissues (see Section 6.6). If abnormal findings are obtained by the pathological dissection, consider to perform these examinations. Consider to perform urinalysis when scientifically indicated (see Table 2).

4.4.5 Evaluation methods
Acute systemic toxicity is judged as absent when there is no severe biological reaction in all animals of the test group compared to those of the control group across the entire observation period.

Acute systemic toxicity is judged as present when 2 or more animals in the test group have died, when marked toxic symptoms such as convulsions or general weakness have been observed in 2 or more animals, or in 3 or more animals decreased the final body weight by more than 10 %when compared to the body weight measured at the time of administration. Conduct a re-test in 10 animals each in the test and control groups when the animals in the test groups showed slight biological reactions compared to the control animals, or only 1 animal showed severe biological reaction or died.

Acute systemic toxicity is judged as absent when no scientifically significant biological reaction is found in the test animals compared to those in the control group across the entire

する．

4.5　試験報告書

　　試験報告書には，少なくとも以下の事項を記載する．
1)　試験実施機関及び試験責任者
2)　試験実施期間
3)　試験試料（最終製品又は原材料）を特定する要素
　　（例：医療機器の名称，製造販売業者名，製造番号，材料，滅菌方法，形状，物理学的特性など）
4)　用いた媒体（抽出溶媒）など，試験液の調製方法
5)　試験に用いた動物
6)　試験条件
7)　試験結果
　　表：一般状態，死亡率（必要に応じて），体重集計，病理組織学的検査集計
　　写真：病理解剖学的検査（毒性学上問題と考えられる所見が認められた場合のみ）
8)　結果の評価と考察
9)　参考文献

5．反復投与による全身毒性試験（亜急性・亜慢性・慢性全身毒性試験）

5.1　目的

　　本試験は，試験試料（最終製品又は原材料）から抽出した抽出液（以下「試験液」とする．）中に，亜急性（亜慢性）全身毒性を有する物質が存在しないことを確認するための試験である．本ガイダンスに示した試験法は，引用規格に基づいたものである．全身毒性を検出するための投与方法や評価（検査・観察）項目は，引用規格の Annex A，B，C，D，E，F 及び H などを参考に，試験試料の種類や想定される医療機器の種類を勘案して，試験計画にあたり個々に検討すべきである．

5.2　試験の要約

　　試験試料から生理食塩液を用いて抽出した試験液を，雌雄のラットの静脈内に 14 日間（亜慢性全身毒性試験の場合は 14〜28 日間，慢性毒性試験の場合はそれ以上の期間）反復投与し，対照液投与群との間で毒性を比較して評価を行う．1 群の動物数は亜急性全身毒性試験の場合は雌雄各 5 匹とし，亜慢性，慢性全身毒性試験の場合は試験期間中の動物の死亡の可能性などを考慮して動物数を増やす（表 1 参照）．技術的に可能であり，想定される医療機器の適用経路としても適切であるならば，埋植試験又は血液適合性試験と一体化させてもよい（6.5 項参照）．また医療機器として臨床で用いられる期間・形態に合わせた投与期間及び評価期間が求められるが，その必要性については，実施した全身毒性試験結果及び試験試料の構成材料・成分などに関する既知の成績などを検証し，科学的に判断すべきである．

observation period as a result of the re-test.

4.5   Test report

The test report shall include at least the following details:

1) Name of the testing facility and study director
2) Test period
3) Elements to identify test samples (final products or raw materials)
   (e.g., name of the medical device, manufacturer'sname, manufacturing number, materials, sterilization process, shape, physical properties, etc.)
4) Method employed in preparing the test solutions such as the vehicle (extraction solvent)
5) Test animals
6) Test conditions
7) Test results
   Tables: Data may be summarized in tabular form, observations of general conditions, mortality rate (if required), body weights and pathological examination
   Photographs: Photograph given pathological observations (only when toxicologically significant findings are obtained)
8) Interpretation of results and discussion
9) References

5.   Repeated exposure systemic toxicity (subacute, subchronic and chronic systemic toxicity)

5.1   Objectives

These test methods are intended to confirm absence of a substance exhibiting subacute (subchronic) systemic toxicity in the extract from the test sample (final products or raw materials) (hereinafter referred to as "test solution"). These test methods described in this Part are based on the normative reference. The administration method and evaluation (examination and observation) parameters to detect systemic toxicity should be discussed individually in planning the test by referring to Annexes A, B, C, D, E, F and H of the normative reference and in consideration of the types of the test sample or the intended medical device.

5.2   Summary of test

The physiological saline extract is administered intravenously in male and female rats for 14 continual days (14 to 28 days in a subchronic systemic toxicity test and a longer period in a chronic toxicity test) and toxicity is evaluated by comparison with the control. Five male and 5 female animals are used per group in the subacute systemic toxicity test while the number of animals is increased in the subchronic or chronic systemic toxicity test taking possible deaths of animals during the test period into consideration (see Table 1). The test may be integrated with the implantation test or the hemocompatibility test if it is technically possible and is appropriate as the planned route of application of the medical device (see Section 6.5). While it is required to set the administration period and evaluation period corresponding to the period and form of clinical application as a medical device, their setting should be decided scientifically through verification of systemic toxicity results conducted and known results relating to the constituting materials and ingredients of the test sample.

5.3　試験液の調製

抽出溶媒には，生理食塩液（日局又は同等品）を用いることとし，その他の条件は4.3項に従う．

5.4　試験法

5.4.1　試験動物

原則としてラットを用いるが，全身毒性試験の動物として適切であるならば，他の動物種を用いてもよい．また基本的に雌雄の動物について試験を行い，片性で行う場合は一用量当たりの動物数を増やす．動物数は表1を参考とする．投与開始時の体重の幅は平均体重の±20％以内とする．

表1　1群当たりの最小動物数（推奨）

	げっ歯類	非げっ歯類
急性全身毒性試験[a]	5	3
亜急性全身毒性試験	10（雌雄各5）[a]	6（雌雄各3）[a]
亜慢性全身毒性試験	20（雌雄各10）[a]	8（雌雄各4）[a]
慢性全身毒性試験	30（雌雄各15）[b, c]	[c]

a　雌雄いずれかの性で試験を実施してもよい．その医療機器がいずれかの性に臨床適用されるものならば，試験はその性の動物で実施するのがよい．
b　一つの用量群で構成される試験において推奨される動物数．過剰投与の用量群を追加する場合には，各用量群当たり雌雄各10匹まで減らしてもよい．
c　試験動物数は，その試験が意義あるデータを提供するための必要最低限の数とする．動物評価期間の終了時に，試験結果の統計学的評価に充分な数の動物が残るよう設定しなければならない．

5.4.2　投与液量

ラット静脈内反復投与による試験の場合，試験液の投与液量は，原則として，試験動物の体重1kg当たり20mLとする．他の動物及び他の投与経路を選択する場合は，引用規格のAnnex Bを参考にする．この場合，投与液量は，想定される医療機器によるばく露量から充分に安全率を見込んだものである必要がある（6.7項参照）．

5.4.3　投与経路及び投与期間

静脈内投与が汎用されるが，想定される医療機器の適用経路を勘案して決定することが望ましい．標準的投与期間は，亜急性全身毒性試験では3.2項に，亜慢性全身毒性試験では3.3項に，慢性全身毒性試験では3.4項にそれぞれ従うものとする（6.8項参照）．

5.4.4　観察及び測定項目

表2と，引用規格のAnnex C，D及びEなどを参考に設定する．尿検査及び眼科的検査は定型的に行う必要はないが，他の検査結果や文献情報などから毒性が示唆される場合には実施することが望ましい．

5.3   Preparation of test solution

Use physiological saline (JP or equivalent) as an extraction solvent and follow Section 4.3 for other conditions.

5.4   Test methods

5.4.1   Test animals

Generally, rats are used but other animal species may be used if they are appropriate as the test animals for systemic toxicity. Perform the test basically in male and female animals. If the test is conducted in either sex, increase the number of animals per dose level. Refer to Table 1 for the number of animals. The body weight range at the start of administration should be within ± 20 % of the mean body weight.

Table 1   Recommended minimum group sizes

	Rodent	Non-rodent
Acute[a]	5	3
Subacute	10 (5 per sex)[a]	6 (3 per sex)[a]
Subchronic	20 (10 per sex)[a]	8 (4 per sex)[a]
Chronic	30 (15 per sex)[b, c]	[c]

a   Testing in a single sex is acceptable. When a device is intended for use in only one sex, testing should be done in that sex.
b   The recommendation for rodents refers to one dose-level group testing. Where additional exaggerated dose groups are included the recommended group size may be reduced to 10 per sex.
c   The number of animals tested should be based on the minimum required to provide meaningful data. Enough animals shall remain at the termination of the study to ensure proper statistical evaluation of the results.

5.4.2   Dosing volume

Generally, the dosing volume of the test solution is 20 mL per kg body weight in the test by repeated intravenous administration in rats. Refer to Annex B of the normative reference if other animals and/or other routes of administration are selected. In the latter case, the dosing volume should be determined with adequate safety margin considering the amount of exposure expected by the medical device (see Section 6.7).

5.4.3   Route and duration of administration

While the intravenous administration is frequently used, it is advised to decide the route of administration in consideration of the planned route of application of the medical device. The standard administration period should be set based on Sections 3.2, 3.3 and 3.4 for subacute systemic toxicity, subchronic systemic toxicity and chronic systemic toxicity, respectively (see Section 6.8).

5.4.4   Observations and parameters

Set observations and parameters by referring to Table 2 of this guidance and Annexes C, D and E of the normative reference. Routine urinalysis and ophthalmologic examination are not necessary. However, they should be carried out when toxicities about these parameters are suggested by the results from other examinations, literature information, etc.

表 2　全身毒性試験の観察項目

評価項目	急性全身毒性	亜急性全身毒性 / 亜慢性全身毒性	慢性全身毒性[a]
体重変化	要	要	要
一般症状観察	要	要	要
血液検査・尿検査	b	a, b	要
病理解剖学的検査	要	要	要
臓器重量	b	要	要
病理組織学的検査	b	a, b, c	要, c

a　慢性全身毒性試験は，通常，亜慢性全身毒性試験の期間延長であり，その期間は臨床ばく露期間を根拠に設定する．評価項目はできる限り共通化する．測定を行う目的のためにサテライト群を設けることが必要となって，一群当たりの動物数が増えることもあり得る．
b　臨床症状が認められた場合や，当該試験より長期の試験が予定されていない場合には，ここに挙げた項目の評価も考慮するとよい．推奨される測定項目は，引用規格 Annex D，E 及び F に示されている．
c　試験液を投与する群を複数設定した試験の場合，全臓器に関する病理組織学的検査は，まず対照群と最高用量群について実施し，より低い投与量群に対しては肺及び影響が認められた臓器についてのみの実施でもよい．

5.5　試験報告書

　4.5 項参照．ただし，ここでは，7) 試験結果については，表として，一般状態，死亡率（必要に応じて），平均体重集計，血液検査集計，病理検査集計を，写真としては，病理解剖学的検査（毒性学上特に問題と考えられる所見が認められた場合のみ）及び病理組織学的検査（毒性学上特に問題と考えられる所見が認められた場合のみ）を含むこと．

6．参考情報
6.1　動物福祉

　ISO 10993-2 及び動物福祉に関する国内規制を参照し，試験の開始から実験の終了まで動物福祉に配慮した全身毒性試験の実施が求められる．試験液の pH，浸透圧などの物理化学的性状は試験計画時に充分に考慮すべき要因である．試験液の刺激性，腐食性が強く，投与にあたり試験動物に著しい苦痛を与える可能性が考えられる場合などには，その試験液を用いて全身毒性試験を実施してはならない．6.9 項に示す試験液調製法の工夫や，ICCVAM や ECVAM による動物実験代替法（細胞毒性試験）の成績から全身毒性を評価する．

6.2　急性全身毒性試験の観察期間

　急性全身毒性試験の観察期間は，標準的には投与後 72 時間までとする．ただし，試験試料の特性や試験中の動物の状態に応じて，観察期間を延長してもよい．この場合，観察期間を通じて一般状態は毎日観察し，体重は 1 週間に 1 回以上，並びに投与最終日と病理解剖実施日に測定する．

Table 2   Summary of observations

Evaluation item	Acute	Subacute/subchronic	Chronic[a]
Body weight	+	+	+
Clinical observations	+	+	+
Haematology and clinical chemistry/ urinalysis	b	a, b	+
Gross pathologicalexamination	+	+	+
Organ weights	b	+	+
Histopathology	b	a, b, c	+, c

+   Data should be provided.

a   Chronic systemic toxicity testing is generally the test elongated the test period of subacute/subchronic testing, justified by the human exposure period. Parameters should be standardized between the test as much as possible. The number of animals per group may be increased to include satellite groups for the purpose of measurement.

b   Consideration should be given to these measurements when clinically indicated or if longer exposure testing is not anticipated. Lists of suggested parameters are included in Annex D, Annex E and Annex F of the normative reference.

c   In a test where there are multiple dose groups, perform histopathology of all organs first for the control and highest dose group. For animals treated with lower doses, histopathological examinations may be performed only on the lungs and the organs in which toxic effects have been observed.

5.5   Test report

See Section 4.5. However, Item 7) Test results include tables of clinical observations, moratlity rate (if required), mean body weights, haematology and clinical chemistry and photographs of gross and histo-pathological changes (only when toxicologically significant finding is noted).

6.   Reference information

6.1   Animal welfare

Systemic toxicity tests need to be performed with consideration to animal welfare from the initiation of the test to the completion of animal experimentation by referring to ISO 10993 -2 and domestic regulations on animal welfare. Physical and chemical properties of the test solution including the pH and osmotic pressure are the factors thoroughly investigated in planning the test. A systemic toxicity test with the test solution, strongly irritating and/or corrosive, and its administration could cause marked pain in test animals is prohibited. Systemic toxicity shall be evaluated based on the results being obtained through adjusting test solution preparation methods as described in Section 6.9 or by alternative methods for animal testing (*in vitro* cytotoxicity test) validated by the Interagency Coordinating Committee on the Validation of Alternative Methods (ICCVAM) and the European Centre for the Validation of Alternative Methods (ECVAM).

6.2   Observation period in acute systemic toxicity test

The standard observation period in an acute systemic toxicity test is 72 hours after administration. However, it may be extended depending on the characteristics of the test sample or conditions of animals during the test. In this case, clinical observations should be performed every day through the observation period and the body weight be measured at once a week or more as well as on the days of last administration and pathological dissection.

6.3　急性全身毒性試験の投与液量及び投与速度

　　急性全身毒性試験の投与液量は，充分な実績を持つ米国薬局方[1]及び ASTM Standard F 750-87[2] に採用されている量を標準とした．毒性検出の目的から判断すると，投与液量を大きくすることが望ましいが，一時的な循環血液量の増大と血液希釈による試験動物への影響や動物福祉の観点から，充分に考慮すべき試験条件の一つである[3]．原則として，試験動物の体重 1 kg 当たり試験液，対照液とも，マウスの静脈内及び腹腔内投与にあっては 50 mL，ラットの場合は，静脈内投与 40 mL，腹腔内投与では 20 mL とする（引用規格 Annex B 参照）が，試験試料の臨床適用形態などにより，充分な安全係数を確保した投与液量を一回で投与する事が不可能な場合には，24 時間を超えない期間で分割して投与してもよい．投与経路や投与液量，投与の間隔を変更する場合，その科学的根拠を示すことが必要である．また急性全身毒性試験の投与速度は特に静脈内投与において試験成績に影響を与える因子の 1 つである．引用規格 4.8.2 項に従い，静脈内投与に当たっては，投与速度は 1 分間につき 2 mL を超えないものとする．なお，引用規格 Annex B に従い，投与速度は 1 分間につき 1 mL を超えないことが望ましく，投与時には投与速度が速すぎることによる影響が表れないよう充分に注意して投与を行う．

6.4　急性全身毒性の評価について

　　体重変化は全身毒性評価の重要な目安となる．米国薬局方[1]のマウスを用いた急性全身毒性試験の基準では，5 匹中 3 匹以上の動物に 2 g 以上の体重減少を認めた場合，不適合（全身毒性有り）と判定する規定がある．OLAW ガイダンス[4]では，著しい毒性症状とは，痙攣や衰弱，継続的な背臥や側臥，明確な呼吸困難，ラ音呼吸，4〜6 ℃以上の体温低下を挙げている．動物福祉[5]の面から，これらの症状を最低限の humane endpoints と考え，該当する動物は安楽死させるなどの対応が望ましい．

6.5　埋植試験の利用

　　「5. 反復投与による全身毒性試験（亜急性・亜慢性・慢性全身毒性試験）」には試験液の投与による亜急性全身毒性試験の方法を示したが，適当な動物（ラット以外の試験動物でもよい）に試験試料の埋植が可能な場合で，かつ，本ガイダンスに挙げた評価項目が適切に評価された 3.2〜3.4 項記載の期間の埋植試験の結果を亜急性 / 亜慢性 / 慢性全身毒性試験の結果として用いることができる．吸収性の試験試料による亜急性，亜慢性，慢性全身毒性を埋植によって評価する場合で，極めて速やかな吸収が想定される場合には，埋植のための手術による局所の反応が終息し，試験試料による生体への影響が評価可能となった段階で速やかに剖検を行い，評価を実施する．試験試料全量が吸収されると想定される期間と，投与期間の関係については根拠を示して考察する必要がある．

6.6　急性全身毒性試験の試験動物及び代替

　　急性全身毒性試験で血液・血液生化学検査を行う場合には，ラットを用いるとよい．

6.3   Dosing volume and rate of injection in the acute systemic toxicity test

The dosing volume adopted in the two traditional authoritative regulations, US Pharmacopoeia[1] and ASTM Standard F 750-87[2] has been determined as the standard dosing volume in an acute systemic toxicity test. While a large dosing volume is preferred considering from the objective of detecting toxicity, from the standpoints of animal welfare[3], it is one of the important test conditions to be thoroughly considered during protocol plannning in terms of the effects of temporary increase in circulating blood volume and blood dilution on the test animals. Generally, the dosing volume per kg body weight of mouse is 50 mL for both the test solutions and control solutions by intravenous and intraperitoneal administrations, and 40 mL by intravenous administration and 20 mL by intraperitoneal administration in rats (see Annex B of the normative reference). However, the dosing volumes may be administered in divided doses within a period of 24 hours if it is difficult to administer the dosing volume with an adequate safety margin in one dose depending on the form of clinical use of the test sample. Any change in the route of administration, dosing volume, or dosing frequency should be rationalized scientifically. The rate of injection in an acute systemic toxicity test is one of the factors affecting the test results particularly by the intravenous administration. As described in Section 4.8.2 of the normative reference, the rate shall not exceed 2 mL/min for intravenous administration. The rate of less than 1 mL/min is desirable as described in the normative reference Annex B. Administration should be performed very carefully, so that it does not result in any effects associated with administering too rapidly.

6.4   Evaluation of acute systemic toxicity

Body weight changes are important indicator for evaluation of systemic toxicity. In the standard acute systemic toxicity test using mice in the US Pharmacopoeia[1], the result is judged incompatible (presence of systemic toxicity) if the body weight showed 2 g or more decrease in 3 or more animals among 5. In the OLAW guidance[4], severe toxic symptoms include convulsion andgeneral weakness, persistent supine posture or prolonged recumbency, rapid or labored breathing, rales and decrease of 4 to 6 ℃ or more in body temperature. It is advised to euthanize the relevant animals considering that these symptoms are minimum humane endpoints in terms of animal welfare[5].

6.5   Utilization of implantation test

While the procedure for the subacute systemic toxicity test by the administration of the test solution is described in Section 5, "Repeated exposure systemic toxicity (subacute, subchronic and chronic systemic toxicity)". However, the results of the implantation test described in Sections 3.2 through 3.4 may be appropriate as the results of the subacute, subchronic or chronic systemic toxicity tests, under conditions if the test sample is implantable in a suitable species of animals (including non-rats) and the parameters descrive in this guidance are evaluate appropriately. When subacute, subchronic or chronic systemic toxicity of an absorbable test sample is assessed by implantation and extremely quick absorption is assumed, autopsy is performed immediately in the stage disappeared the local reactions due to operation for implantation and able to evaluate the effects of the test sample. It is necessary to discuss the relationship between the period expected for complete absorption of the test sample and the administration period with rationales.

6.6   Test animals and alternatives in acute systemic toxicity test

For the acute systemic toxicity test, rat is preferred, to perform haematology and clinical

一般的に体重 150〜300 g の動物が汎用される．また 5. 項に示した反復投与による全身毒性試験の実施が計画されている場合，急性全身毒性の評価も合わせて行うことが可能と考えられる．

6.7　反復投与における投与液量

5. 項では，引用文献[6]に基づき，ラットにおける投与液量を 20 mL/kg とした．一方，引用規格においては静脈内投与の最大投与液量は 40 mL/kg である．投与液量，投与経路を決定する場合には，当該医療機器の臨床での使用を考慮し，妥当性のある投与液量を設定し，根拠を説明することが重要である．

6.8　投与期間及び観察期間

投与期間及び観察期間は，当該医療機器の臨床での使用時間を考慮して設定し，その根拠を記載する．

6.9　試験液の調製

生理食塩液を抽出溶媒として試験液を調製する際，試験試料がポリ乳酸など加水分解性のポリマーの場合には，試験液の pH が酸性に傾くことがある．このような場合には，少量のアルカリを使用して中和する，リン酸緩衝生理食塩液を抽出溶媒に用いるなどの対応が考えられる．

被験物質細切時の破片などが不溶性異物として抽出液に含まれる場合がある．このような抽出液の性状観察（色調変化や微粒子の有無）は投与前の確認として重要である．全身毒性試験の投与経路が静脈内の場合には，不溶性異物ができる限り入り込まないような調製方法が推奨される．一方，ナノマテリアルの含まれる医療機器の場合には，抽出液の濾過は避けた方がよい（ISO/TR 10993-22 参照）．

6.10　血液適合性評価との併用試験

血管内に留置する医療機器の全身毒性試験では，臨床適用部位に被験物質を留置して全身毒性及び血液適合性評価を行うことがある．例えば冠動脈ステントの評価では，ブタを実験動物として用い，被験物質を冠動脈に留置して，亜急性期以降の全身毒性評価を実施すると同時に，末梢臓器の病理組織学的検査で血栓症リスクを確認し血液適合性評価を行うことが可能となる．

6.11　ISO 10993-11: 2017 に追加された参考情報
6.11.1　段階的病理組織学的検査

全身毒性試験では全身臓器を網羅的に病理組織学的検査して，総合的な毒性評価を行うのが基本である．ISO 10993-11: 2017 Annex F（参考情報）には全身臓器を機能ごとに 12 に分類し，その代表臓器に異常があった場合にその所属の組織や臓器を評価する段階的な病理組織学的検査の提案がなされている．ただし，この方法は原材料や滅菌条件など軽微変更が実施された際のようにおおむね安全性の確認できている医療機器の全身毒性を再評価する場合など，限定的に活用すべき方法と考えられる．

chemistry. Animals weighing 150 to 300 g are commonly used. When a repeated exposure study for the systemic toxicity as shown in Section 5 is planned, it is possible to evaluate acute systemic toxicity at the same time.

6.7 Dosing volume in repeated administration

In Section 5, the dosing volume in rats is determined as 20 mL/kg based on the reference[6]. This normative reference describes the maximum limit for intravenous administration at 40 mL/kg. It is important for deciding the dosing volume and route of administration to provide justifiable dosing volumes based on the clinical use of the medical device and give rationales and noted for the setting.

6.8 Administration and observation periods

The administration and observation periods should be determined in consideration of the duration of clinical use of the medical device and the rationales for setting should be given.

6.9 Preparation of test solution

In the preparation of a test solution using physiological saline as the extraction solvent, the pH of the test solution may become acidic when the test sample is a hydrolyzable polymer such as polylactic acid. If this occurs, measures such as neutralization with a small amount of alkali and use of phosphate-buffered physiological saline as the extraction solvent may be taken.

The test solution may be included insoluble foreign matter such as debris and other particulates of the test substance generated from cutting it into small pieces. Observation of physical properties of such extract (color change and presence of particulates) is a critical part of pre-application assessment. When evaluating intravenous systemic toxicity, it is recommended to use a preparation method where insoluble foreign matter contamination can be avoided as much as possible. It is better to avoid filtering extract from any medical device containing nanomaterials (see ISO/TR 10993-22).

6.10 Tests being performed in conjunction with hemocompatibility evaluation

In systemic toxicity tests of medical devices being inserted into a blood vessel, evaluation of systemic toxicity and hemocompatibility may be performed by placing test substances in a clinical application site. For the evaluation of coronary artery stents for example, systemic toxicity that may appear on and after the subacute phase is evaluated in pigs implanted with a test article in the coronary artery. This procedure enables hemocompatibility evaluation at the same time by checking the thrombosis risk through histopathological assessment of the peripheral organs.

6.11 General information being added to ISO 10993-11: 2017
6.11.1 Two-tier histopathological analysis

Systemic toxicity tests are fundamentally performed in full through comprehensive histopathological examinations of body organs. In Annex F (informative) of ISO 10993-11: 2017, body organs are classified into 12 organ systems. Two-tier histopathological examinations are suggested that "Organs/tissue (when species applicable) of system" are examined only when abnormalities are found in the "tier I tissues". However, use of this method should be limited to medical devices whose general safety has been verified, if for example, re-evaluation of such device is needed for a minor change being made to a material or sterilization condition.

6.11.2　二重投与経路による亜急性 / 亜慢性毒性試験

　　4 項の急性全身毒性試験に示したように，極性と非極性の 2 種類の溶媒で抽出液を調製した場合，それぞれ異なる動物に投与して行う評価が一般的である．本ガイダンスでは反復投与全身毒性試験を，2 種類の溶媒で抽出する必要性を求めていないが，ISO 10993-11: 2017 の Annex H（参考情報）では同一動物に極性溶媒は静脈内投与を非極性溶媒は腹腔内投与を行う試験法が新しく追加された．被験物質からの極性 / 非極性抽出化学成分の複合的評価が可能になるなど二重投与のメリットを勘案して ISO/TC 194/WG 7 の賛成が得られたが，現状は一部の試験施設に限られた実施に留まっている．初めて実施する施設は，評価法を確立し基礎データを取得の上，評価を行うことが肝要である．

7．薬食機発 0301 第 20 号からの変更点

　　ISO 10993-11: 2017 との調和を考慮し，主として以下の改正を行った．
1)　急性毒性から慢性毒性までの全身毒性試験実施にあたり，動物福祉などの配慮事項を示した．
2)　慢性全身毒性試験に用いる推奨動物数を改訂した．
3)　亜慢性全身毒性試験における観察・検査項目を改訂した．
4)　ISO 10993-11: 2017 に追加された参考情報を追記した．

　　以上により，全身毒性試験の実施指針及び参考情報が最新化され，指針が明確になったと考えられる．

8．引用文献

1)　USP General Chapters: ⟨88⟩ Biological Reactivity Tests, *In vivo*-Systemic Injection Test
2)　ASTM Standard F 750-87（Reapproved 2012）: Standard Practice for Evaluating Material Extracts by Systemic Injection in the Mouse
3)　Diehl, K.-H., Hull, R., Morton, D., Pfister, R., Rabemampianina, Y., Smith, D., Vidal, J.-M., van de Vorstenbosch C.: A Good Practice Guide to the Administration of Substances and Removal of Blood, Including Routes and Volumes. J. Appl. Toxicol. 21, 15-23（2001）
4)　Office of Laboratory Animal Welfare, National Institutes of Health: Institutional Animal Care and Use Committee Guidebook 2nd Edition, pp.103（2002）
5)　ISO 10993-2: 2006, Biological evaluation of medical devices-Part 2: Animal welfare requirements
6)　Derelanko, M.J., Hollinger, M.A.: CRC Handbook of Toxicology. CRC Press, New York, pp.78（1995）

6.11.2   Subacute/subchronic toxicity tests using dual routes of administration

As described in Section 4, "Acute systemic toxicity", the extract being prepared using polar and non-polar solvents is generally administered to different animals for evaluation. This guidance does not require extraction using two types of solvents for repeated exposure systemic toxicity studies. However, Annex H (informative) of ISO 10993-11: 2017 newly introduces one approach to concurrent parenteral (intravenous and intraperitoneal) administration of polar and nonpolar extracts into the same animal. This method was approved by the ISO/TC 194/WG 7 for the advantages of dual routes, including the capability of multiple evaluations of polar/non-polar extract chemical component from the test substance. Currently, only a limited number of laboratories use this method. If the laboratory decided to use this model, establish effective parameters and collect basic data for the first time.

7.   Points changed from MHLW Notification, YAKUSHOKUKI-HATSU 0301 No. 20

The following revisions were mainly made to harmonize with ISO 10993-11: 2017.

1) Animal welfare and other concerns have been included for acute to chronic systemic toxicity tests.

2) Number of animals recommended for the chronic systemic toxicity test has been changed.

3) Observation and parameters in the subchronic systemic toxicity test have been changed.

4) The general information added to ISO 10993-11: 2017 has been added.

   Principles have been made clearer by the above after updating the systemic toxicity test policy and general information.

8.   References cited

1) US Pharmacopoeia General Chapters: ⟨88⟩ Biological Reactivity Tests, *In vivo*-Systemic Injection Test

2) ASTM Standard F 750-87 (Reapproved 2012): Standard Practice for Evaluating Material Extracts by Systemic Injection in the Mouse

3) Diehl, K.-H., Hull, R., Morton, D., Pfister, R., Rabemampianina, Y., Smith, D., Vidal, J.-M., van de Vorstenbosch C.: A Good Practice Guide to the Administration of Substances and Removal of Blood, Including Routes and Volumes. J. Appi. Toxicol. 21, 15-23 (2001)

4) Office of Laboratory Animal Welfare, National Institutes of Health: Institutional Animal Care and Use Committee Guidebook 2nd Edition, pp.103 (2002)

5) ISO 10993-2: 2006, Biological evaluation of medical devices-Part 2: Animal welfare requirements

6) Derelanko, M.J., Hollinger, M.A.: CRC Handbook of Toxicology. CRC Press, New York, pp.78 (1995)

第7部　発熱性物質試験

1．適用範囲

本試験の目的は，医療機器又は原材料中に存在する発熱性物質（エンドトキシン及び非エンドトキシン性発熱性物質）の有無を調べることにある（5.1，5.2 項参照）．ただし，コラーゲン，ゼラチン，アルギン酸塩などの天然由来材料から構成される医療機器の場合には，材料に由来するエンドトキシン汚染の可能性があることから，発熱性物質試験の一環としてエンドトキシン試験も実施して，エンドトキシン量を測定することが望ましい．

ISO 10993 シリーズでは，発熱性物質試験は Part 11: Systemic toxicity に含まれ，米国薬局方（USP），欧州薬局方（EP）及び日本薬局方（JP）の発熱性物質試験を推奨している．これらの試験法は，本ガイダンスと試験感度的にほぼ同等と考えられることから，ISO 10993-11 あるいは各国薬局方に従って実施された試験結果が存在する場合には，改めて本試験を実施する必要はない．

2．引用規格

2.1　第十七改正日本薬局方　一般試験法　4.04 発熱性物質試験法

2.2　第十七改正日本薬局方　一般試験法　4.01 エンドトキシン試験法

2.3　JIS K 8008: 1992　4.3 エンドトキシン試験

2.4　ISO 10993-11: 2017, Biological evaluation of medical devices–Part 11: Tests for systemic toxicity

3．発熱性物質試験

3.1　目的

本試験は，試験試料（最終製品又は原材料）から抽出した抽出液（以下「試験液」とする）中に，原材料に由来するエンドトキシン及び非エンドトキシン性発熱性物質が存在しないことを確認するための試験である（5.3 項参照）．

3.2　試験の要約

試験試料から生理食塩液（日局）を用いて抽出した試験液を，JP の発熱性物質試験に準拠して，3匹のウサギに静脈注射し，直腸温を注射後3時間測定し，注射直前の体温との比較により，発熱性物質の存在を評価する．

3.3　試験液の調製

3.3.1　抽出溶媒

抽出には，生理食塩液（日局）を用いる．

Part 7 Pyrogen Test

1. Scope

The purpose of this test is to determine the presence of pyrogens (bacterial endotoxins and non-endotoxin pyrogens) in medical devices or their raw materials (refer to 5.1 and 5.2). However, when a medical device is made of naturally derived materials such as collagen, gelatin, and alginate, the device may be contaminated with endotoxins that originate from the natural materials. In such cases, it is desirable to also perform an endotoxin test as part of the pyrogen test to measure the endotoxin level.

In the ISO 10993 series of standards, the pyrogen test is included in Part 11: Systemic toxicity, which recommends the pyrogen tests found in the United States Pharmacopeia (USP), European Pharmacopoeia (EP), and Japanese Pharmacopoeia (JP). The sensitivity of these testing methods is considered to be practically equivalent to that of the method in this guideline. Accordingly, it is not necessary to repeat this test if a result is available from another test that was conducted in accordance with ISO 10993-11 or national pharmacopoeias.

2. Normative references

2.1 The Japanese Pharmacopoeia, Seventeenth Edition; General Tests, 4.04 Pyrogen Test

2.2 The Japanese Pharmacopoeia, Seventeenth Edition; General Tests, 4.01 Bacterial Endotoxins Test

2.3 JIS K 8008: 1992; 4.3 Bacterial endotoxins test

2.4 ISO 10993-11; Biological evaluation of medical devices-Part 11: Tests for systemic toxicity (2017)

3. Pyrogen test

3.1 Purpose

This test is designed to confirm the absence of endotoxins and non-endotoxin pyrogens derived from raw materials in the extracts (referred to below as "test solutions") that are prepared by extraction from test samples (final products or their raw materials) (refer to 5.3).

3.2 A brief description of the test

The test is to determine if pyrogens are present. First, the test solution is prepared by extraction from test sample with physiological saline (JP), then an intravenous injection is administered to three rabbits in accordance with the pyrogen test in the JP, their rectal temperature is measured for 3 hours after injection, and finally this temperature is compared with the temperature shortly before injection.

3.3 Preparation of test solution
3.3.1 Extraction medium

Use physiological saline (JP) for extraction.

3.3.2　抽出溶媒と試験試料量の比

原則として，付録1の規定に従うものとする．

3.3.3　抽出条件

付録2に示した温度・時間条件の中から，適切な条件を選んで抽出する（5.4項参照）．

3.3.4　試験液の取扱い

抽出後，直ちに室温（25℃以下にならないよう）に冷却する．次いで，容器の内容液を無菌的に別の乾燥した滅菌容器に集め，付録3に従い，25℃前後で保存し，これを試験液として24時間以内に発熱性物質試験を実施する．なお，試験を実施する直前に，試験液を超音波処理することが望ましい（5.5項参照）．

3.4　発熱性物質試験法（5.6項参照）

3.3で調製した試験液を用いて，第十七改正日本薬局方・発熱性物質試験法に準拠して，試験を実施する（5.1，5.7項参照）．

3.4.1　試験動物（5.8項参照）

体重1.5 kg以上の健康なウサギで，1週間以上の馴化後，体重の減少をみなかった3匹を試験動物とする．ウサギは個別ケージに入れ，興奮させないよう刺激のない環境で飼育する．試験前48時間以上及び試験中は室温を20～27℃の範囲内で一定に保つ．初めて試験に用いるウサギは，試験前1～3日間以内に注射を除く全操作を含む偽試験を行い，試験に馴化させる．ウサギを再使用する場合には，48時間以上休養させる．ただし，発熱性物質陽性と判定された試料を投与されたウサギ，又は以前に試験試料と共通な抗原物質を含む試料を投与されたウサギは再使用しない．

3.4.2　装置及び器具（5.9項参照）

温度計は，測定精度±0.1℃以内の直腸体温計又は体温測定装置を用いる．試験に用いるガラス器具，容器，注射筒，注射針などは，あらかじめ250℃で30分間以上加熱して，発熱性物質を除去する．発熱性物質が検出されないことが確認された製品を用いてもよい．

3.4.3　投与液量（5.10項参照）

原則として，試験動物体重1 kg当たり試験液10 mLを投与する．

3.4.4　試験方法（5.11項参照）

試験は，飼育室と同じ室温の部屋で，刺激のない環境で行う．飼料は対照体温測定の数時間前から試験終了まで与えない．試験動物は，通例，自然な座姿勢のとれる穏やかな首枷固定器に固定する．体温は，直腸体温計又は体温測定装置の測温部分を直腸内に60～90 mmの範囲内で一定の深さに挿入して測定する．試験液注射の40分前から注射

3.3.2   Extraction medium/test sample ratio

Follow the specifications in Annex 1 unless otherwise justified.

3.3.3   Extraction conditions

Choose appropriate conditions from the temperature and time conditions given in Annex 2 (also refer to section 5.4).

3.3.4   Handling of test solution

Cool the extract to ambient temperature (not below 25 ℃) immediately after extraction. Then, aseptically transfer the liquid into a separate, dry, sterile container, store it at around 25 ℃ in accordance with Annex 3, and perform the pyrogen test within 24 hours using it as the test solution. In addition, ultrasonication of the test solution is recommended shortly before its use in the test (also refer to section 5.5).

3.4   Pyrogen test procedures (refer to 5.6)

The test is conducted using the test solution prepared as in described in 3.3 in accordance with the pyrogen test described in the JP, XVII (refer to 5.1 and 5.7).

3.4.1   Test animals (refer to 5.8)

For test animals, use three healthy rabbits, each weighing not less than 1.5 kg, which have not lost weight after acclimation for a period of at least one week. House the rabbits individually in cages and keep them in an environment free from disturbances likely to excite them. Maintain a constant room temperature between 20 ℃ and 27 ℃ for at least 48 hours before and throughout the test. Before using a rabbit in the test for the first time, condition it for 1 to 3 days before the actual test by conducting a sham test that includes all procedures except for injection. Before using the same rabbit, allow it to rest for at least 48 hours. However, do not re-use a rabbit that has previously been given a test specimen that was judged pyrogen-positive or that contained an antigenic substance also present in the specimen to be examined.

3.4.2   Apparatus and instruments (refer to 5.9)

Use a rectal thermometer or temperature measuring apparatus with an accuracy of ±0.1 ℃ or better.
Render the glassware, containers, syringes and needles that are used in the test free from pyrogens by heating at 250 ℃ for not less than 30 minutes. Alternatively, products that have been verified to be free of detectable pyrogens may also be used.

3.4.3   Volume of test solution (refer to 5.10)

Unless otherwise specified, administer 10 mL of test solution per kg body weight of the test animal.

3.4.4   Testing procedures (refer to 5.11)

Perform the test in a room kept at the same temperature as the room for housing and free from disturbances. Withhold food for several hours before measurement of the control (baseline) body temperature and until the test is completed. The test animals are usually restrained with light-fitting neck stocks that allow them to assume a natural resting posture. Measure body temperature by inserting the rectal thermometer or temperature-

までの間に，30 分の間隔をとって 2 回測温し，それらの平均値を対照体温とする．これら 2 回の体温測定値の間に 0.2 ℃を超える差がある動物，又は対照体温が 39.8 ℃を超える動物は使用しない．

　試験液は 37 ± 2 ℃に加温し，試験動物の耳静脈に緩徐に注射する．ただし 1 匹への注射は 10 分以内に完了させる．低張な試験液には，発熱性物質を含まない塩化ナトリウムを加えて等張としてもよい．注射後 3 時間まで，30 分以内の間隔で体温を測定する．対照体温と最高体温との差を体温上昇度とする．体温が対照体温より低下した場合，体温上昇度を 0 ℃とする．

3.4.5　判定（5.12 項参照）

　3 匹の試験動物を用いて試験を行い，3 匹の体温上昇度の合計により判定する．ただし，試験結果により試験動物を 3 匹単位で追加する．初めの 3 匹の体温上昇度の合計が 1.3 ℃以下のとき発熱性物質陰性，2.5 ℃以上のとき発熱性物質陽性とする．体温上昇度の合計が 1.3 ℃と 2.5 ℃の間にあるとき，3 匹による試験を追加する．計 6 匹の体温上昇度の合計が 3.0 ℃以下のとき発熱性物質陰性，4.2 ℃以上のとき発熱性物質陽性とする．6 匹の体温上昇度の合計が 3.0 ℃と 4.2 ℃の間にあるとき，さらに 3 匹による試験を追加する．計 9 匹の体温上昇度の合計が 5.0 ℃未満のとき発熱性物質陰性，5.0 ℃以上のとき発熱性物質陽性とする．発熱性物質陰性のとき，試験試料は発熱性物質試験に適合する．

　付録 2．(1)～(4)のいずれかの条件で得た試験液について陽性と判定された場合は，室温又は氷冷下，適切な抽出方法により調製した試験液を用いて，エンドトキシン特異的ライセート試薬を用いた試験（例：JIS K 8008 4.3）を実施し，エンドトキシンの有無を確認する（4，5.4，5.13，5.14 項参照）．これらの結果を総合して発熱性物質の由来を考察する．

3.5　試験報告書

　試験報告書には，少なくとも以下の事項を記載する．
1)　試験実施機関及び試験責任者
2)　試験実施期間
3)　試験試料（最終製品又は原材料）を特定する要素
　　（例：医療機器の名称，製造販売業者名，製造番号，原材料名など）
4)　試験液の調製方法
5)　試験方法
6)　試験結果
　　表：個体ごとの体温値
7)　結果の評価及び考察
8)　参考文献

measuring probe into the rectum at a constant depth between 60 and 90 mm. Measure body temperature twice with a 30-minute interval during a 40-minute period prior to injection of the test solution. Determine the control temperature as the mean of two readings. Do not use any animal showing a difference greater than 0.2 ℃ between two temperature readings or having a control body temperature exceeding 39.8 ℃.

Warm the test solution to a temperature of 37 ± 2 ℃ and inject it slowly into the ear vein of each test animal. The injection time for each animal must not exceed 10 minutes. Pyrogen-free sodium chloride may be added to a hypotonic test solution to make it isotonic. Measure the body temperature at 30-minute or shorter intervals until 3 hours after injection. A rise in body temperature is defined as the difference between the control body temperature and the highest body temperature. Consider any temperature decrease as a zero body temperature rise.

3.4.5   Interpretation (refer to 5.12)

Conduct the test using a group of three test animals and make a judgment based on the sum of the temperature rise in the three animals. However, the test may be extended to add another three animals if the criteria below are met. The test result is judged to be pyrogen-negative or pyrogen-positive when the sum of temperature rise in the first three animals is ≤1.3 ℃ or ≥2.5 ℃, respectively. Repeat the test using another three animals if the sum of temperature rise is between 1.3 ℃ and 2.5 ℃. The result is judged to be pyrogen-negative or pyrogen-positive when the sum of temperature rise in all six animals is ≤ 3.0 ℃ or ≥4.2 ℃, respectively. Repeat the test using three more animals if the sum of temperature rises in these six animals is between 3.0 ℃ and 4.2 ℃. The result is judged to be pyrogen-negative or pyrogen-positive when the sum of temperature rises in all nine animals is ＜5.0 ℃ or ≥5.0 ℃, respectively. The test specimen passes the pyrogen test when the test result is pyrogen-negative.

When the result is positive for a test solution prepared in accordance with the condition (1) to (4) given in Annex 2, check for the presence of endotoxins by preparing another test solution by extraction at ambient temperature or 4 ℃ with an appropriate method and test it by an assay using an endotoxin-specific lysate reagent (e.g., JIS K 8008 4.3). Undertake a comprehensive evaluation of the origin of the pyrogen(s) from these results. Also refer to the references in Section 7 for an endotoxin test using an endotoxin-specific lysate reagent (refer to 4, 5.4, 5.13 and 5.14).

3.5   Test report

The test report shall include the following:

1) Names of the testing agency and study director
2) Test period
3) Identity of the test specimen (medical device or its material)
   (e.g., name of the medical device, manufacturer's name, serial number, and names of raw materials)
4) Preparation method for test solution
5) Test method
6) Test result
   Table: body temperatures of individual animals
7) Evaluation of the result and discussion
8) References

4．エンドトキシン試験（5.13項参照）

　天然由来の医用材料（例：キチン，キトサン，植物ガム，ペクチン，アルギン酸塩，コラーゲン，ゼラチン）は，原材料に由来するエンドトキシン汚染の可能性が否定できないことから，室温下，可能なら連続振とう又は氷冷下で超音波処理を行って適切な時間抽出し，エンドトキシン特異的ライセート試薬によるエンドトキシン試験（第十七改正日本薬局方エンドトキシン試験又はJIS K 8008 4.3）を実施する（3.4.5，5.4，5.13，5.14項参照）．

5．参考情報

5.1　発熱性物質の分類と体温調節・発熱機序

　発熱性物質は，最も強力な発熱性を示すエンドトキシンとその他の非エンドトキシン性発熱性物質に大別される．さらに後者は，化学物質に相当するMaterial-mediated pyrogenとエンドトキシンを除く各種の微生物由来成分に分類される．ウサギを用いた試験では，基本的に全ての発熱性物質の存在の有無を評価できるが，エンドトキシン試験により検出できる発熱性物質はエンドトキシンのみである．ただし，医療機器又はその材料に微生物汚染が生じる場合，通常，グラム陰性細菌以外の微生物汚染も同時に起こるため，エンドトキシン試験の結果から，その他の微生物由来成分の混入の有無を推定することは可能である．

　発熱性物質は，その作用機序から，(1)サイトカインネットワークを介して発熱を惹起する物質，(2)体温調節に関与する中枢神経系に直接作用する物質，(3)酸化的リン酸化の脱共役剤，(4)その他，作用機序の不明な物質に大別される．エンドトキシンをはじめとした各種微生物成分は(1)に該当する発熱性物質である．一方，化学物質であるMaterial-mediated pyrogenは(2)〜(4)に相当する発熱性物質である（5.7項参照）．

　ウサギを用いた発熱性物質試験法は，かつてはエンドトキシンの検出を主目的として，ヒトとの反応相関性を見ながら開発された試験法である．恒温動物における体温調節機構の研究は，その多くがウサギを用いた本試験法の手技により行われている．体温調節は，なお未解明のところも多いが，視床下部，脊髄及び皮膚粘膜の関与するものであり，視床下部の体温調節神経回路網における中枢モノアミン（ノルアドレナリン，セロトニン）やアセチルコリンなどの神経伝達物質の作用によって行われていると考えられている．

　Toll-like receptor（TLR）familyは微生物感染に対する宿主の初期免疫応答を制御する生体防御蛋白質[1]であり，肺，胃腸管のような外部環境に接する組織やマクロファージのような免疫応答細胞に優先的に発現している．生体内におけるエンドトキシンの一次標的はマクロファージであり，血中に投与されたエンドトキシンはLBP（LPS Binding Protein）及びCD14分子と複合体を形成し，TLR4/MD-2を介して発熱をはじめとした様々な生理活性を発現する．多くのTLRはホモ二量体を形成して機能を発現するが，TLR2はTLR1又はTLR6とヘテロ二量体を形成することにより，グラム陽性細菌の細胞外膜に局在するリポタイコ酸や細胞膜の構成成分であるリポ蛋白質などを認識する．その他，ウイルス由来の二本鎖RNA，細菌鞭毛及び細菌DNAはそれぞれTLR3，TLR5及びTLR9を介して生物活性を発現することが知られている．TLR7及びTLR8は合成抗ウイルス分子に対する親和性を持つことが知られている[2]．また細菌類の細胞壁成分であるペプチドグリカンはTLR2アゴニストとして作用すると考えられていたが，近年，

4.　Endotoxin test (refer to 5.13)

For naturally derived biomedical materials (e.g., chitin, chitosan, plant gum, pectin, alginate, collagen, and gelatin), the possibility of endotoxin contamination originating from raw materials cannot be excluded. Consequently, an endotoxin test using an endotoxin-specific lysate reagent (Bacterial Endotoxins Test in JP XVII or JIS K 8008 4.3) shall be performed on extracts prepared at ambient temperature for an appropriate period of time, and when possible, with continuous shaking or by ultrasonication at 4 ℃ (refer to 3.4.5, 5.4, 5.13 and 5.14).

5.　Reference information

5.1　Classification of pyrogens and the mechanisms of thermoregulation and fever

Pyrogens are broadly classified into endotoxins, which are the most potent pyrogens, and other non-endotoxin pyrogens. The latter are further divided into material-mediated pyrogens, which are chemicals, and various types of microorganism-derived components excluding endotoxins. While testing in rabbits can detect the presence of basically any pyrogen, an endotoxin test can detect endotoxins but not other pyrogens. However, in case of the contamination of medical devices or their materials by microorganisms, contaminations by Gram-negative bacteria and other microorganisms usually occur together. Therefore, the result of an endotoxin test can predict contamination with other microorganism-derived components.

Pyrogens are classified according to their mechanisms of action into (1) substances that induce fever through cytokine networks, (2) substances that have a direct effect on the central nervous system (CNS) that controls the body temperature, (3) uncouplers of oxidative phosphorylation, and (4) others with unknown mechanisms of action. Endotoxins and other microbial components are pyrogens belonging to the category (1). In contrast, material-mediated pyrogens, which are chemicals, are classified into (2), (3) or (4) (refer to 5.7).

The rabbit pyrogen test was initially developed primarily for detection of endotoxins, through the study of the correlation between the response in rabbits and in humans. The mechanisms of thermoregulation in homeotherms have been studied mostly in rabbits using this testing method. Although the mechanisms of thermoregulation are not completely revealed yet, it involves the hypothalamus, spinal cord, and skin/mucosa and it is thought to be mediated by neurotransmitters such as central monoamines (noradrenaline and serotonin) and acetylcholine in the hypothalamic thermoregulatory neural circuit.

The Toll-like receptor (TLR) family is a class of proteins involved in the host defense mechanism[1] that regulate the primary immune response of the host upon microbial infection. TLR expression is preferential in tissues in contact with the external environment such as the lung and gastrointestinal tract and in immunocompetent cells such as macrophages. Macrophages are primary targets for endotoxins in the body. When released into the blood stream, endotoxins form complexes with lipopolysaccharide (LPS)-binding protein (LBP) and CD14 and express various physiological activities such as febrile response via TLR4/MD-2 complex. While many TLRs function by forming homodimers, TLR2 forms a heterodimer with TLR1 or TLR6 to recognize lipoteichoic acid that are localized in the cell wall of Gram-positive bacteria and lipoproteins that are constituents of the cell membrane. In addition, it is known that TLR3, TLR5 and TLR9 are required for expression of biological activities of virus-derived double-stranded RNA, bacterial flagellum, and bacterial DNA, respectively. TLR7 and TLR8 have been reported to have an affinity for synthetic antiviral molecules[2]. Previously, peptidoglycans, which are components of bacterial cell walls, were considered to function as the TLR2 agonists. However, recent studies have

精製したペプチドグリカンは TLR2 を介さずに活性を発現することが報告され，NOD1 や NOD2 などのその他の蛋白質の関与が示唆されている[3,4]．これらの菌体成分が TLR に認識されると，セリンキナーゼ（IL-1-R-associated kinase, IRAK）の活性化や NF-κ-B 転写因子の活性化など，一連のシグナルカスケードを経て，IL-1β，TNFα，IL-6 などの炎症性サイトカインの産生が誘導される．これらのサイトカインは COX-2 の発現を介して，体温調節に関与する最終的なメディエーターと考えられている PGE$_2$ 合成を促進することにより発熱作用を誘導する．活性発現の強度はそれぞれ異なるが，TLR family に認識されるこれらの菌体成分はいずれも発熱性物質となる．

5.2　ISO/TC 194/WG 16 の設立と新規 *in vitro* 発熱性物質試験法

　発熱性物質試験について個別に協議するため，2007 年に ISO/TC 194/WG 16 が新設された．近い将来，ISO 10993-11 とは独立した形として，発熱性物質試験に利用できる各手法の特徴などを概説したテクニカルレポートが取りまとめられる予定である．

　同テクニカルレポートには，ウサギを用いた発熱性物質試験法及びエンドトキシン試験法のほか，ヒト細胞を使用した新規 *in vitro* 発熱性物質試験法（Human-cell based pyrogen test, HCPT）に関する情報も収載されている．HCPT はヨーロッパを中心にウサギを用いた発熱性物質試験の代替として開発された試験法である．ヨーロッパにおいては，医薬品及び医療機器ともに検証実験が終了しており，動物試験代替法として既に利用されている[5,6]．国内における検証試験としては，平成 28 年度医療研究開発推進事業費補助金 / 創薬基盤推進事業（16ak0101029j2603）において，可塑剤及び医用材料を検体とした 4 機関によるラウンドロビンテストが実施され，良好な成績が得られている．

　HCPT は固形試料を用いる直接法（direct HCPT）と，従来同様，抽出液を試料として用いる間接法（indirect HCPT）に大別される．ヒト細胞としては，ヒト血液（全血）のほか，THP-1，MM6，MM6-CA8，U937，HL-60 などの株化細胞を利用することができる[5-9]．いずれの測定系も，(1)ヒトに対する発熱性を直接予測できる，(2)エンドトキシン以外の発熱性物質（主に微生物成分）を比較的感度よく広範囲に探知できる，(3)直接法においては，煩雑な抽出を必要とせず，発熱性物質の回収率に留意する必要がない，(4)動物を使用しないなどの利点があるため，HCPT はウサギを用いた発熱性物質試験法とエンドトキシン試験法に次ぐ，第 3 の試験法として有用であると思われる．

　HCPT においては，単球やマクロファージなどの免疫応答細胞の細胞膜上に発現している TLR をはじめとした生体防御に関与する受容体を介して認識される全ての発熱性物質が探知される（5.1 項参照）．HCPT では，各種の TLR アゴニストによって活性化されたマクロファージなどの免疫応答細胞が産生する炎症性サイトカイン（IL-1β，IL-6，TNFαなど）を発熱マーカーとして ELISA により検出・定量する．HCPT では，マクロファージなどに貪食される摩耗粉などの微粒子が生体に及ぼす影響も評価できる可能性があるが，その原理上，サイトカインネットワークを介することなく発熱を惹起する物質（Material-mediated pyrogen）は探知されない可能性が非常に高い（5.1 項参照）．また HCPT では，細胞に影響を及ぼす物質を含む検体や生きた細胞から成る再生医療品などの発熱性を評価できないほか，直接法に適用できる検体の大きさに制限があるな

reported the TLR2-independent activity of purified peptidoglycans and suggest the involvement of other proteins such as NOD1 and NOD2[3, 4]. When these bacterial components are recognized by TLRs, through a series of signaling cascades involving activation of serine kinases (interleukin-1R-associated kinases (IRAKs)) and NF-κ-B transcription factors, production of pro-inflammatory cytokines such as interleukin-1 beta (IL-1β), tumor necrosis factor-alpha (TNFα), and interleukin-6 (IL-6) is induced. These cytokines, through expression of cyclooxigenase-2 (COX-2), then induce a febrile response by promoting the synthesis of prostaglandin E2 (PGE$_2$), which is considered to be the ultimate mediator of thermoregulation. All of these bacterial components that are recognized by the TLR family are pyrogens although the intensity of their pyrogenic activity differs from each other.

5.2 Establishment of ISO/TC 194/WG 16 and novel methods of *in vitro* pyrogen testing

A new working group, ISO/TC 194/WG 16, was established in 2007 to focus specifically on pyrogen testing. A technical report that outlines the features and other aspects of each method that can be used for pyrogen testing is soon to be assembled independently of ISO 10993-11.

This technical report will include information on novel *in vitro* pyrogen tests based on human cells (human-cell based pyrogen test, HCPT) as well as the rabbit pyrogen test and endotoxin assay. HCPT is testing methods that have been developed primarily in Europe to replace the pyrogen test using rabbits. Verification tests have been completed for drugs and medical devices, and it has already been used as an alternative method in Europe[5, 6]. As for a verification test in Japan, the Round Robin Study was performed by four institutions using plasticizers and medical materials as samples in the Research on Basic Medicinal Sciences (16ak0101029j2603) supported by the Japan Agency for Medical Research and Development (2016), and a good outcome was obtained.

HCPT is divided into direct method (direct HCPT) that use solid specimens and indirect method (indirect HCPT) that use extracts as specimens as in the conventional method. Human cells that can be used in HCPT include human blood (whole blood) as well as human cell lines such as THP-1, MM6, MM6-CA8, U937, and HL-60[5 - 9]. All of these measurement systems have the following advantages: (1) direct prediction of the pyrogenicity in humans; (2) relatively sensitive and broad detection of pyrogens other than endotoxins (mainly microbial components); (3) in case of direct method, no need for complicated extraction process and consideration of the pyrogen yield; and (4) no requirement for animals. Accordingly, HCPT is considered to be useful as the third testing method after the rabbit pyrogen test and endotoxin assay.

HCPT can detect any pyrogen that is recognized by receptors involved in the host defense mechanism such as TLRs, which are expressed on the cytoplasmic membrane of immunocompetent cells including monocytes and macrophages (refer to 5.1). In HCPT, ELISA is used for detection and quantification of proinflammatory cytokines (e.g., IL-1β, IL-6 and TNFα), which are produced by immunocompetent cells such as macrophages when they are activated by various TLR agonists, as markers of pyrogenic activity. It may be possible to use HCPT to evaluate the effect of microparticles on the body, such as wear debris, which are removed by macrophage phagocytosis. However, because of their characteristics, HCPT is highly unlikely to detect materials that induce fever independently of cytokine networks; namely, material-mediated pyrogens (refer to 5.1). Furthermore, HCPT has certain disadvantages. For example, they cannot be used to evaluate the pyrogenicity of specimens containing materials that affect cells or regenerative medicine products con-

どの欠点が存在する.

　ウサギを用いた発熱性物質試験法, エンドトキシン試験法及び HCPT にはそれぞれ特徴があるため, 目的に応じて適切な試験法を選択することが重要である.

5.3　試験の目的

　本試験は品質管理に用いることを目的としたものではなく, 試験試料中に存在する発熱性物質の有無を測定することを主目的としたものである. 品質マネジメントシステム (Quality Management System, QMS) において, 原材料の受入れ時や製品製造過程における微生物汚染又はエンドトキシンをはじめとした菌体成分の残存をチェックすることが必要になることは当然であるが, この場合に用いる試験法は個別の製品の QMS 中や規格・基準中で定められるべきものである.

　いわゆる合成ポリマーなどの場合, 非常にまれではあっても添加された化学物質による発熱の可能性を否定できず, Material-mediated pyrogen の有無も調べるために, ウサギを用いた試験を実施する必要がある.

　一方, コラーゲン, ゼラチン, アルギン酸塩などの天然由来の生体材料は, その製造過程においてエンドトキシン汚染が避けられず, またエンドトキシンの除去も容易でないため, 設計段階でエンドトキシン量を測定しておく必要がある. このような認識に基づいて, 本試験のスキームが組み立てられた.

　本試験は, 試験試料中から抽出された物質の発熱性を検出する試験である. 試験試料中に低濃度のエンドトキシンが存在していても, 付録2.(1)～(3)の条件で抽出すると, 発熱活性が検出できないことがある (5.4項参照).

5.4　抽出温度

　従来の試験液の調製は付録2.の「抽出温度・時間」のうち(1)～(3)のような高温かつ長時間の条件で行われていた. この場合, エンドトキシンが極めて強い耐熱性を有するリポ多糖であるという根拠に基づいて, 試験液中に認められた発熱性物質は, 「エンドトキシン」であるとの判定がなされてきた. しかし, 引用文献[10-12]及びその他の報告にもあるように, エンドトキシン溶液を加熱処理すると活性が失われることがあり, その現象はエンドトキシン濃度, 加熱の温度並びに時間の3因子に依存することが示された. 特に, 低濃度のエンドトキシンであれば付録2.(1)～(3)のような条件下ではかなり活性が下がる可能性があることが明らかにされた. エンドトキシンの血清型 (O-抗原性) を決定する多糖体部分は非常に強い耐熱性を示すが, エンドトキシンの生物活性を担うリピドA部分は弱酸性及びアルカリ性条件下では容易に加水分解 (リピドA遊離による溶解度低下, 活性低下に直接関係するグリコシド結合型リン酸又は脂肪酸残基の脱離) を受ける. またエンドトキシンの活性は緩衝液中で加温・加熱した場合でも低下することが確認されている. そのため, 付録2.(1)～(3)に規定した加温条件で抽出した場合, 材料表面に存在する活性基又は材料から遊離する化学物質の影響による抽出液の pH 変動のほか, エンドトキシン自体の物性 (酸性) により, リピドA部分の分解が起こり得る. エンドトキシン濃度が低い場合は, 材料表面への非特異的吸着やイオン結合による回収損失も無視できない. 引用文献[10-12]及びその他の報告に見られた活性低下は, お

sisting of live cells. They also have limitations in terms of the size of specimens that can be examined using direct method.

The rabbit pyrogen test, endotoxin assay, and HCPT each have their own properties. Therefore, it is important to choose the appropriate test method depending on the purpose.

5.3　Purpose of the test

This test is not intended for use in quality control. Instead, the test is primarily designed to determine the presence or absence of pyrogens in test specimens. There is no question that a quality management system (QMS) must include checks for microbial contamination and residual bacterial components such as endotoxins when receiving raw materials and throughout the manufacturing process. However, test methods for such purposes should be determined in the QMS or specifications and standards for each product.

In the case of so-called synthetic polymers, although extremely rare, the possibility that pyrogenicity may result from chemical substances as well as natural pyrogens cannot be excluded. Therefore, in order to determine if material-mediated pyrogens are also present, the rabbit pyrogen test must be conducted.

On the other hand, naturally derived biomaterials such as collagen, gelatin, and alginate cannot be kept completely free of endotoxin contamination during the production process. In addition, removal of endotoxins is not easy. Therefore, it is necessary to measure their endotoxin content during the design stage. The scheme for this test was devised based on this understanding.

This test is designed to detect the pyrogenicity of substances extracted from test specimens. Pyrogenic activity due to a small concentration of endotoxins in the test specimen may not be detected in some cases when extracts are prepared under the condition (1), (2), or (3) in Annex 2, (refer to 5.4).

5.4　Extraction temperature

Previously, test solutions were prepared using high temperatures and long durations such as conditions (1), (2), and (3) of "extraction temperature and time" in Annex 2. When pyrogens were detected in test solutions prepared under such conditions, the pyrogenicity has been attributed to "endotoxins" based on the rationale that endotoxins are extremely heat-resistant LPS. However, as demonstrated in the literature[10–12] included in the References and other reports, an endotoxin solution can lose its activity through heat treatment depending on three factors: endotoxin concentration, heating temperature, and time. In particular, endotoxins present in a low concentration may lose a significant portion of their activity under conditions (1), (2), and (3) in Annex 2. Whereas the polysaccharide portion of endotoxins that determines their serotype (O-antigenic) is extremely heat resistant, the lipid A portion responsible for their biological activity is fairly susceptible to hydrolysis under basic or weakly acidic conditions (resulting in the removal of lipid A, which reduces their solubility, and the removal of phosphate in a glycosidic linkage or fatty acid residue, which directly causes a reduction in their activity). Additionally, reduction in endotoxin activity was observed under warming or heating even in buffer solutions. As a consequence, extraction under the warming conditions specified in (1), (2) or (3) in Annex 2 may result in degradation of the lipid A portion because of the pH shift of the extract caused by active groups on the material surface or chemical substances released from the materials or because of the properties (acidity) of the endotoxins themselves. Yield loss from nonspecific binding to or ionic interaction with the material surface cannot be disregarded for endotoxins present at a low concentration. These factors may have been part of the reason for the

そらくこれらの要因も関与しているものと思われる．またエンドトキシンの LAL 活性は，水中下 25℃又は 37℃で 24 時間保存することにより，それぞれ 40％又は 80％程度低下するが，4℃下では保持されることが報告されている[13]．エンドトキシン回収率は超音波処理により向上するが，同処理に伴い超音波浴槽の水温が顕著に上昇するため，超音波抽出を用いる場合は氷水中で行う必要がある．超音波処理を利用しない場合は，エンドトキシンの溶解性と失活度合を考慮して，室温下で抽出することを基本とする．最適な抽出時間は材料の種類によって異なるが，室温下 8 時間を越える場合，LAL 活性が 40％程度低下する可能性があることに留意する[13]．なお，エンドトキシン標品の LAL 活性は，5±3℃で 72 時間静置膨潤後，室温下，ボルテックスミキサーで 10 分間攪拌することにより向上することが報告されていることから[14]，材料からの抽出についても，この知見が参考になる可能性がある．

エンドトキシンの抽出に当たっては，容器表面への非特異的吸着を回避するため，ガラス製器具を用いることが望ましい（5.13 項参照）．また調製した試験液を保存する場合は，ガラス製容器中，期間に応じて 4℃下又は凍結保存し，試験実施前に十分攪拌して再分散する必要がある．可能であれば，氷冷下で超音波処理することが望ましい．

5.5 抽出条件

抽出では，抽出溶媒とサンプル表面との接触，その時間と温度，冷却，振とう（例：超音波処理），無菌的取扱い，保存が重要な要素である．高温で抽出する場合に，抽出時には溶解性が良くても，保存時の温度が低下すると溶解度が低下して不溶性物質が生成されてくる場合がある．抽出液は 20℃以下にならないよう冷却した後，無菌的にエンドトキシンフリーの容器に移す必要がある．抽出液の採取はデカンテーション又はその他の適切な方法により行い，もし，肉眼観察により不溶性の物質が認められる場合は，遠心して，これを除去する．不溶性物質の除去の目的で，除菌用のメンブランフィルターなどを用いることは避けることが望ましい（エンドトキシンが存在する場合，エンドトキシンはメンブランに吸着される可能性があるため）．また無菌的取扱い（抽出及び保存）に可能な限り注意し，抽出後 24 時間以内に，発熱性物質試験を実施することと定めている．なお，容器壁に吸着したエンドトキシンを再溶解させるとともに，均一にミセル化するため，ウサギに投与する前に超音波処理することを推奨する．

なお，抽出後あるいは注射前に抽出液に認められる不溶性物質を遠心により除去した場合は，試験報告書に遠心分離の理由及び遠心条件を明記する必要がある．やむを得ずメンブランフィルターを使用する場合には，同様に，その理由と使用したメンブランフィルターの名称も記載する必要がある．

5.6 発熱性物質試験法

本ガイダンスに記載されている発熱性物質試験法は，JP の方法に準じたものである．本試験法は，後述するように各国薬局方において試験液の投与液量や試験動物の再使用などに関して若干の相違があるが，多くの部分は共通しているため，現行の USP あるいは EP の方法を参考に実施してもよい（5.8 項参照）．

reduction in activity reported in the literature[10-12] in the References and other reports. In addition, although Limulus amebocyte lysate (LAL) coagulation activity of endotoxins decreases by approximately 40 % and 80 % respectively after keeping in water at 25 ℃ and 37 ℃ for 24 hours, it has been reported that LAL activity is maintained at 4 ℃[13]. Recovery ration of endotoxin is improved by treatment with ultrasonication. However, ultrasonic extraction needs to be performed in ice water (4 ℃), because water temperature in ultrasonic bath drastically increases by the treatment. If ultrasonication is not performed, extraction should be basically conducted at room temperature, taking the solubility and degree of inactivation of the endotoxin into consideration. The optimal extraction time is different from the type of material. It should be noted, however, that LAL activity potentially decreases by approximately 40 % in case of extraction at room temperature for more than 8 hours[13]. This information may be useful, since it has been reported that LAL activity of reference standard endotoxin improves by agitating with a vortex mixer at room temperature for 10 minutes after allowing to stand and swell at 5 ± 3 ℃ for 72 hours[14].

The use of glassware is desirable for extraction of endotoxins to avoid nonspecific binding to the container surface (refer to 5.13). In addition, when storing a prepared test solution, use a glass container and keep it at 4 ℃ or freeze, depending on the storage period. It must be sufficiently agitated and re-dispersed before testing. If possible, it is desirable to sonicate at 4 ℃.

5.5   Extraction conditions

In the process of extraction, important factors include contact between the extraction medium and the specimen surface, extraction time and temperature, cooling, shaking or agitation (e.g., ultrasonication), aseptic handling, and storage. When extraction is performed at a high temperature, materials with good solubility during extraction may become insoluble as the storage temperature goes down because of their reduced solubility. The extract must be cooled at temperatures that do not drop below 20 ℃ and then aseptically transferred to an endotoxin-free container. Collect the extract by decantation or by another appropriate method. If insoluble materials are detected by visual inspection, remove them by centrifugation. Whenever possible, avoid using bacterial removal membrane filters for the removal of insoluble materials because endotoxins, if present, may bind to the membrane. Specimens must be handled aseptically (during extraction and storage) with as much care as possible and shall be used for the pyrogen test within 24 hours after extraction. In addition, ultrasonication before administration to rabbits is recommended for redissolving endotoxins that have bound to the container wall and for uniform micellization.

When insoluble materials observed in the extract are removed by centrifugation after extraction or before injection, the reason and conditions for centrifugation must be recorded in the test report. Similarly, when membrane filters must be used for some reason, the reason and name of the membrane filters must be recorded.

5.6   Pyrogen assay

The pyrogen assay described in this guideline is based on the method in the JP. Most parts of this assay are common to the assays described in other national pharmacopoeias although there are some differences in the administration volume of the test solution and repeated use of test animals, as described later. Therefore, the assay can be also conducted following the methods in the current editions of the USP or EP (refer to 5.8).

5.7　化学物質による発熱事例

　　医療機器に関連した化学物質による発熱についての報告数は，決して多くはないが，例えば，下平らは，ゴムの老化防止剤として用いられていた N-フェニル-β-ナフチルアミン及びアルドール-α-ナフチルアミンは，いずれもウサギに対して発熱性がみられ，体温上昇のピークは注射後 1 ～ 2 時間であったと報告している[15]．また実際に食道カテーテル用のゴムからは N-フェニル-β-ナフチルアミンが検出されたと報告されている．しかし，現在ではこれらのナフチルアミンは発がん性を有する疑いがあるために使用されていない．

　　体温上昇を起こすその他の化学物質として次のようなものがある[16]．駆虫剤として使用される 4,6-ジニトロ-o-クレゾールや黒色硫化染料中間体として使われているジニトロフェノールなどは，酸化的リン酸化の脱共役により，高エネルギーのリン酸化物を減少させて酸化的代謝を刺激し，生体の熱産生を促進させるために体温が上昇する．o-ニトロフェノール，m-ニトロフェノール，p-ニトロフェノールなどは有機合成中間体，防黴剤，殺虫剤などに使用されるが，これらは実験的に高体温を起こすことが知られている．また殺菌剤や染料の製造などに使用されるピクリン酸もイヌの実験で体温の上昇がみられている．LSD，モルヒネなどの向神経性物質は，直接中枢系に作用して体温調節機構を撹乱することにより，体温の上昇をもたらすことが知られている．

5.8　試験動物

　　体重 1.5 kg 以上の健康で成熟したウサギを用いる．4 ～ 5 週齢の幼若ウサギではエンドトキシンに対する感受性が低く，また反応の変動が大きいことより成熟したウサギを使用する．伝染病予防の上から，またウサギは同居すれば騒ぐ場合が多いので，個別ケージで 1 匹ずつ飼育する．雌雄いずれのウサギも使用できるが，情緒的刺激を避けるためにいずれかの性に統一して試験を実施することが望ましい．

　　飼育室及び試験室内の温度変化は，各国薬局方ともに ± 3 ℃以内の変動にとどめている．JP では，室温を 20～27 ℃の範囲内で一定に保つこととしているが，USP では 20 ～23 ℃と規定している．飼育室及び試験室の間はドアで区切られていて，両室内の温度・湿度は同じ条件で一定に制御されていることが望ましい．試験時におけるウサギの保定は，首枷固定法により行う．数時間に及ぶ首枷固定での拘束を行うので，できるだけストレスを軽減させるために背中と脚は拘束されないような固定器を使用する．首枷固定時にウサギは騒音その他の刺激に対して動揺して暴れることがあり，このことが原因となってしばしば腰抜け現象を起こして体温が下降することがある．このような状態になったウサギは正常な状態に復帰することはほとんどなく，おおむね数日以内に死亡する．したがって，初めて試験に用いるウサギは，試験前 1 ～ 3 日以内に注射を除く全操作を含む偽試験を行い，試験に馴化させる．USP では試験前 7 日以内に JP と同様の馴化を行うように規定している．EP では，2 週間以上使用していないウサギを用いて，本試験の 1 ～ 3 日前に実際に滅菌生理食塩液を注射する予備試験を行い，注射前 90 分から注射後 3 時間の間に体温上昇度が 0.6 ℃を超えないウサギを本試験に使用することになっている．

　　USP と同様，発熱性物質陰性と判定されたウサギは 48 時間の休養期間をおいた後，再使用できる．EP ではこれが 3 日間と規定されている．

　　発熱性物質陽性と判定されたウサギ又は以前に試験試料と共通な抗原物質を含む試料

5.7   Cases of fever induced by chemical substances

Only a few cases of febrile reaction induced by chemical substances have been reported for medical devices. For example, Shimohira, *et al.* reported that *N*-phenyl-β-naphthylamine and aldol-α-naphthylamine used in rubber as anti-aging agents were both pyrogenic in rabbits and the peak of increase in body temperature was 1 to 2 hours after injection[15]. They also reported that *N*-phenyl-β-naphthylamine was actually detected from the rubber of esophageal catheters. However, these naphthylamines are no longer used because of their potential carcinogenicity.

Other chemical substances that induce an increase in body temperature are as follows[16]. 4,6-Dinitro-*o*-cresol used as a pesticide and dinitrophenols used as intermediates of black sulfur dyes increase body temperature because they uncouple oxidative phosphorylation and reduce high-energy phosphorylated compounds resulting in stimulating oxidative metabolism and promoting thermogenesis in the body. *o*-, *m*-, and *p*-Nitrophenols, used as intermediates in organic synthesis and for antifungal agents and insecticides, have been shown experimentally to induce elevated body temperature. In addition, picric acid used for production of insecticides and dyes was reported to increase body temperature in an experiment on dogs. Neurotropic substances such as LSD and morphine are known to increase body temperature by directly acting on the CNS and disturbing the thermoregulatory mechanisms.

5.8   Test animals

Use healthy, mature rabbits weighing not less than 1.5 kg. Mature rabbits are used because 4- to 5-week old, young rabbits have low sensitivity to endotoxins and show large fluctuations in response. House rabbits individually in cages to protect against infection and also because they tend to become excited when housed together. Although both female and male rabbits can be used, it is desirable to use only one gender in an assay in order to avoid emotional stimulation.

The variation in the temperature in the housing and testing rooms is specified to be kept within ±3 ℃ in any national pharmacopoeia. The JP specifies a constant room temperature between 20 ℃ and 27 ℃ is to be maintained, whereas the USP specifies a range of 20 ℃ to 23 ℃. Ideally, rooms for housing and testing should be separated by a door and the temperature and humidity in both rooms should be uniformly controlled under the same conditions. Use neck stocks to restrain the rabbits during the test. Since rabbits are restrained for several hours using neck stocks, use restraint devices that do not restrict the back or limbs in order to minimize stress. When restrained with neck stocks, rabbits may struggle in response to noise and other kind of stimulation, which often causes a tonic immobility response accompanied by a decrease in body temperature. Once in such a state, rabbits rarely recover and most will die within several days. Therefore, before using a rabbit in a test for the first time, as specified by the JP, condition it for 1 to 3 days before the test by conducting a sham test that includes all procedures except for injection. The USP specifies that the same conditioning procedure as the JP should be performed not more than 7 days before the test. In the EP, if the rabbits have not been used during the previous 2 weeks or longer, a pilot experiment of actually injecting physiological saline is conducted 1 to 3 days before the actual test and rabbits that do not show a rise in body temperature exceeding 0.6 ℃ in a 90-minute period before and 3 hours after injection are used for the actual test. As in the USP, the JP specifies that a rabbit that has been given a test specimen that was adjudged pyrogen-negative can be reused after a 48-hour rest period. The EP specifies that this period should be 3 days.

を投与されたウサギの再使用はできないこととされている．これはエンドトキシンを投与されたウサギはトレランスを生じ，次回のエンドトキシン投与に対する反応が減弱し，時には消失する現象が起こり得ることに基づいている．一方，USPでは2週間，EPでは3週間が経過すれば再使用ができることになっている．

5.9　装置及び器具

温度計としては水銀温度計，熱電対温度計，電気抵抗温度計などが用いられる．しかし，今日では多くの施設でサーミスター温度測定装置（±0.1℃以内の精度を有する）とパーソナルコンピューターなどによる自動測定が行われている．センサーを直腸に留置した状態で平衡温度を測定する場合，あらかじめ試験動物の直腸体温測定に必要な時間を計測する必要はない．直腸温測定にあたり，温度計の挿入はJPでは60～90mmの範囲内としている．これは，USP（7.5cm以上）やEP（5cm）の規定にほぼ対応したものであるが，熱電対温度計及び電気抵抗温度計においては，ある一点のみの温度を示すものの他，ある一定面積に感知される温度の代数平均を記録計に示すものがあるので，これらの電気的連続測温の普及とともに挿入深度の幅を考慮することも必要となり，上記の挿入範囲が定められた．

耐熱性のガラス器具，容器，注射筒及び注射針などは，環境中に存在するグラム陰性細菌によって汚染されている可能性があるため，あらかじめ250℃で30分間以上の乾熱滅菌により，グラム陰性細菌由来のエンドトキシンの生物活性を不活化させる．EPでは，200℃，1時間の加熱処理も利用できることになっている．またリポ多糖体であるエンドトキシンは通常の滅菌法ではほとんど分解を受けないため，試験に使用する器具類の脱パイロジェンには強い加熱処理が必要である．エンドトキシン試験のための試験液を調製する際に用いるガラス製の器具・容器の乾熱滅菌は，エンドトキシンによるリムルス反応が発熱性物質試験よりも数百倍も感度が高いことより，250℃での30分間では充分でなく，250℃で少なくとも60分間の加熱処理を行う方が安全である．注射筒及び注射針は発熱性物質が検出されない（パイロジェンフリー）ことが保証された単回使用の市販製品を用いることもできる．

抽出及び希釈には生理食塩液を用いるが，JPの生理食塩液を用いればパイロジェンフリーであることが保証されている．

5.10　投与液量

USPと同様に投与液量は，通例，体重1kgにつき試験液10mLとしており，1匹への注射は10分間以内に完了させる．EPでの規定では，投与液量が0.5mL/kg～10mL/kgの範囲内となっており，4分以内に注射を完了させるように規定されている．少量の投与液量の場合は試験液の加温は特に必要ではないと考えられる．また試験液の注射器への充填の際には，試験液のエンドトキシンによる汚染がないように，特に，手指などが試験液と接触することがないようにして行う必要がある．ただし試験液の注射器への充填を手早く無菌的に実施すれば，室内での落下細菌などの影響は無視できるので，必ずしもクリーンベンチなどの無菌環境下で行う必要はないと考えられる．

Rabbits that have been given a test specimen that was adjudged pyrogen-positive or that contained an antigenic substance also present in the specimen to be examined cannot be reused. This is because endotoxin tolerance develops in rabbits that have been exposed to endotoxins, which attenuates or sometimes even eliminates the response to the next endotoxin administration. In contrast, reuse of such rabbits is allowed in the USP and EP after 2 weeks and 3 weeks, respectively.

5.9　Apparatus and instruments

Mercury, thermocouple, electrical resistance, and other types of thermometers can be used. However, in many facilities today, automatic measurement is conducted with thermistor temperature sensors (with an accuracy of $\pm 0.1\,^{\circ}\mathrm{C}$ or better) connected to compuyter software that automatically records temperatures. When the equilibrium temperature is measured by the sensor situated in the rectum, it is not necessary to measure the time required for rectal temperature measurement of the test animal in advance. The JP specifies insertion of a thermometer probe for rectal temperature measurement to be in the range of 60 to 90 mm. This range is roughly equivalent to the specifications in the USP (not less than 7.5 cm) and EP (5 cm). However, in addition to thermometers that display the temperature for one point, some types of thermocouple thermometers and electrical resistance thermometers display the arithmetic mean of the temperature detected for a certain area in the recorder. As this form of continuous electronic temperature measurement became increasingly popular, the range of the insertion depth had to be considered and was defined as the range above.

Since heat-resistant glassware, containers, syringes, and needles may be contaminated by Gram-negative bacteria present in the atmosphere, inactivate the biological activity of endotoxins derived from Gram-negative bacteria in advance by dry heat sterilization at $250\,^{\circ}\mathrm{C}$ for not less than 30 minutes. In the EP, heat treatment at $200\,^{\circ}\mathrm{C}$ for 1 hour is also acceptable. Pyrogen removal from instruments for the test requires excessive heat treatment because endotoxins are LPSs, which are difficult to destroy under general sterilization conditions.

For heat sterilization of glass instruments and containers used for preparation of test solutions for the endotoxin test, treatment at $250\,^{\circ}\mathrm{C}$ for 30 minutes is not sufficient and it is safer to perform heat treatment at $250\,^{\circ}\mathrm{C}$ for at least 60 minutes. This is because the Limulus test for endotoxins is several hundred-fold more sensitive than the pyrogen test. For syringes and needles, single-use commercial products that are validated to be free of detectable pyrogens (pyrogen-free products) can also be used.

Physiological saline is used for extraction and dilution. It is validated to be pyrogen free when using JP grade physiological saline.

5.10　Volume of test solution

In the same manner as the USP, unless otherwise specified, the volume of the test solution is set at 10 mL per kg body weight and injection to one rabbit shall be completed within a period of not more than 10 minutes. The EP specifies the test solution volume to be in the range of 0.5 to 10 mL/kg and injection to be completed within 4 minutes. Warming of the test solution is not considered to be necessary for administration of a small volume. In addition, when filling a syringe with the test solution, it is necessary to avoid endotoxin contamination, especially by avoiding contact between the fingers and the test solution. However, this procedure does not always have to be performed under a sterile environment such as on a clean bench because the effects of indoor airborne bacteria and other sources of contamination can be eliminated by filling the syringe with test solution quickly and aseptically.

5.11　試験方法

　　従来は対照体温の測定だけに3時間以上を要していたが，現在はEPと同様，試験液注射の40分前から注射までの間に，30分の間隔をとって2回測温し，それらの平均値を対照体温とするように改正された．USPでは試験液を注射する30分前までに対照体温を測定すればよいことになっている．

　　対照体温の規定は，従来（第七改正日本薬局方）38.9〜39.8℃であった．ウサギを固定器に固定するときは38.9〜39.8℃の範囲に収まるものは，通常使用ウサギの約30％にとどまるに過ぎないが，この下限を著しく逸脱しない限り，発熱性物質に対する感受性は変化しないことが観察されたので，第八改正日本薬局方以降は39.8℃以下と改められている．USPはJPと同じ規定だが，EPは38.0℃以下と39.8℃以上の個体を除外するように規定している．またJPでは，2回の体温測定値の間に0.2℃を超える差がある動物は使用できないことになっている．一方，USPとEPでは，個体間で1℃以上の差異があるウサギは使用できないと定められている．

　　JPとUSPは試験液の加温温度を37±2℃と定めているが，EPは38.5℃と規定している．以前，試験液投与後の体温の測定は，1時間間隔で3回行うことになっていたが，現在はUSP及びEPと同様，注射後3時間まで，30分以内の間隔で体温を測定するように改正されている．現在では，ほとんどの施設で電気的連続測温記録計が用いられており，2〜3分間隔で温度の記録が可能となっているので，発熱を観察する3時間の間で最も高い発熱度を検知する方法を採用してもよい．例えば，エンドトキシンによる発熱の場合は，エンドトキシン投与後ほぼ1.5時間後に発熱のピークがみられ，投与量が多い場合にはさらに3〜3.5時間後に第2のピークがみられることが分かっている．このように，3時間の体温をできるだけ狭い間隔で測定することにも意味があるので，本法に従い30分以内の間隔で測定した値を採用する場合であっても，試験液投与後3時間の体温変化に注意して，発熱性の判定を行うことが勧められる．

5.12　判定

　　本試験での判定が，極めて変動を受けやすいウサギの体温のわずかな上昇によるものなので，体温上昇の程度によっては，再試験を行って最終的に判定するという慎重な手段がとられている．本試験法は現行の第十七改正日本薬局方の方法である．基本的にEPも同様の判定方法を採用しているが，判定温度に若干の相違がある．またJPは最終判定に至るまで必要に応じて3段階の試験を実施するように規定しているが，EPはこれが4段階である．一方，USPでは，3匹のウサギを使用した初回の試験において，0.5℃以上の体温上昇が認められた場合，5匹のウサギを使用した再試験を実施することになっており，初回の試験を含めた8匹のウサギ中3匹の体温上昇度が0.5℃未満又は8匹のウサギの体温上昇度の合計が3.3℃未満のとき，試験に適合すると規定されている．

5.11 Test procedures

It used to take 3 hours or longer solely for measurement of the control body temperature. However, the procedure was revised and the control body temperature is now defined in the same way as in the EP as the mean of two temperature readings with a 30-minute interval during a 40-minute period prior to injection of the test solution. The USP specifies the control body temperature to be measured not less than 30 minutes before the injection of the test solution.

Previously, the control body temperature was specified to be between 38.9 °C and 39.8 °C (JP VII). When rabbits are restrained with restraint devices, only ~30 % of the rabbits used usually have a body temperature between 38.9 °C and 39.8 °C. It was revised in JP VIII and later to not exceed 39.8 °C because it was found that their sensitivity to pyrogens does not change unless the body temperature was much lower than the previous lower limit. The USP uses the same specification as the JP, whereas in the EP, animals with a body temperature of ≤38.0 °C or ≥39.8 °C are excluded. In addition, the JP does not allow use of animals showing a difference greater than 0.2 °C between two body temperature readings. On the other hand, the USP and EP specify that a rabbit should not be used if the animal shows a difference of not less than 1 °C.

The JP and USP specify that the temperature of warmed test solution should be 37 ± 2 °C, whereas in the EP it is 38.5 °C. Previously in the JP, body temperature after administration of the test solution was to be measured three times at one-hour intervals. However, this has now been revised to conform to the USP and EP; i.e., body temperature is measured at intervals not exceeding 30 minutes until 3 hours after injection. Currently, continuous electronic temperature recorders are used in most facilities, allowing temperature recording at intervals of 2 to 3 minutes. Therefore, it is acceptable to choose a method capable of detecting the highest degree of fever during a 3-hour period of fever monitoring. For example, fever caused by endotoxins is known to peak at approximately 1.5 hours after endotoxin administration with a second peak, if a large amount was administered, at 3 to 3.5 hours after administration. Accordingly, it could be meaningful to measure temperature over a 3-hour period with the intervals between measurements kept as short as possible. Therefore, it is recommended that pyrogenicity be assessed while remaining cognizant of the pattern of body temperature change in the 3 hours after administration of the test solution even when taking readings at intervals not exceeding 30 minutes in accordance with the method described in this guideline.

5.12 Interpretation

Interpretation of this test is based on a slight increase in the body temperature of the rabbit. Because the body temperature fluctuates very readily, the final interpretation needs to be made carefully after repeating the test depending on the degree of temperature increase. The test method in this guideline is the same as that described in the current edition of JP XVII. Although the EP generally uses the same method of interpretation, there are some differences in the temperature criteria. In addition, the JP specifies that test is to be conducted in three stages before the final interpretation when necessary, whereas the EP specifies four stages. On the other hand, the USP requires the second test to be conducted using 5 rabbits when a rise in temperature not less than 0.5 °C is observed in the first test using 3 rabbits. It specifies that the test shows absence of pyrogenicity when 3 of 8 rabbits including those in the first test show a temperature rise of less than 0.5 °C or the sum of temperature rises in 8 rabbits is less than 3.3 °C.

5.13　エンドトキシン試験法

　エンドトキシン試験法に関しては，第十七改正日本薬局方・一般試験法のエンドトキシン試験法と JIS K 8008 4.3 が参考となる．その他，JP の技術情報誌 JPTI1[7]及びその他の資料[18-20]には，測定手法，試験例，注意事項，分析法バリデーションなどが記載されている．

　エンドトキシン試験法は，グラム陰性細菌由来のエンドトキシンがカブトガニ（*Limulus polyphemus* 又は *Tachypleus tridentatus* など）の血球抽出成分 LAL（Limulus Amebocyte Lysate）を活性化し，ゲル化を引き起こす反応に基づき，エンドトキシンを検出又は定量する *in vitro* 試験法である．試験法としては，ゲル形成を指標とするゲル化法，ゲル形成時の濁度変化を指標とする比濁法及び発色合成基質の加水分解による発色を指標とする比色法がある．エンドトキシン試験法は，エンドトキシンに対する反応特異性が高く，またウサギによる発熱試験に比較して数百倍もの高感度であることより，エンドトキシンを対象とした発熱性物質試験法の代替法として製薬，臨床，医療機器の分野で汎用されている．

　別に規定するもののほか，エンドトキシン試験用の試料は水（注射用蒸留水）抽出により調製するが，エンドトキシンの回収率は材料の種類により大きく異なる．水抽出により 100 ％近い回収率を得ることができる材料も存在するが，プラスチック，金属，ハイドロキシアパタイトのほか，コラーゲン，キチン，キトサンなどの天然医用材料から効率良くエンドトキシンを回収するためには工夫を要する．プラスチックからのエンドトキシン回収率は，EDTA，PEG/Tween 20/EDTA 又はヒト血清アルブミンなどの溶媒を利用することにより改善されることがある．金属からの回収には EDTA 溶液が有効である．ハイドロキシアパタイト，コラーゲン，キチン，キトサンからのエンドトキシン回収には塩酸抽出を利用することができる．またハイドロキシアパタイトについては EDTA 抽出，コラーゲンの場合は精製コラゲナーゼ / 塩酸抽出を行うことによりさらに回収率を改善することができる．

　なお，製造工程中の微生物汚染をチェックする意味で最終製品の規格としてエンドトキシン試験が設定されることがあり，その場合にも本試験法を適用できる．

5.14　エンドトキシン特異的ライセート試薬

　従来，エンドトキシン試験に使用する試薬は，その起原から LAL 試薬と呼ばれていたが，*Tachypleus tridentatus* の追加により，ライセート試薬と改称された．真菌の細胞壁構成成分である β-グルカンやセルロース系の物質（キュプロファン膜による人工腎臓抽出物など）などは発熱活性を示さないとされているが，LAL に対して強く反応することがわかり，現在では，β-グルカン類によって活性化される LAL 成分である Factor G を除去又はその機能を飽和させることにより，エンドトキシンと特異的に反応するライセート試薬が開発・市販されている[21]．またβ-グルカンはエンドトキシンが示す生物活性やアレルギー反応を増強する可能性があることが知られている[22]．

　数年前より，カブトガニの保護，試薬の安定供給，製品ロット間差の解消及び試験の安定性の向上を目的として，組換えタンパク質から構成されるエンドトキシン測定試薬（組換え試薬）が開発され，現時点で 3 種類の組換え試薬が上市されている．三薬局方（JP，USP，EP）の調和合意に基づいて規定されたエンドトキシン試験法では，カブトガニ血球抽出成分より調製されたライセート試薬を用いることとされているため，現時

5.13 Endotoxin assay

For endotoxin assay, Bacterial Endotoxins Test in General Tests of JP XVII and JIS K 8008 4.3 can be referenced. In addition, The Japanese Pharmacopoeia Technical Information (JPTI)[17] and other materials[18–20] cover the assay method, testing examples, important notes, validation of analytical procedures, and so on.

Endotoxin assay refers to *in vitro* testing methods for detection or quantification of endotoxins based on the reaction of endotoxins derived from Gram-negative bacteria to activate LAL, which is an extract of blood cells of horseshoe crabs (*Limulus polyphemus* or *Tachypleus tridentatus*), and to cause gel clotting. Assay methods include gel clot, turbidimetric, and chromogenic methods, indicators for which are gel clotting, change in turbidity by gel clotting, and color development by hydrolysis of synthetic chromogenic substrates, respectively. Since endotoxin assay has high reaction specificity to endotoxins and sensitivity several hundred-fold higher than the rabbit pyrogen test, the assay is widely used in the fields of pharmaceuticals, medical practice, and medical device as an alternative method for pyrogen assay targeting endotoxins.

Unless otherwise specified, specimens for endotoxin assay are prepared by extraction with water (distilled water for injection) although the yield of endotoxin recovery varies widely depending on the material. The yield from some materials is nearly 100 %, whereas modifications are required for efficient recovery of endotoxins from plastics, metals, and hydroxyapatite, as well as naturally derived biomedical materials such as collagen, chitin, and chitosan. Endotoxin recovery from plastics may be improved by using media that includes EDTA, PEG/Tween 20/EDTA, or human serum albumin. EDTA solution can be used for recovery from metals. Hydrochloric acid extraction can be used for endotoxin recovery from hydroxyapatite, collagen, chitin, and chitosan. Furthermore, additional improvement in the yield can be achieved by using EDTA extraction for hydroxyapatite and purified collagenase/hydrochloric acid extraction for collagen.

This assay can be applied to the endotoxin test for the final product, which is sometimes included in the specifications of the final product for checking microbial contamination during the manufacturing process.

5.14 Endotoxin-specific lysate reagent

Previously, the reagent used in the endotoxin assay was called the LAL reagent due to its source, but later was referred to as the lysate reagent following the addition of *Tachypleus tridentatus*. Materials such as β-glucans, which is a component of the fungal cell wall, and cellulosic materials (such as extracts from artificial kidney using cuprophan membranes) were found to strongly react with LAL, although they are considered to be nonpyrogenic. Accordingly, by removing or saturating the function of Factor G, which is the LAL component that is activated by β-glucans, lysate reagents that react specifically with endotoxins were developed and they are now commercially available[21]. In addition, β-glucans is known to enhance the biological activity of and allergic response to endotoxins[22].

Since several years ago, reagents for endotoxin assay (recombinant reagents) composed of recombinant proteins have been developed in order to protect horseshoe crabs, ensure stable supply of reagents, eliminate differences among product lots and improve stability of tests. Three kinds of the recombinant reagents are commercially available at present. The endotoxin test specified based on the harmonization agreement among the three Pharmacopoeias (JP, USP and EP) requires the use of a lysate reagent prepared from extract of

点では組換え試薬を代替品として使用することはできない．ただし，第十七改正日本薬局方通則 14 に記載されているように，規定の方法以上の真度及び精度が得られることを使用者が検証すれば組換え試薬を用いることができる．現在，組換え試薬の局方収載へ向けた検証実験として，各組換え試薬間並びに既存のライセート試薬との性能比較に係る国内ラウンドロビンテストが実施されている[14]．

6．薬食機発 0301 第 20 号からの変更点

1) 引用規格の一つである日本薬局方と ISO 10993-11 をそれぞれの最新版に更新した．
2) エンドトキシンの抽出及び試験液の保存について，3.4.5 項，4 項，5.4 項の該当箇所を修正した．
3) HCPT に関する最新情報を参考情報 5.2 項に追加した．
4) 参考情報 5.14 項に組換えタンパク質から構成されるエンドトキシン測定試薬（組換え試薬）に関する情報を追記した．
5) これらに伴う変更として，引用文献 13 と 14 を追加し，番号を整理した．

7．引用文献

1) 三宅健介：エンドトキシン（LPS）認識分子機構，エンドトキシン研究 6，pp.23-30，医学図書出版株式会社（2003）
2) Hemmi, H., Kasiho, T., Takeuchi, O. et al.: Small anti-viral compounds activate immune cells via the TLR 7 MyD88-dependent signaling pathway. Nat. Immunol. 3, 196-200 (2002)
3) Travassos, L.H., Girardin, S.E., Philpott, D.J. et al.: Toll-like receptor 2-dependent bacterial sensing does not occure via peptidoglycan recognition. EMBO Rep. 5, 1000-1006 (2004)
4) Girardin, S.E., Jehanno, M., Mengin-Lecreulx, D. et al.: Identification of the critical residues involved in peptidoglycan detection by Nod1. J. Biol. Chem. 18, 38648-38656 (2005)
5) Hofmann, S., Peterbauer, A., Schindler, S. et al.: International validation of novel pyrogen tests based on human monocytoid cells. J. Immunol. Methods 298, 191-173 (2005)
6) Jahnke, M., Weigand, M., Sonntag, H.G.: Comparative testing for pyrogens in parenteral drugs using the human whole blood pyrogen test, the rabbit in vivo pyrogen test and the LAL test. Eur. J. Paren. Sci. 5, 39-44 (2000)
7) Hasiwa, M., Kullmann, K., Aulock, V.S., Klein, C., Hartung, T.: An in vitro pyrogen test for immune-stimulating components on surfaces. Biomaterials 28, 1367-1375 (2007)
8) Nakagawa, Y., Maeda, H., Murai, T.: Evaluation of the in vitro pyrogen test system based on proinflammatory cytokine release from human monocytes: Comparison with a human whole blood culture test system and with the rabbit pyrogen test. Clin. Diagno. Lab. Immunol. 9, 588-597 (2002)
9) Nakagawa, Y., Murai, T., Hasegawa, C., Hirata, M., Tsuchiya, T., Yagami, T., Haishima, Y.: Endotoxin contamination in wound dressings made of natural biomaterials. J. Biomed. Mater. Res. Part B: Appl. Biomater. 66, 347-355 (2003)

horseshoe crab blood cells, and it is not allowed to use a recombinant reagent as an alternative. However, as described in Article 14, General Notices of the JP XVII, a recombinant reagent can be used if it provides better accuracy and precision than the specified method. As validation study to list recombinant reagents to the JP[14], the Round Robin Study in Japan is now in progress to compare performance among different recombinant reagents and with existing lysate reagents.

6. Points changed from MHLW Notification, YAKUSHOKUKI-HATSU 0301 No. 20

1) JP and ISO 10993-11, one of the normative references, were updated to the latest versions.

2) The descriptions of endotoxin extraction and test solution storage in Sections 3.4.5, 4 and 5.4 have been corrected.

3) The latest information on HCPT has been added to Section 5.2 of General Information.

4) Information on reagents for endotoxin assay consisting of recombinant proteins (recombinant reagents) has been added to Section 5.14 of General Information.

5) Accordingly, references 13 and 14 have been added and citation numbers have been rearranged.

7. References cited

1) Miyake, K.: Molecular mechanism for the recognition of endotoxin (LPS). Endotoxin Research vol. 6, p.23 30, Igakutosho shuppan Ltd. (2003), in Japanese.

2) Hemmi, H., Kasiho, T., Takeuchi, O. *et al.*: Small anti-viral compounds activate immune cells via the TLR7 MyD88-dependent signaling pathway. Nat. Immunol., 3, 196-200 (2002)

3) Travassos, LH., Girardin, SE., Philpott, DJ. *et al.*: Toll-like receptor 2-dependent bacterial sensing does not occure via peptidoglycan recognition. EMBO Rep., 5, 1000-1006 (2004)

4) Girardin, SE., Jehanno, M., Mengin-Lecreulx, D. *et al.*: Identification of the critical residues involved in peptidoglycan detection by Nod1. J. Biol. Chem., 18, 38648-38656 (2005)

5) Hofmann, S., Peterbauer, A., Schindler, S. *et al.*: International validation of novel pyrogen tests based on human monocytoid cells. J. Immunol. Methods, 298, 191-173 (2005)

6) Jahnke, M., Weigand, M., Sonntag, HG: Comparative testing for pyrogens in parenteral drugs using the human whole blood pyrogen test, the rabbit *in vivo* pyrogen test and the LAL test. Eur. J. Paren. Sci., 5, 39-44 (2000)

7) Hasiwa, M., Kullmann, K., Aulock, VS., Klein, C., Hartung, T.: An *in vitro* pyrogen test for immune-stimulating components on surfaces. Biomaterials, 28, 1367-1375 (2007)

8) Nakagawa, Y., Maeda, H., Murai, T.: Evaluation of the *in vitro* pyrogen test system based on proinflammatory cytokine release from human monocytes: Comparison with a human whole blood culture test system and with the rabbit pyrogen test. Clin. Diagno. Lab. Immunol., 9, 588-597 (2002)

9) Nakagawa, Y., Murai, T., Hasegawa, C., Hirata, M., Tsuchiya, T., Yagami, T., Haishima, Y.: Endotoxin contamination in wound dressings made of natural biomaterials. J. Biomed. Mater. Res. Part B: Appl. Biomater., 66B, 347-355 (2003)

10) Ogawa, Y., Murai, T., Kawasaki, H.: Endotoxin test for medical devices. The correlation of the LAL test with the pyrogen test. J. Antibact., 19, 561-566 (1991), in Japanese.

11) Kanoh, S., Mochida, K, Ogawa, Y.: Studies on heat-inactivation of pyrogen from *Escherichia coli*. Biken Journal, 13, 233-239 (1970)

10)　小川義之，村井敏美，川崎浩之進：医療用具のエンドトキシン試験法―リムルス試験と発熱試験の関係―，防菌防黴 19，561-566（1991）

11)　Kanoh, S., Mochida, K, Ogawa, Y.: Studies on heat-inactivation of pyrogen from *Escherichia coli*. Biken Journal 13, 233-239（1970）

12)　Miyamoto, T., Okano, S., Kasai, N.: Inactivation of *Escherichia coli* endotoxin by soft hydrothermal processing. Appl. Environ. Microbiol. 75, 5058-5063（2009）

13)　藤原雄太，福田誠，明田川純，益田多満喜：エンドトキシン低濃度溶液の測定値に与える保存環境の影響，Clinical Engineering 22(10)，983-990（2011）

14)　菊池裕他：エンドトキシン試験法に用いる組換え試薬の評価に関する研究，医薬品医療機器レギュラトリーサイエンス 48(4)，252-260（2017）

15)　下平彰男，風間成孔，松本茂：発熱性物質に関する研究（Ⅲ）輸血セット類の発熱性と理化学試験，東京都立衛生研究所年報 22，147-152（1970）

16)　毒性試験講座：産業化学物質，環境化学物質，和田攻編，pp.129-151，地人書館（1993）

17)　第十七改正日本薬局方：4．生物学的試験法/生化学的試験法/微生物学的試験法，4.01. エンドトキシン試験法，厚生労働省，pp.99-102（2016）

18)　田中重則：検査材料からの直接検査法（エンドトキシン検査法）臨床と微生物 18，81-87（1991）

19)　田中重則：血中エンドトキシンの微量定量法；エンドトキシンの試験法（細菌学技術叢書 11 巻）日本細菌学会教育委員会編，pp.128-147，菜根出版，東京（1990）

20)　Haishima, Y., Hasegawa, C., Yagami, T. *et al.*: Estimation of uncertainty in kinetic-colorimetric assay of bacterial endotoxins. J. Pharm. Biomed. Anal. 32, 495-503（2003）

21)　土谷正和他：大過剰のカルボキシメチル化カードランによる G 因子系阻害作用を利用したエンドトキシン特異的リムルステストの開発とその応用，日本細菌学雑誌 45，903-911（1990）

22)　Adachi, Y., Okazaki, M., Ohno, N., Yadomae, T.: Enhancement of cytokine production by macrophages stimulated with（1-3）-beta-D-glucan, grifolan（GRN）isolated from *Grifola frondosa*. Biol. Pharm. Bull. 17, 1554-1560（1994）

8．参考文献

1)　USP General Chapters:〈151〉Pyrogen test
2)　EP Methods of Analysis: 2.6.8 Pyrogens

12) Miyamoto, T., Okano, S., Kasai, N.: Inactivation of *Escherichia coli* endotoxin by soft hydrothermal processing. Appl. Environ. Microbiol., 75, 5058–5063 (2009)

13) Fujiwara, Y., Fukuda, M., Aketagawa, J., Masuda, T.: Impact of storage conditions on measurements of low–concentration solutions of endotoxins. Clinical Engineering 22(10), 983–990 (2011)

14) Kikuchi, Y., Haishima, Y., Fukui, C., Murai, T., Nakagawa, Y., Ebisawa, A., Matsumura, K., Ouchi, K., Oda, T., Mukai, M., Masuda, T., Kato, Y., Takasuga, Y., Takaoka, A.: Collaborative study on the bacterial endotoxins test using recombinant factor c–based procedure for detection of lipopolysaccharides. Pharmaceutical and Medical Device Regulatory Science, 48(4), 252–260 (2017)

15) Shimohira, A., Kazama, M., Matsumoto, S.: Studies on fever–producing substances (III). Pyrogenicity and physical chemical experiments on disposable transfusion assemblies. Annual Report of Tokyo Metropolitan Research Laboratory of Public Health, 22, 147–152 (1970), in Japanese.

16) Toxicity test course, Industrial chemical substances, Environmental chemical substances, p.129–151, Chijin Shokan Co., LTD (1993), in Japanese.

17) Japanese Pharmacopoeia 17th edition English version. General tests, processes and apparatus. Section 4 Biological tests/biochemical tests/microbial test. Section 4.01 Bacterial endotoxin test, The Ministry of Health, Labour and Welfare, pp.99–102 (2016).

18) Tanaka, S.: Direct estimation of endotoxin from test materials. Clinical Microbiology, 18, 81–87 (1991), in Japanese.

19) Tanaka, S.: Micro quantification method of endotoxin in blood. Endotoxin test. Technical Report of Bacteriology, p128–147, Saikon Shuppan Co. Ltd (1990), in Japanese.

20) Haishima, Y., Hasegawa, C., Yagami, T. *et al.*: Estimation of uncertainty in kinetic–colorimetric assay of bacterial endotoxins. J. Pharm. Biomed. Anal., 32, 495–503 (2003)

21) Tsuchiya, M., Takaoka, A., Tokioka, N., Matsuura, S.: Development of an endotoxin–specific Limulus amebocyte lysate test blocking β–glucan–mediated pathway by carboxymethylated curdlan and its application. Jpn. J. Bacteriol., 45, 903–911 (1990), in Japanese.

22) Adachi, Y., Okazaki, M., Ohno, N., Yadomae, T.: Enhancement of cytokine production by macrophages stimulated with (1–3)–beta–D–glucan, grifolan (GRN) isolated from *Grifola frondosa*." Biol. Pharm. Bull., 17, 1554–1560 (1994)

8.　References

1) USP General Chapters: ⟨151⟩ Pyrogen test
2) EP Methods of Analysis: 2.6.8 Pyrogens

第8部　血液適合性試験

1．適用範囲

　　本試験は，医療機器の血液適合性を評価するためのものである．

　　ISO 10993-4 では，血液適合性を「医療機器が目的とする機能を発揮するうえで，血液に関連する有害事象（健康被害）を引き起こすことなく血液と接触できる能力」と定義している．医療機器と血液との相互作用の結果生じる健康被害は，以下に示す2つに大別される．本項ではこれらのリスク評価を実施するための試験項目，試験実施における一般的要求事項，試験法及びその参考情報を提示する．

1）　医療機器が血液に損傷や活性化の影響を与えることで生じる溶血，出血及び塞栓などの健康被害
2）　血液が医療機器に血液成分の付着などの影響を与えることで医療機器に不具合が発生し，その結果生じる健康被害

2．引用規格

　　ISO 10993-4: 2017, Biological evaluation of medical devices-Part 4: Selection of tests for interactions with blood（以下，ISO 10993-4 と記載）

3．試験項目

　　血液適合性の要求事項は，当該医療機器の使用方法，形状，大きさ及び接触形態（体内／体外，接触期間など）により異なるため，それらを考慮して，必要な試験項目を設定する（8.1 項参照）．

4．評価項目

　　本ガイダンスでは，国際規格 ISO 10993-4 で記載されている一般的な評価方法（下表

試験項目		評価項目
溶血	材料起因	遊離ヘモグロビン測定（ASTM[1]，NIH[2]）
	機械的因子起因	遊離ヘモグロビン測定
血栓形成 （*In vivo/Ex vivo*）		肉眼的観察，閉塞率，解剖学的検査，病理組織学的検査，走査型電子顕微鏡検査
血栓形成（*In vitro*）		
血液凝固		トロンビン-抗トロンビン複合体（TAT），フィブリノペプタイド A（FPA），部分トロンボプラスチン時間（PTT）
血小板活性化		血小板数及び活性化マーカー（血小板放出因子及び活性化マーカー（β-トロンボグロブリン（β-TG），血小板第4因子（PF4），トロンボキサン B2（TxB2）），又は走査型電子顕微鏡検査による血小板形態観察
血液学		全血算（CBC），白血球活性化因子
補体		SC5b-9（C3a を追加してもよい）

Part 8　Tests for hemocompatibility

1.　Scope

The tests and their relevant information in this Section are for evaluating the hemocompatibility of medical devices.

Hemocompatibility is defined as "ability of a medical device to come into contact with blood without any blood-associated adverse event occurring, when carrying out its performance". That has been mentioned in a part of ISO 10993-4. The adverse events resulting from medical device/blood interactions are roughly classified into the two types below.

1) Adverse events, where the medical device mainly affects the blood to induce events; such as hemolysis, bleeding and embolism, which are caused by the damage and activation of blood cells or components

2) Adverse events occurring as a result of medical device malfunction, where blood mainly affects the medical device to induce events; such as blood components attaching to the device

Test categories, general requirements, testing methods and their corresponding information for risk assessment are provided in this Section.

2.　Normative reference

ISO 10993-4: 2017, Biological evaluation of medical devices-Part 4: Selection of tests for interactions with blood (hereinafter referred to as ISO 10993-4)

3.　Test categories

The requirements for hemocompatibility of a medical devices depend on how it is to be used, its shape and size, and the nature of its blood contact (implanted/external, duration of contact, etc.). Test categories shall be determined, considering these factors (see Clause 8.1).

4.　Tests

This section recommends using "Common tests used to assess interaction with blood",

Test categories		Tests
Hemo -lysis	Material-induced	Plasma-free hemoglobin detection (ASTM[1], NIH[2])
	Mechanically-induced	Plasma-free hemoglobin detection
Thrombosis (*In vivo / ex vivo*)		Gross analysis, percentage occlusion, necropsy, light microscopy, scanning electron microscopy (SEM)
Thrombosis (*In vitro*)		
Coagulation		Thrombin-antithrombin complex (TAT), fibrinopeptide A (FPA), partial thromboplastin time (PTT)
Platelet activation		Platelet count and some indicator of activation (release products or platelets surface markers such as β-thromboglobulin [β-TG], platelet factor 4 [PF4] and thromboxane B2 [TxB2]) or platelet morphology through SEM
Hematology		Complete blood count (CBC), leucocyte activation
Complement system		SC5b-9 (C3a optional)

参照）を推奨する．これらの項目は，医療機器の血液適合性試験において，精度や汎用性の観点から提示されている．3項で選択した試験項目に対して，これらの中から一つ以上の適切な評価項目を選択する．ISO 10993-4 には，一般的ではない評価方法（Less common laboratory tests）及び推奨されない評価方法（Test which are not recommended）が，それぞれ Annex F 及び Annex G に記載されている．これらの評価方法は，試験目的によって有用な評価項目となり得るため，妥当性を示したうえで使用する．

5．一般的要求事項

5.1　試験試料

　　最終製品又は最終製品の一部を試験試料に用いる．最終製品の血液適合性について評価可能と判断される場合は，最終製品を模擬した試料を用いることができるが，医療機器表面の材質，性状，形状が血液適合性に影響を与えることを考慮して試験試料を設定する必要がある．

　　必要に応じて，無処置対照，陰性対照，陽性対照又は試験試料のリスク評価を容易にするための比較対照（既承認 / 認証品など）を設定する．既承認 / 認証品を設定する場合は，国内で同じ用途で使用実績があり，安全性が確立されている材料を設定することが望ましい．

5.2　検体数

　　統計解析を可能とするなど，陽性と陰性を適切に判別することが可能な検体数を用いて実施する．ただし，*in vivo* 試験については，動物福祉を考慮しなければならない．このため，統計学的解析に必要な検体（動物）数は必須でなく，リスク評価が可能な動物数を設定する．

5.3　試験系

　　In vivo 試験において，ウサギ，ブタ，ウシ，ヒツジ及びイヌなどを使用することができる．動物モデルは，試験される医療機器の大きさや使用方法と，動物の解剖学的又は血液の特性を考慮して設定する．ヒトとの解剖学的な類似点から，ブタやヒツジが選択されることが多い．この他，イヌはヒトより血栓症が生じやすい傾向があることから，血栓症の試験に汎用されている．

　　In vitro 試験においては，ヒト血液を使用することが推奨される．その利点は，動物種差の影響を考慮しなくてよい外挿性の有利さに加え，臨床診断に用いられるマーカーが活用可能であることも挙げられる．ただし，溶血性試験のように動物血液を用いた試験法が確立されている試験もある．使用方法，試験目的，試験方法や評価方法を検討して適切な試験系を選択する．

5.4　試験方法

　　試験試料の使用方法，本ガイダンスに記載した試験法（6項参照）若しくは参考情報（8項参照），ISO 10993-4 及びその他の関連 ISO 規格に記載又は引用されている試験方法に準じて実施する．妥当性が示されれば，文献など広く報告されている試験方法を選択してもよい．原則として，循環血液と直接接触する医療機器や材料については，血液

presented in ISO 10993-4 (see Table above). These tests have been discussed and presented in view of precision and versatility for hemocompatibility of medical devices. Set at least one test for the test categories determined in Clause 3. "Less common laboratory tests" and "Tests which are not recommended" are also presented in the Annex F and Annex G of ISO 10993-4. These tests sometimes serve as useful endpoints depending on the purpose of testing, and therefore should be used following the justification.

5.　General requirements

5.1　Test samples

The final product or a part of the final product shall be used as test samples. Samples mimicking final product may be also applicable when hemocompatibility of the final product is ensured to evaluate appropriately. However, the test samples shall be determined with careful consideration that the material, characteristics and shape of medical device surface affect hemocompatibility.

Controls, untreated, negative, positive or other reference controls as needed, shall be used. A typical reference control is medical devices already approved or certified by the authority. The use of such a reference control can make the risk of test sample clear. In that case, it is preferable to select a device that has been already used in Japan with the established safety for the same application.

5.2　Number of samples

A sufficient number of samples shall be determined to allow to distinguish between positive and negative responses. For example, testing may be performed with the number of samples to permit statistical analysis. For *in vivo* tests, animal welfare shall be also considered. Accordingly, it is not always essential to design the number of samples for statistical analysis in *in vivo* tests, but it shall be sufficient to conduct the risk assessment.

5.3　Test systems

For *in vivo* tests, rabbits, pigs, calves, sheep or dogs are available. Animal model is primarily determined based on the size and method of use of the medical device being tested and the anatomical and hematological characteristics of animal. Pigs and sheep are often used because of their anatomical similarities to humans. Dogs are commonly used for thrombosis testing, as thrombosis tends to occur more readily in canines than in humans.

For *in vitro* tests, human blood is preferable as the test system. This is because it has the advantages in the ease of extrapolation without species differences in blood reactivity, as well as ready use of markers for clinical diagnosis. There are some already established test methods with animal blood, such as some hemolysis tests. Such tests are exempt from this recommendation. A suitable test system should be determined based on the method of use, purpose, test method and evaluation method.

5.4　Test methods

Tests should be designed according to the method of use of test samples (or the final device), test methods described in Clauses 6 of this Section and reference information in Clause 8 of this Section and test methods described or cited in ISO 10993-4 and other related ISO standards. Widely used tests found in literature are also available with the justification provided. In principle, testing should be performed by exposing test samples to contact with blood or blood components for medical devices and materials that directly contact

又は血液成分と直接的に接触させて試験を実施する．間接的に血液と接触する医療機器については，抽出液を使用する．

6．材料起因の溶血性試験
本項では，材料起因の溶血性試験の 1 つである ASTM F756 に記載されている試験法を提示する．

6.1 試験目的
材料起因の溶血は，医療機器又は材料表面の化学物質又はそれから溶出する化学物質が，赤血球膜に傷害を与えることで引き起こす溶血である．本試験は，この化学物質に起因する溶血リスクを評価する（8.2.1 項参照）．

6.2 試験試料，陰性対照及び陽性対照
試験試料の他，陰性対照，陽性対照及び無処置対照を設定する．

補足：陰性及び陽性対照（8.2.1 項参照）
陰性対照：ブランク補正溶血率が 2 ％未満である材料を設定する
陽性対照：陰性対照補正溶血率（6.6.5 項参照）が 5 ％以上である材料を設定する．

6.3 試薬
・カルシウム，マグネシウム不含リン酸緩衝生理食塩液：PBS（−）
・ヘモグロビン標準品
・シアンメトヘモグロビン試薬（Drabkin's 試薬も使用可）

シアンメトヘモグロビン試薬		Drabkin's 試薬	
リン酸カリウム	0.14 g	重炭酸ナトリウム	1 g
シアン化カリウム	0.05 g	シアン化カリウム	0.05 g
フェリシアン化カリウム	0.2 g	フェリシアン化カリウム	0.2 g
非イオン性界面活性剤	0.5〜1.0 mL	蒸留水	
蒸留水			
	1 L		1 L

補足：ASTM F756-17[1]では，シアンメトヘモグロビン試薬によるヘモグロビンの検出が提示されているが，バリデートされていればその他の方法も可能である．シアン化物を必要とせずかつバリデートされたヘモグロビン測定法を参考文献[3]に示す．

6.4 試料の準備と試験液の調製
・直接接触法：試験試料，陽性対照及び陰性対照をそれぞれ 3 試料準備する．
・抽出液法：試験試料，陽性対照及び陰性対照をそれぞれ 3 試料準備し，いずれも PBS（−）を用いて抽出する．抽出条件については付録の規定に従う．
・無処置対照：直接接触法及び抽出液法ともに PBS（−）3 試料を試験試料，陽性対照

with circulating blood. For medical devices that will contact blood indirectly, extracts from the device should be used.

6. Tests for material-induced hemolysis

The test described in ASTM F756 is presented in this Clause, as representative of material-induced hemolysis testing.

6.1 Purpose

Material-induced hemolysis in this Section is designated as hemolytic properties which is induced by the damage that chemicals on the surface of and/or leaching from medical device have on the erythrocyte membrane. This test is intended to evaluate the risk of hemolysis related to the chemicals (see Clause 8.2.1).

6.2 Test samples and controls

Test samples as well as a negative, positive and untreated controls shall be prepared.

Supplementary: Information on negative and positive controls is presented in Clause 8.2.1.

Negative control: Use a material with a blank corrected percent hemolysis of less than 2 %

Positive control: Use a material producing a hemolytic index above negative control of 5 % or more (see Clause 6.6.5)

6.3 Reagents

- Calcium and magnesium-free phosphate-buffered saline (PBS [−])
- Hemoglobin reference standard
- Cyanmethemoglobin reagent (Drabkin's reagent is also acceptable)

Cyanmethemoglobin reagent		Drabkin's reagent	
Potassium phosphate	0.14 g	Sodium bicarbonate	1 g
Potassium cyanide	0.05 g	Potassium cyanide	0.05 g
Potassium ferricyanide	0.2 g	Potassium ferricyanide	0.2 g
Nonionic detergent	0.5–1.0 mL	Distilled water	
Distilled water			
Total	1 L	Total	1 L

Supplementary: Hemoglobin detection using a cyanmethemoglobin reagent is provided in ASTM F756-17[1]. In addition, the other detection techniques are also available if validated. For example, a validated cyanides-free hemoglobin detection technique is provided in Bibliography[3] of this Section.

6.4 Preparation of test samples and test solutions (extract)

- Direct contact method: Prepare three replicates for each test sample, positive control and negative control.
- Extracts contact method: Prepare an extract of each of three replicates for each test sample, positive control and negative control. Extraction shall be performed using PBS (−) under the condition specified in the Attachment.

及び陰性対照と同じ条件で処理し，準備する．

6.5 血液の調製

　3匹以上の健康なウサギから血液を採取し，抗凝固剤としてクエン酸ナトリウムを添加する．プール血液は，各動物から得た血液を等量ずつ混合して調製する．

　ヘモグロビン標準品を用いて吸光度を測定して得られた検量線を基に，採取したプール血液の遊離ヘモグロビン濃度を測定し，2 mg/mL 未満であれば試験に使用可能とする．

　また採取したプール血液の総ヘモグロビン量を測定し，PBS（−）により，総ヘモグロビン濃度 10±1 mg/mL となるように希釈する（調製血液）．希釈後，再度吸光度を測定し，調製血液の総ヘモグロビン濃度（10±1 mg/mL）を確認する．

　補足1：検量線の作成

　　ヘモグロビン標準品を用いて6濃度の希釈液を調製して，0.03～0.7 mg/mL の範囲を含む検量線を作成する．シアンメトヘモグロビン試薬希釈液をゼロ補正に使用する．

　補足2：遊離ヘモグロビン濃度の測定

　　採取したプール血液3 mL を 700～800×g で約15分間遠心する．シアンメトヘモグロビン試薬で上清を1：1若しくは適切な比率で希釈し，15分後に吸光度（λ 540 nm）を測定する．以下の計算式により，採取したプール血液の遊離ヘモグロビン濃度を算出する．

　　遊離ヘモグロビン濃度＝吸光度（λ540 nm）×F×2（希釈比率）
　　　F：吸光度を x 軸に濃度を y 軸にプロットして作成した検量線の傾き

　補足3：採取したプール血液の総ヘモグロビン濃度

　　採取したプール血液20 μL とシアンメトヘモグロビン溶液5.0 mL を混合して5分間静置（Drabkin's 試薬；15分間）後，吸光度（λ540 nm）を測定する．この操作を2回繰り返し行い，以下の計算式により，総ヘモグロビン濃度を算出する．

　　総ヘモグロビン濃度＝吸光度（λ540 nm）×F×251

　補足4：調製血液の総ヘモグロビン濃度の測定

　　希釈した血液300 μL とシアンメトヘモグロビン溶液4.5 mL を混合して5分間静置（Drabkin's 試薬；15分間）後，吸光度（λ540 nm）を測定する．この操作を3回繰り返す．以下の計算式により，総ヘモグロビン濃度を算出する．

· Untreated control: Prepare three replicates of untreated control for direct and extracts contact methods, respectively. Add PBS(−) to individual tubes without the materials and proceed with them under the same conditions as the test sample, positive control and negative control.

6.5   Preparation of blood

Collect blood from at least three healthy rabbits and add sodium citrate as an anticoagulant to it. Mix the same amount of the blood collected from each animal to prepare a pooled blood. Calculate free hemoglobin concentration of the pooled blood based on the standard curve prepared by measuring the absorbance of hemoglobin reference standard. It is acceptable if the concentration is less than 2 mg/mL.

Calculate total hemoglobin concentration of the pooled blood and adjust the concentration by diluting with PBS(−) to make a total hemoglobin concentration of 10 ± 1 mg/mL. After the dilution, re-measure the absorbance to verify the hemoglobin concentration (10 ± 1 mg/mL) of the diluted blood. Hereafter, it is cited as prepared blood for this testing.

Supplementary 1: Preparation of standard curve
Prepare a standard curve using the dilutions at 6 different concentrations, which are prepared by diluting a hemoglobin reference standard to accommodate the range of 0.03 to 0.7 mg/mL. The cyanmethemoglobin reagent diluent serves as a zero blank in the spectrophotometer.

Supplementary 2: Measurement of free hemoglobin concentration
Centrifuge 3 mL of the pooled blood at 700 to $800 \times g$ for about 15 minutes. Dilute the supernatant with the cyanmethemoglobin reagent in a 1:1 ratio or another suitable ratio. After 15 minutes, measure the absorbance at 540 nm. Calculate the free hemoglobin concentration by the following formula:

Free hemoglobin concentration (plasma free hemoglobin) = Absorbance (at 540 nm) × F × 2 (dilution ratio)
F = Slope of the calibration curve drawn by plotting absorbances on the x-axis and concentrations on the y-axis

Supplementary 3: Total hemoglobin concentration of pooled blood
Mix 20 μL of the pooled blood and 5.0 mL of cyanmethemoglobin reagent and leave to stand for 5 minutes (or 15 minutes when Drabkin's reagent is used). Then measure the absorbance at 540 nm. Repeat this procedure twice, and calculate the total hemoglobin concentration by the following formula:

Total hemoglobin concentration = Absorbance (at 540 nm) × F × 251

Supplementary 4: Determination of total hemoglobin concentration of prepared blood
Mix 300 μL of the diluted blood and 4.5 mL of cyanmethemoglobin reagent and leave to stand for 5 minutes (15 minutes when Drabkin's reagent is used). Then measure the absorbance at 540 nm. Repeat this procedure three times. Calculate the total hemoglobin concentration by the following formula:

$$調製血液の総ヘモグロビン濃度 = 吸光度（\lambda540\,nm） \times F \times 16$$

6.6　試験方法

6.6.1　試料又は抽出液と血液の接触比

直接接触法：試料と PBS（-）及び調製血液の添加比

試料	試料 / PBS（-）※	血液接触比
試験試料	PBS（-）を添加 付録の規定に合わせた試料 / PBS（-） 比を用いて算出	調製血液を添加 ※で添加した PBS（-）/ 調製血液比を 7：1 になるよう添加
陰性対照		
陽性対照		
無処置対照	-	

抽出液法：抽出液と調製血液の添加比

抽出液	血液接触比
試験試料抽出液	調製血液を添加 （抽出液 7 mL に対して調製血液 1 mL を添加）
陰性対照抽出液	
陽性対照抽出液	
無処置対照（PBS（-））（空抽出液）	

6.6.2　接触時間

　6.6.1 項で作製した各試験液を 37 ± 2℃の水浴中で少なくとも 3 時間インキュベートする．30 分ごとに緩やかに撹拌又は転倒混和を 1 回（反転を連続 2 回）する．

6.6.3　肉眼観察

　インキュベート終了後，各試験液を試験管に回収し，各試験液を 700〜800 xg で約 15 分間遠心する．上清を新しい試験管に回収して，上清の色調や沈殿物の有無を観察する．

6.6.4　溶血率の算出

　6.6.3 項の上清 1.0 mL に対してシアンメトヘモグロビン溶液 1.0 mL を添加し，3 〜 5 分間静置（Drabkin's 試薬；15〜30 分間）後，吸光度（$\lambda540\,nm$）を測定する．測定した吸光度を基に以下の式から溶血率を算出する．

$$溶血率（\%） = \frac{試験液上清のヘモグロビン濃度}{試験管中の総ヘモグロビン濃度} \times 100$$

$$ブランク補正溶血率（\%） = \frac{試験液上清のヘモグロビン濃度 - 無処置対照の上清ヘモグロビン濃度の平均値}{調製血液の総ヘモグロビン濃度 - 無処置対照の上清ヘモグロビン濃度の平均値} \times 100$$

$$\text{Total hemoglobin concentration of prepared blood} = \text{Absorbance (at 540 nm)} \times F \times 16$$

6.6   Test methods

6.6.1   Ratio of sample or extracts to blood

Direct contact method:

Sample	Sample/PBS ($-$)*	Prepared blood contact ratio
Test sample	Calculate and add the volume of PBS($-$) at the ratio of sample to solvent specified in the Attachment	Add the volume of prepared blood at the ratio of 1:7 of prepared blood to the PBS($-$) being added*
Negative control		
Positive control		
Untreated control	$-$	

Extracts contact method:

Extract	Prepared blood contact ratio
Test sample extract	
Negative control extract	Add the volume of prepared blood at the ratio of 1 mL of prepared blood to 7 mL of extracts.
Positive control extract	
Untreated control (PBS [$-$]) (blank extract)	

6.6.2   Duration of contact

Incubate the tubes which contain the solution prepared in Clause 6.6.1 in a water bath for at least 3 hours at $37 \pm 2\ ^{\circ}\text{C}$. Gently agitate/invert each test tube twice approximately every 30 minutes.

6.6.3   Gross examination

At the end of the incubation, transfer the solution to a suitable tube and centrifuge at 700 to $800 \times g$ for approximately 15 minutes. Collect the supernatant in a new test tube and observe the color in the supernatant and the presence of any precipitate.

6.6.4   Calculation of percent hemolysis

Add 1.0 mL of cyanmethemoglobin reagent to 1.0 mL of the supernatant obtained in Clause 6.6.3 and leave to stand for 3 to 5 minutes (15 to 30 minutes when Drabkin's reagent is used). Then measure the absorbance at 540 nm. Calculate the percent hemolysis by the following formula based on the absorbance:

$$\% \text{ hemolysis} = \frac{\text{Hemoglobin concentration of the supernatant}}{\text{Total hemoglobin concentration in the test tube}} \times 100$$

$$\substack{\text{Blank-corrected} \\ \% \text{ hemolysis}} = \frac{\substack{\text{Hemoglobin concentration} \\ \text{of the supernatant}} - \substack{\text{Mean hemoglobin concentra-} \\ \text{tion of the supernatants of the} \\ \text{untreated control}}}{\substack{\text{Total hemoglobin concentra-} \\ \text{tion of prepared blood}} - \substack{\text{Mean hemoglobin concentra-} \\ \text{tion of the supernatants of the} \\ \text{untreated control}}} \times 100$$

又は

$$\text{ブランク補正溶血率（％）} = \frac{\text{試験液上清の吸光度} - \text{無処置対照上清の吸光度の平均値}}{\text{調製血液の吸光度} - \text{無処置対照上清の吸光度の平均値}} \times 100$$

6.6.5　結果の判定

　下表を用いて試験試料の溶血グレード付けをする．陰性対照補正溶血率は，試験試料の平均ブランク補正溶血率から陰性対照の平均ブランク補正溶血率を差し引いた値とする．試験試料の陰性対照補正溶血率が5％以上の場合を溶血性ありと判断する．

　また試験試料の平均溶血率が5％未満の場合でも，1例ないし2例に5％以上の溶血率が認められた場合には，新たに試験試料を6試料に増やして再試験を行う．

試験試料の陰性対照 補正溶血率（％）	溶血グレード
0以上2未満	非溶血
2以上5未満	軽度の溶血
5以上	溶血性あり

7.　試験報告書

　血液適合性試験の試験報告書には，以下の事項を記載する．

1)　試験実施機関及び試験責任者
2)　試験実施期間
3)　試験試料を特定する要素
　　（例：医療機器の名称，製造販売業者名，製造番号，原材料，形状など）
4)　対照材料を特定する要素
　　（例：対照材料の名称，入手先，製造番号など）
5)　試験方法
　　（例：試験項目，評価方法，それらの妥当性説明など）
6)　試験結果
　　表：個体ごとの評価結果，必要に応じて統計学的解析結果
　　写真：外観写真（血栓の付着状態），顕微鏡写真など
　　（必要に応じて）
7)　結果の評価及び考察
8)　参考文献

Alternative formula:

$$\text{Blank-corrected \% hemolysis} = \frac{\text{Absorbance of the supernatant} - \text{Mean absorbance of the supernatants of the untreated control}}{\text{Absorbance of prepared blood} - \text{Mean absorbance of the supernatants of the untreated control}} \times 100$$

6.6.5　Evaluation of the results

The hemolytic properties of the test sample is graded, using the following table as a guide. The hemolytic index above the negative control is obtained by subtracting the mean blank-corrected percent hemolysis of the negative control from the mean blank-corrected percent hemolysis of the test sample. The test sample is considered hemolytic when the hemolytic index above the negative control is 5 % or more. If the mean % hemolysis of the test samples is less than 5 %, but one or two of the three replicates gave a % hemolysis of more than 5 %, the test should be repeated with 6 samples of the test samples.

Hemolytic index above the negative control (%)	Hemolytic grade
0 to <2	Non-hemolytic
2 to <5	Mild hemolytic
≥5	Hemolytic

7.　Test report

The test report shall include at least the following details:

1)　Name of the testing facility and study director
2)　Test period
3)　Elements identifying the test sample
　　(e.g., name of the medical device, name of the marketing authorization holder, manufacturing number, materials, shape, etc.)
4)　Elements identifying the control materials
　　(e.g., name of the control material, supplier, manufacturing number, etc.)
5)　Test procedures
　　(e.g., test categories, evaluation methods, their justification, etc.)
6)　Test results
　　Data may be summarized in tabular form, showing results of individual evaluations and results from the statistical analysis (if required)
　　Photographs: macro photographs (appearance of thrombus attached), photomicrographs, etc. (if required)
7)　Interpretation of results and discussion
8)　Bibliography

8. 参考情報

8.1 各医療機器に適切とされる血液適合性の試験項目 (ISO 10993-4 より抜粋)

循環血液と直接的に接触する医療機器について、適切とされる血液適合性の試験項目を下表に示す。この表を参考に試験項目を設定するとよい。

血液と間接的に接触する医療機器については、材料起因の溶血性試験を実施して、溶出される化学物質の血球 (赤血球) への傷害の有無を確認する。材料やその他の情報から、さらなる血液との相互作用が考えられる場合は、下表に示す試験項目の中から適切な項目を追加する。

医療機器例	溶血 — 材料起因	溶血 — 物理的影響起因	血栓症 in vitro — 凝固	血栓症 in vitro — 血小板活性化	血栓症 in vitro — 補体活性[d]	血栓症 in vitro — 血液学	血栓症 — In vivo/Ex vivo[a]
体外連結医療機器							
血液モニター (一時的 (ex vivo))[b]	X		X	X		X	
血液保存・投与用具 (例：輸血セット)、採血用具 (例：採血セット)、延長セット	X		X	X		X	
血管内留置カテーテル (24時間未満) (例：アテレクトミー用具、血管内超音波診断カテーテル、冠動脈灌流カテーテル) 及びカニューレ	X		X[c]	X[c]		X[c]	X[c]
血管内留置カテーテル (24時間以上) (例：中心静脈栄養カテーテル) 及びカニューレ[b]	X		X[c]	X[c]	X	X[c]	X[c]
細胞セーバー[b]	X	X	X	X			
血液から特定の物質を吸着させる医療機器[b]	X	X	X	X	X		
アフェレーシス機器及び血球分離用具[b]	X	X	X[c]	X[c]	X	X[c]	
人工肺バイパスシステム[b]	X		X[c]	X[c]	X	X[c]	X[c]
血液透析器/血液ろ過器[b]	X	X	X[c]	X[c]	X[c]	X[c]	X[c]
白血球除去フィルター[b]	X		X[c]	X[c]	X	X[c]	X[c]
経皮的循環補助装置[b]	X	X	X[c]	X[c]	X	X[c]	X[c]
インプラント							
人工弁輪、機械弁	X	X					X
塞栓材料	X						X
エンドバスキュラーグラフト	X						X
体内植込み除細動器及びリード[b]	X	X					X
大動脈内バルーンポンプ	X	X					X
ペースメーカーリード	X						X
人工血管、血管パッチ (動静脈シャントグラフト含む)	X						X
血管内ステント	X						X
生体弁、人工血管及びパッチ、動静脈シャント	X	X					X
完全人工心臓	X	X					X
大静脈フィルター[b]	X						X
心室補助装置	X	X					X

a 血栓症は in vitro 又は in vivo 若しくは ex vivo の現象であるが、in vitro で模擬できることもある。臨床を適切に反映させた in vivo の血栓性試験が実施されていれば、in vivo 又は ex vivo 試験は不要な場合がある。

b 直接又は間接的に血液に接触する部材のみ実施する。間接的に接触する部材については、in vivo 血栓症、力学的因子に起因した溶血及び補体の評価は不要な場合がある。

c 血栓形成に関与する部材の評価を行う場合は、血小板及び白血球の反応が関与する。血液凝固、血小板及び白血球の反応を確認する。材料起因の溶血については主に血液凝固。

d アナフィラキシーショックのような他のエンドポイントに対しても評価する。ISO/TS 10993-20 も参考にして評価する。

注記 血液と長時間接触する医療機器の血栓症リスクの評価に in vitro の評価を用いることは不適切な場合があるため (8.3.2 項参照)、血小板及び血液適合性の各試験項目の in vivo 試験の代替法として適切。一般的には in vitro 試験が推奨される。

8.   Reference information

8.1   Medical devices and the categories of appropriate testing for hemocompatibility evaluation

For medical devices that contact circulating blood directly, the categories of appropriate hemocompatibility testing are shown in the table below, which is excerpted from Table 1 in ISO 10993-4.

For medical devices that contact circulating blood indirectly, material-induced hemolysis testing should be conducted primarily to examine if the chemical substances from the medical device cause any injury to blood cells, using erythrocytes. In addition, appropriate categories listed below should be determined, when more interactions with blood are concerned based on the materials and other information.

Device examples	Test category						
	Haemolysis		Thrombosis				
			in vitro				
	Material-induced	Mechanically-induced	Coagulation	Platelet activation	Complement[d]	Haematology	In vivo/ Ex vivo[a]
External communicating devices[b]							
Blood monitors (temporary/ex vivo)[b]	X		X	X		X	
Blood storage and administration equipment (e.g. infusion/transfusion sets), blood collection devices, extension sets	X		X	X		X	
Catheters in place for less than 24 h (e.g. atherectomy devices, intravascular ultrasound catheters, antegrade/retrograde coronary perfusion catheters, guide wires): cannulae	X		X[c]	Xc		X[c]	X[c]
Catheters in place for more than 24 h (e.g. parenteral nutrition catheters, central venous catheters): cannulae	X		X[c]	X[c]		X[c]	X[c]
Cell savers[b]	X		X	X			
Devices for adsorption of specific substances from blood[b]	X	X	X	X	X		
Donor and therapeutic apheresis equipment and cell separation systems[b]	X	X	X	X	X		
Cardiopulmonary bypass system[b]	X	X	X[c]	X[c]	X	X[c]	X[c]
Haemodialysis/haemofiltration equipment[b]	X	X	X[c]	X[c]	X	X[c]	X[c]
Leukocyte removal filter[b]	X		X[c]	X[c]	X	X[c]	X[c]
Percutaneous circulatory support devices[b]	X	X	X[c]	X[c]	X	X[c]	X[c]
Implant devices							
Annuloplasty rings, mechanical heart valves	X	X					X
Embolization devices	X						X
Endovascular grafts	X						X
Implantable defibrillator and cardioverter leads	X						X
Intra-aortic balloon pumps[b]	X	X					X
Pacemaker leads	X						X
Prosthetic (synthetic) vascular grafts and patches, including arteriovenous shunts	X						X
Stents (vascular)	X						X
Tissue heart valves, vascular grafts and patches and AV shunts	X						X
Total artificial hearts	X	X					X
Vena cava filters	X						X
Ventricular-assist devices[b]	X	X					X

a   Thrombosis is an in vivo or ex vivo phenomenon, but can be simulated with in vitro conditions. In vivo or ex vivo testing might not be necessary if clinically relevant in vitro thrombosis testing is performed.

b   Direct or indirect blood-contacting components only. For components that have only indirect blood contact, in vitro thrombogenesis and mechanical hemolysis or complement activation might not be necessary.

c   It is recognized that coagulation, platelet and leucocyte responses are primarily involved in the process of thrombosis. Therefore, it is up to the manufacturer to decide if specific testing in the coagulation, platelet and hematology test categories is appropriate as an alternate to in vitro testing.

d   See also ISO/TS 10993-20 for information on when complement activation should be considered for other end points such as anaphylaxis.

Note: In vitro testing may not be appropriate for the thrombosis risk assessment of medical devices that come in contact with circulating blood for a long period of time (see Clause 8.3.2). In vivo testing is generally recommended in such cases.

8.2　溶血

　　医療機器には，主に材料に起因する溶血の他，一部の医療機器では機械的因子に起因する溶血のリスクが考えられる．

8.2.1　材料起因の溶血

　　材料起因の溶血は，医療機器表面の化学物質又は溶出する化学物質との化学的相互作用による溶血リスクを評価する．材料の血球への化学的傷害作用は，医療機器と血液との相互作用の基本的な情報と考えられている．このため，材料起因の溶血性試験は，循環血液と接触するほとんどの医療機器で求められている．

（試験に関する情報）

　　本試験においては，使用条件に合わせて試験条件を設定するのではなく，4 項「評価項目」に示す確立された試験法で実施するのが望ましい．

　　通常，材料と赤血球を直接接触させる方法（直接接触法）と，抽出液と赤血球を接触させる方法（抽出液法）の 2 つの方法を用いて高分子材料の溶血性を評価する．循環血液と直接接触しない医療機器（間接接触医療機器）については，血液と接触するのは溶出物と考えられるため，抽出液法のみで評価してもよい．

　　ASTM F756-17[1] では，溶血指数と溶血グレードを示す表が提示されている．これを用いて溶血性を判定する．その他の試験法を用いる場合は，判定基準とその妥当性を示す必要がある．

　　試験には，陰性及び陽性対照材料を用いて，試験系の感度や精度を確認する．陰性対照材料には，高密度ポリエチレンシートが用いられている．陽性対照材料についての情報を下表に示す．

参考表 1　溶血性試験（材料起因の溶血）に使用可能な陽性対照材料リスト

材料	その他の情報
0.91 ％非イオン界面活性剤含有軟質ポリ塩化ビニルペレット（Y-3）	Y-3 は，ISO/TC 194/WG9 が実施した溶血性試験に関する国際ラウンドロビンテストにおいて標準材料の一つとして使用され，溶血性を有することが確認されている． 　Y-3 に含まれる非イオン界面活性剤（Genapol X-080）は曇点が 74～76 ℃であり，当該温度を境にして溶解度が大きく低下するため，抽出液法による試験において抽出温度が曇点近く若しくは上回ると Y-3 の溶血性が低下することに留意する．参考情報として，試験施設で ASTM F756-17 に従って実施した時の各抽出温度における Y-3 のブランク補正溶血率が 20～80 ％となる溶媒抽出比を以下に示す． 　　抽出温度（時間）　　　　　　試料 / 溶媒抽出比※ 　　　　37 ℃（72 時間）　　　　0.08 g/mL 　　　　50 ℃（72 時間）　　　　0.08 g/mL 　　　　70 ℃（24 時間）　　　　0.24 g/mL 　　　121 ℃（1 時間）　　　　　0.80 g/mL 　直接接触法においては，付録で提示された抽出条件（0.2 g/mL）で実施したところ，Y-3 のブランク補正溶血率が 20～80 ％の範囲内にあった． 　※抽出完了後，室温放冷した場合に中陽性が得られる試料/溶媒抽出比である．

8.2 Hemolysis

Medical devices have the hemolysis risk induced by materials. Some medical devices also have the risk of mechanically-induced hemolysis.

8.2.1 Material-induced hemolysis

Tests of material-induced hemolysis are intended to evaluate the risk of hemolysis which is induced by chemical interactions with the chemical substances on the surface of or leachable from the medical device. The chemical injury action to blood cells can provide a fundamental information on medical device/blood interactions. Therefore, testing for material-induced hemolysis is required for most of all medical devices that contact circulating blood.

Information related to testing

It is preferable to use the established method presented in Clause 4 "Tests", rather than determining or changing the test condition according to the clinical use .

Hemolytic properties of materials such as polymers are usually investigated using two methods: a direct contact method, in which materials directly expose to contact with erythrocytes, and an extracts contact method, in which the extracts from materials have a contact with erythrocytes. For medical devices that do not directly contact circulating blood, but indirectly, the risk of hemolysis may be evaluated using the extracts contact method only, as any substance contacting blood is deemed to be the leachables from the device.

A hemolytic index and grade are presented in the table of ASTM F756-17[1], which can be applied to pass/fail criteria for the hemolytic properties of material or medical device. When another test method is used, its criteria should be clarified and justified.

Negative and positive controls shall be designed to ensure the sensitivity and precision of the test system. High-density polyethylene sheet is used as the negative control material. Information on positive control materials is shown in the table below.

Reference Table 1 A list of positive control materials available to material-induced hemolysis testing

Material	Information
Plasticized polyvinyl chloride pellet containing 0.91 % non-ionic surfactant (Y-3)	The hemolytic properties of Y-3 has been ensured in the international Round Robin Study conducted by ISO/TC 194/WG 9. The cloud point of non-ionic surfactant (Genapol X-080) in Y-3 is 74 ℃ to 76 ℃, and the solubility decreases greatly from this point on. Consequently, the hemolytic properties of Y-3 drops sharply when it is extracted at around the cloud point or higher. This point should be taken into consideration when it is used for extracts contact method. The followings are informative data for Y-3 when the testing was conducted in test facilities. They are focused on the extraction solvent to sample ratios to achieve 20 % to 80 % of blank-corrected hemolysis at each extraction temperature. Extracts contact method Extraction temperature (hour)　　Sample/ extraction solvent ratio[*] 　　　37 ℃ (72 hours)　　　　　　0.08 g/mL 　　　50 ℃ (72 hours)　　　　　　0.08 g/mL 　　　70 ℃ (24 hours)　　　　　　0.24 g/mL 　　　121 ℃ (1 hour)　　　　　　0.80 g/mL Direct contact method The blank-corrected hemolysis of Y-3 was within a range of 20 % to 80 % when the testing was conducted at the extraction solvent to sample ratios of 0.2 g/mL. [*]The information above shows the sample/extraction solvent ratio with a medium

	付録2/(1)項の特例に従い，冷却処理を施した場合は，中陽性を得るために抽出比を若干増加させる必要がある．50℃及び70℃抽出時の抽出比は，それぞれ0.5 g/mL，1.2 g/mL 程度となる． 　これらの抽出比はあくまでも参考値である．各試験施設でY-3を使用する前に適切な条件を設定し，その溶血性を確認したうえで試験に使用する．
Buna N rubber	Aero Rubber Company; ARC-45010, 0.031 inch thick sheet（ASTM F756-17[1]で例示）
Vinyl plastisol	Plasti-Coat; 0.025～0.075 inch thick sheet（ASTMF756-17[1]で例示）

Y-3の入手先
（一財）食品薬品安全センター秦野研究所　対照材料担当
　電話 0463-82-4751，FAX 0463-82-9627
　e-mail: rm.office@fdsc.or.jp

8.2.2　機械的因子起因の溶血

　機械的因子に起因する溶血は，主に血流速度や乱流のような物理的因子により引き起こされる．血流自体も赤血球を変形させ赤血球膜を破壊させるリスク因子であるが，医療機器側の複雑な形状が関与することで重度の溶血を引き起こす可能性がある．本試験は，この物理的相互作用による溶血リスクを評価する．対象となる医療機器としては，血液アフェレーシス機器，血液フィルタ，血液ポンプ，人工肺システム，血液透析器，機械弁などがあげられる．

（試験に関する情報）
　臨床使用時における血液との接触状態を模擬した試験モデルを設定する．遊離したヘモグロビン量又は医療機器との接触前後の赤血球数の変動により溶血の程度を評価する．

　主に *in vitro* 試験が設定される．臨床使用時における血液との接触状態のうち最大流量の条件でリスク評価することが望ましい．例えば，国際規格では，ISO 7199[4]に，人工肺の血球損傷試験が提示されており，人工肺システムについては，この規格を参考に試験を行う．

　通常，機械的因子に起因する溶血リスクを評価する目的のみで *in vivo* 試験を実施する必要はない．ただし，その他の項目を含めた使用時の安全性又は機能評価として *in vivo* で使用模擬試験を行う場合，この試験で赤血球数や遊離ヘモグロビンを測定して機械的因子に起因した溶血リスクを評価することができる．例えば，ISO 5840-2[5]に人工弁の動物試験が提示されており，この試験で得られた血液学検査値を基に機械的因子に起因する溶血リスクを評価することができる．

	hemolysis based on the results of the tests which were conducted using the extracts cooled to room temperature following extraction. When it is cooled down once according to the exceptions shown in Clause 1 of the Attachment 2, the extraction ratio may be slightly high to obtain the result of a medium hemolysis. The extraction ratio could be around 0.5 g/mL and 1.2 g/mL when extracted at 50 ℃ and 70 ℃, respectively. These extraction ratios are just informative. Each laboratory should determine and confirm an appropriate extraction condition and the hemolytic properties of Y-3 to use it.
Buna N rubber	Aero Rubber Company; ARC-45010, 0.031 inch thick sheet (example is shown in ASTM F756-17[1])
Vinyl plastisol	Plasti-Coat; 0.025-0.075 inch thick sheet (example is shown in ASTM F756-17[1])

Y-3 supplier:
Person in charge of Reference Materials: Hatano Research Institute, Food and Drug Safety Center
  Telephone: +81-463-82-4751, Facsimile: +81-463-82-9627
  E-mail: rm.office@fdsc.or.jp

8.2.2   Mechanically-induced hemolysis

Mechanically-induced hemolysis is mainly caused by physical or dynamic factors, such as blood flow rate and turbulence. Blood flow itself is a risk factor of erythrocyte deformation and rupture of the membrane. Additionally, the factors of non-physiological forces, being involved with the complicated shape or operation of medical device, potentially exacerbate the hemolysis. The information in this Clause is intended to evaluate the risk of hemolysis associated with such a physical interaction. Medical devices to be assessed include apheresis and cell separation systems, blood filters, blood pumps, cardiopulmonary bypass systems, hemodialysis systems and mechanical heart valves.

Information related to testing

A test should be designed to simulate the nature of device/blood interactions which will occur during the clinical application. The hemolytic potentials of medical device are determined by detecting the change in the amount of free hemoglobin or number of erythrocytes from the values before and after the device/blood contact.

It is common to use *in vitro* test system, where testing should be performed at the highest flow rate experienced in the clinical applications to evaluate the risk of mechanically-induced hemolysis. For example, a blood cell damage test for artificial lungs is provided in the international standard ISO 7199[4]. The testing for cardiopulmonary bypass systems can be conducted referring to the standard.

Usually, *in vivo* testing is not necessary just for the risk assessment of mechanically-induced hemolysis. However, for some devices, the animal study, which is usually designed to simulate the clinical usage of the device, is often conducted to evaluate the non-clinical safety comprehensively. The primary purpose is to ensure that the medical device can work well in/on body without causing any significant adverse events. Such a study can also provide important information on the risk assessment of mechanically-induced hemolysis by detecting the amount of free-hemoglobin or the number of erythrocytes. Therefore, where conducting such an animal study appropriately, consideration should be taken to make the most of the result for the risk assessment. For cardiac valve prosthesis, the requirements for animal study (or a preclinical *in vivo* study) are provided by ISO 5840-2[5]. The study can be also used for the risk assessment of mechanically-induced hemolysis based on the hematology data.

　臨床使用を模擬して実施される試験では，試験試料と同等の血液接触形態（時間・面積など）でその臨床実績から安全性が確立している類似製品の臨床情報や試験結果などの既知情報から許容値を設定することにより，人体に与える影響を評価することができる．またそのような製品を既承認/認証対照として同時に試験し，結果を比較することでリスクを評価してもよい．

8.3　血栓形成

　医療機器に起因する血栓症のリスクを評価するために実施する．以下に考えられるリスクを示す．なお，医療機器の用途や使用方法により考慮すべきリスクは異なることに留意する．
1)　医療機器内の血栓狭窄又は閉塞及び医療機器の機能不良
2)　医療機器に起因して形成した血栓の遊離による末梢側血管の閉塞
3)　医療機器が血液又は血液成分に影響（活性化，傷害など）を与えることで体内の微小血管の各所で生じる血栓形成

　補足：本項では，使用する血栓形成，血栓症及び血栓性を以下に定義している．
　・血栓形成：血栓が形成される事象
　・血栓症：血栓が形成されることによる健康被害．
　　血栓形成の項目では，血栓症の有無を直接観察する他，血栓形成や試験試料の血栓性を調べて，最終製品の血栓症リスクを評価する．
　・血栓性：最終製品若しくは材料が血栓を形成させる能力又は性質．
　　試験試料の血栓形成やその程度を調べることにより試験試料の血栓性を評価する．

　血栓形成に影響を与える因子を以下に示す．
　　a.　血流（血流量，乱流，血圧）
　　b.　血管径
　　c.　血液の性状や取扱い（血液の粘度，凝固因子及び血小板の活性化程度など）
　　d.　薬剤の使用の有無（薬剤の種類及び量）
　　e.　血液との接触期間
　　f.　血液との接触面積
　　g.　試験試料やその取扱いによる周囲組織や血管損傷，感染症などの炎症の有無
　上記因子と医療機器の使用方法や使用条件を考慮して試験方法を設定する．体内で循環血液に接触する医療機器では *in vivo* 又は *ex vivo* 試験を，体外で血液と接触する医療機器の場合は，*in vitro* 又は *ex vivo* 試験が推奨される．

A test will be designed to simulate conditions of clinical use. In such a test, the impact on the human body can be evaluated by defining the acceptable range based on known information, such as clinically accepted level and clinical data and test results of a marketed product with the equivalent nature of blood contact (contact duration and area, etc.) and the established safety. Alternatively, testing can be performed simultaneously with the reference material of the marketed device above. In that case, the hemolysis risk of test sample can be evaluated by comparing with the reference.

8.3   Thrombus formation (Thrombosis in ISO 10993-4)

The information in this Clause is intended to evaluate the risk of device-associated thrombosis. A list of possible risks is presented below. Consideration should be taken that the risks below depend on the intended use and operation of medical devices.

1) Stenosis or occlusion inside medical device due to thrombus formation and the subsequent malfunction of the medical device
2) Thromboembolism in downstream vessels due to thrombus peeled off or induced by the medical device
3) Disseminated microvascular thromboembolism, systemic impacts induced by the medical device, such as activation or injury, on blood and/or blood component causes thromboembolism in various parts of the body. (Like disseminated intravascular coagulation [DIC])

> **Supplementary:** Definition of thrombus formation, thrombosis and thrombogenicity is defined as follows in this Clause:
> · Thrombus formation: Phenomenon in which a thrombus is being formed.
> · Thrombosis: Adverse event caused by thrombus formation.
>   The test category of thrombus formation in this Section is to evaluate the risk of thrombosis associated with medical devices by direct examination for the presence of thrombosis, examination for thrombus formation or characteristics of the thrombogenicity of test samples.
> · Thrombogenicity: Ability or tendency of the final product or material to form and promote thrombus formation. Thrombogenicity of the test sample is determined by examining the thrombus formation and its extent which it has induced.

Factors that affect thrombus formation are shown below:
a. Blood flow (flow rate, turbulence, blood pressure)
b. Vessel diameter
c. Blood characteristics and handling (e.g., blood viscosity, coagulation factors, platelet activation level)
d. Medication (e,g., anticoagulant type and dose)
e. Blood contacting time
f. Blood contacting area
g. Factors related to inflammation associated with the test sample itself or its handling (e.g., injury of blood vessels and the surrounding tissues, infection)

A test should be designed, considering the factors above, based on what kind of conditions and how a medical device is used. *In vivo* or *ex vivo* test is recommended for the devices which have a contact with circulating blood in the body, and *in vitro* or *ex vivo* test should be considered for the devices which contact circulating blood outside body.

8.3.1 *In vivo/ex vivo* 血栓症

医療機器表面における血栓形成程度，末梢側血管の血栓閉塞や狭窄の有無，又は全身的な微小血管血栓症発生の有無を検出して，血栓症リスクを評価する．対象となる医療機器としては，インプラント，血管用カテーテルなどがあげられる．

In vivo/ex vivo 血栓症のリスク評価のための基本的な試験デザインとして，以下の2つが考えられる．

1) 8.3項のa〜gの条件を使用環境に合わせて十分な試験検体数で試験を実施し，全身状態や末梢組織，臓器の詳細な肉眼観察，病理組織学的検査など様々な方法を用いて血栓症を検出する．使用環境での血栓症の有無を検査するのみでなく様々な検査手法を用いて血栓症を引き起こす可能性のある変化まで詳細に検査して血栓症のリスクを評価する．

2) 8.3項のa〜gの条件よりさらに血栓が形成しやすい条件で試験を実施して，血栓が生じにくいことを示すことで血栓症のリスクが低いことを確認する．

上記1)，2)に対する代表的な試験モデルを以下に示す．

8.3.1.1 *In vivo* 使用模擬試験

8.3.1項の1)は，血栓症のリスク評価に最も好ましい評価方法と考えられている．例えば，ISO 5840-2[5]（人工弁），ISO 7198[6]（人工血管），ISO 25539-1[7]（血管内埋込み機器），ISO 25539-2[8]（血管内ステント）など，循環血液と直接接触するインプラントの多くは，使用模擬試験による性能確認試験が国際規格で求められている．これらの国際規格には，試験の要求事項が記載されている．またいくつかの文献で，これらに合わせて実施された試験の結果も報告されており，参考にすることができる．適切な理由を基に，一部を省略又は変更して試験を実施することも可能である．

（試験に関する情報）

適切な動物を用いて，適用部位又は類似した部位に臨床使用時と同様の方法で試験試料を留置する．抗凝固薬の種類や投与量についても，臨床使用時を想定して設定する．留置期間は，医療機器や評価目的に合わせる．

補足1：*In vivo* 使用模擬試験では，インプラントごとに一般的に使用されている動物種がある．これらの動物種は，解剖学的にヒトに近いインプラントに適切なサイズである，豊富な背景情報があるなど利点があり使用されている．したがって，各インプラントの国際規格に記載されている又は文献で頻繁に報告されている動物種を参考にして選択する．

補足2：留置期間は，4週間や26週間の中長期間が一般的である．また急性期（数時間〜3日間）の評価も重要な情報となる場合がある．

8.3.1   *In vivo/ex vivo* tests

The tests shall be designed to evaluate the risk of thrombosis by detecting the following:

· The extent of thrombus formation on the blood contacting surface of device,

· The presence/absence of thromboembolism and stenosis in downstream vessels,

· The presence/absence of disseminated intravascular (microvascular) thromboembolism.

Medical devices to be tested include implant devices and intravascular catheters.

There are two strategies to evaluate the risk of thrombosis with *in vivo/ex vivo* tests:

1) Design a test with a sufficient sample size to simulate the relevant clinical applications by adjusting the conditions a to g of Clause 8.3. Detect the findings related to thrombosis carefully through various methods, including general condition observation, gross examination of peripheral tissue and organs and light microscopy. Detailed analysis is necessary to detect any changes and signs which have a potential to cause thrombosis, in addition to clarify the presence/absence of thrombosis in the test.

2) Design a test with a few samples to simulate the conditions which tend to form and promote thrombus formation i.e, ‘worst-case scenario’, by adjusting the conditions a to g of Clause 8.3. If the test result shows that the device has little thrombus formation, it can demonstrate that the thrombosis risk is low in the clinical application.

Typical test models of 1) and 2) above are described as follows:

8.3.1.1   *In vivo* non-clinical study (also called "animal study or *in vivo* performance testing")

Test strategy 1) in Clause 8.3.1 is accepted to be the most relevant strategy to evaluate thrombosis risk. An *in vivo* non clinical study is usually required for implant devices contacting circulating blood directly, to ensure that the device can fulfill its performance under the simulated-use conditions, for example, ISO 5840-2[5] (cardiac valve prostheses), ISO 7198[6] (vascular prostheses), ISO 25539-1[7] (endovascular grafts) and ISO 25539-2[8] (vascular stents). These tests may be also available for the purpose in this Clause. The requirements are provided in the international standards above. Some *in vivo* non-clinical studies according to the standards can be also found in the published literature. This information should be referenced. Some of the requirements may be omitted or modified with justification.

Information related to testing

A test device or sample is placed in its intended clinical implant configuration, such as, applying to the same or similar implant site and procedures in an appropriate animal model. The type and dosage of anticoagulant should be used with those anticipated or specified in the clinical application. Implant duration is determined considering the nature of device and the objective of evaluation.

> **Supplementary 1:** There are some animal species used commonly for *in vivo* non-clinical study of implant devices. These species have some advantages, such as anatomical similarity to humans, suitable size for the implant device, and availability of a large stock of background information. For this reason, species should be determined primarily by referring to the international standards relevant to the implant device or the species frequently found in literature.

> **Supplementary 2:** Implant duration is usually determined among short to long-term, i.e., 4 or 26 weeks. Evaluation during acute phase (a few hours to 3 days) may also provide important information.

主な観察項目と評価方法を以下に記載する.

① 試験試料留置部での顕著な狭窄や閉塞の有無

　　主に血管造影や病理組織学的検査などで十分な血流路が確保されているかを観察する.

② 試験試料から飛散した血栓による末梢血管の塞栓の有無

　　解剖学的検査や病理組織学的検査にて，末梢臓器・組織及び主要臓器に虚血による組織変化がないかを観察する. 特に，腎臓は飛散した血栓を捕えやすく虚血による変化も生じやすいことから，腎動脈より中枢側に留置や処置を施した場合には，末梢臓器の観察には腎臓を含めて評価する.

8.3.1.2　NAVI 及び AVI モデル

8.3.1 項の2）における代表的な試験方法は，ISO 10993-4 Annex C で提示されている NAVI（Non-anticoagulated venous implant）又は NAAI（Non-anticoagulated arterial implant）モデルとなる. NAVI や NAAI は，技術的な要因が試験結果に影響を与える可能性を有するが，最も血栓が形成しやすい条件で実施することで，試験試料の血栓性を明確にすることができると考えられている.

抗凝固薬が併用される医療機器については，AVI（Anticoagulated venous implant）又は AAI（Anticoagulated arterial implant）モデルも使用できる. ただし，陽性と陰性を識別できる適切な抗凝固薬の種類や量を設定することが必須である.

血管内に一時的に使用されるカテーテルやガイドワイヤに本試験法を使用することができる. これらの医療機器では，操作中や使用後に体外へ取り出す際に，医療機器表面に付着した血栓が剥がれて飛散し，末梢血管を閉塞させるリスクが考えられる. このモデルで表面に付着した血栓の程度を評価して，使用時の血栓症リスクを評価することができる.

（試験に関する情報）

2～3例の動物を用いる. 左右の血管（頚静（動）脈や大腿静（動）脈など）を用いて，対側血管に対照材料を同時に留置する. 一定時間留置後，過剰量のヘパリンを投与し，試験試料を摘出する.

付着した血栓が剥がれないように注意して，試験試料を摘出し，生理食塩液で緩やかにすすいだ後，試験試料に付着した血栓を肉眼観察する.

肉眼観察を基に，ISO 10993-4 Annex C を参考にグレードを設定する. NAVI や NAAI は，その実績から，血栓形成がない又はわずかであれば血栓性は低く，血栓形成リスクは低いと判定する. AVI や AAI での適否判定では，既に市販され安全性が確立されている医療機器との結果比較だけでなく，血栓形成がないかわずかであることも求められる. これらの試験では，抗凝固薬の用量が，血液適合性の良否を識別できる適切な条件に設定されているかを判断できるよう，陽性対照材料を設定するか，事前に背景データを確認して実施する必要がある.

The main methods and points for evaluation are as follows:

    (1)   The presence/absence of marked stenosis and occlusion at test sample implantation site.

        Observe if blood flow pathways are sufficiently maintained, mainly through angiography and histopathological examination.

    (2)   The presence/absence of downstream vessel embolism associated with a thrombus derived or detached from test sample.

        Observe if ischemia-related changes are found in any downstream organs/tissue from test sample and main organs through careful gross and microscopic examination. The kidneys in particular are prone to trap thrombi detached from a test sample and susceptible to ischemic change. For this reason, the kidneys should be included in the examinations when a test sample is implanted or treated upstream from renal arteries.

8.3.1.2 NAVI and AVI models

Non-anticoagulated venous implant (NAVI) and non-anticoagulated arterial implant (NAAI) are the representative methods employed in test strategy 2) in Clause 8.3.1. NAVI and NAAI models are presented in ISO 10993-4 Annex C. The conditions, which are most likely to induce thrombus, are provided with these models to evoke and clarify the potential thrombogenicity of test samples. On the other side, care should be taken that technical factors might also have some impacts on test results potentially due to the nature of these models.

Anticoagulated venous implant (AVI) and anticoagulated arterial implant (AAI) models are also acceptable for devices that are used with anticoagulants. However, the appropriate type and dosage of anticoagulant shall be determined to allow the test to discern between positive and negative responses.

The models are applicable to catheters and guide wires which are intended to be placed temporarily in the arterial or venous system. For these catheters and guidewires, one of the possible thrombosis risks is that some thrombi formed on the device are stripped off during the operation or removal from body and the released thrombus cause the downstream vessels to embolize. The extent of thrombus on the device surface in the models leads to the assessment of thrombosis risk in the clinical use.

Information related to testing

The test requires two to three animals. A test sample is positioned in one jugular vein (artery) or femoral vein (artery) and a control is placed in the contralateral site simultaneously. At the end of the implantation period, the animal is heparinized with excessive dosing. The samples are removed and followed by gross examination for thrombus on the sample after rinsing gently with saline. Care should be taken not to strip off thrombus on the sample during the procedures.

Determine the grade by referring to the scoring method shown in ISO 10993-4 Annex C based on the gross assessment. In NAVI and NAAl models, the sample with no or minimal is considered to have low thrombogenicity and low risk of thrombus formation or thrombosis. In AVI and AAI models, no or minimal should also be required for the assessment in addition to comparing the test sample with a marketed device with established safety. The type and dose of anticoagulant shall be justified to be able to distinguish between positive and negative responses by using an appropriate positive control or the background data collected preliminarily.

補足 1：留置時間については，使用時間を考慮して設定してよい．30 分〜 4 時間が通常使用される．4 時間以外を設定する場合は，臨床での使用時間や文献情報からその妥当性を示せる時間とする．

補足 2：操作過程で血栓が剥がれた場合は，記録に残してリスク評価に含める．また試験試料側のみでなく，血管側に血栓が残っていればこれも結果に含める．

補足 3：血栓付着状態の肉眼観察は，付着部位，血栓の大きさ（長さ，厚み），色調の記録を残しておく．肉眼観察の他，写真撮影する．

8.3.2　*In vitro* モデル

　医療機器と血液又は血液成分を *in vitro* で接触させて，それらの変化を確認することにより，血栓症リスクを評価する．医療機器局所における血栓形成リスクを評価するほか，凝固能の全身的な亢進，血小板活性化又は炎症反応により血栓が形成しやすい血液となり，微小血管など医療機器が直接影響しない部位で生じる血栓症リスク（全身的な微小血管血栓症誘発リスク）も評価する．

考慮すべき事項
1）　8.3 項の a〜g の条件を可能な限り使用環境に合わせて設定することが望ましい．
2）　使用を模擬しない条件で実施する試験については，バリデーションデータや使用実績のある製品の背景情報などを収集し，設定した試験が陽性 / 陰性を識別できる妥当な条件であることを示す．
3）　使用を模擬しない条件で実施された試験結果については，使用方法を考慮した総合的なリスク評価が必要となる場合がある．使用方法や試験条件によって，各試験項目の血栓形成への寄与度が異なるため，試験項目によっては軽微な変化が使用時の血栓症リスクを鋭敏に反映する場合もあれば，逆にほとんど影響を与えない場合もある．
4）　血液成分は，様々な環境の影響を受けて変化するため，試験に使用するまで適切な管理を行うとともに，血液は採取後速やかに試験に使用する（通常 4 時間以内）．
5）　*In vitro* 試験では，血液性状の変化が生じることや抗凝固薬が必要となるため，長期間血液と接触する医療機器や抗凝固薬を併用することなく使用される場合のある医療機器において，適切なリスク評価が行えない場合があることを考慮する．

8.3.2.1　循環モデル（体外で血液と接触する医療機器）

　使用時に合わせた条件で血液を循環して，医療機器上又は回路内の血栓塞栓リスク及び全身的な血栓症誘発リスクを評価する．対象となる医療機器としては，人工肺システム，血液透析器，血液フィルタ，血液アフェレーシス機器などがあげられる．

Supplementary 1: Implantation period may be determined considering the clinical application, normally 30 minutes to 4 hours. However, when the period except for 4 hours is determined, the rationale, such as the clinical application or literature information, should be provided.

Supplementary 2: Any stripped thrombus shall be recorded and included in the assessment when it happened during the procedures. Additionally, any thrombus on the implanted vessel shall also be included in the results in addition to those on the implanted sample.

Supplementary 3: The information on the formed thrombus should be recorded as the findings of gross examination, including the site, size (length and thickness) and color. Photographs shall be taken in addition to the findings.

8.3.2 *In vitro* tests

The tests are intended to evaluate thrombosis risk by detecting the changes of blood or its components which have been exposed to contact with a device *in vitro*. It is sometimes useful to evaluate the risk of thrombus formation which is induced locally around the device. The tests can be also used to evaluate the risk of disseminated microvascular thromboembolism. A device might have some significant impacts on blood cells or components to make them thrombus-prone. For example, they are blood with hypercoagulation, platelets activation or inflammation. Such blood has a potential risk to induce thromboembolism in small vessels away from the device.

Points to consider
1) The factors of a to g in Clause 8.3 should satisfy the application environment as much as possible.
2) For tests which do not simulate the conditions during the use of device, validation data and background information of marketed devices shall be collected to indicate validity of testing in order to distinguish between positive and negative results.
3) When testing does not simulate the conditions during the use of device, the result should be interpreted comprehensively to conduct the risk assessment, considering the actual clinical use. For some parameters, slight changes have an impact on the thrombosis risk in clinical application, while there are the others that slight changes hardly reflect the risk. This is because the contribution to thrombus formation differs in each parameter, such as coagulation, platelet activation, hematology or complement, depending on the clinical application and test conditions.
4) Blood shall be appropriately managed until testing starts and should be used promptly after collection, usually within 4 hours of blood draw, as many environmental factors alter the components and characteristics of blood.
5) *In vitro* testing will be not appropriate for some devices, such as the devices that have a blood contact for a long period or without any anticoagulants, because of the change of blood properties and need for anticoagulants in *in vitro*.

8.3.2.1 Circulation models for medical devices that have contact with blood *ex vivo*

The models are intended to evaluate the thrombosis risk, such as the risk of thromboembolisim on or inside a device or circuit system and induction of disseminated intravascular thromboembolism, by circulating blood *in vitro* under the actual application conditions. Medical devices to be tested with these models include cardiopulmonary bypass systems, hemodialysis systems, blood filters and apheresis and cell separation systems.

補足：人工肺や血液透析器などの体外循環装置では，使用時において抗凝固薬の厳密な管理や回路にアラーム機能が設けられるなど，医療機器内又は回路内における血栓症リスクが管理されている．このため，上記の医療機器において，既に使用実績のある仕様から軽微な変更をする場合は，医療機器内や回路内の血栓症の試験を必須としなくてもよい．新規性の高い医療機器については，医療機器内又は回路内で血栓症が生じるリスクを評価する．

　またこれらの医療機器は，血液との接触面積が大きいため，血球や血液成分に影響を与え，微小血管などで血栓が生じやすくなることで全身性の健康被害を引き起こす可能性がある．循環後の血球や血液成分の変化を確認することで全身的な血栓症の誘発リスクも評価することができる．またこの目的では，8.3.2.2項の静置モデルを利用することもできる．

（試験に関する情報）

　臨床使用を模擬した回路を作製して血液を循環させる．

　血液には，臨床で使用される範囲内の抗凝固薬を添加し，Activated Clotting Time（ACT）を測定して，使用時と同程度のACT条件で実施する．血流量は予定される平均的な条件又は最低流量を設定することが望ましい．医療機器内又は回路内における血栓の有無については，回路内圧の上昇や循環後の医療機器の肉眼観察によって評価する．血液凝固，血小板活性化，血液学及び補体のいずれか又は両方の評価を行うことで全身的な血栓症誘発リスクを評価してもよい．

8.3.2.2　静置モデル

　静置下で医療機器と血液を接触させて，血液凝固能，血小板活性化，白血球及び補体への影響を調べて，全身的な凝固能亢進又は血小板活性化による全身的な血栓症誘発リスクを評価する．対象となる医療機器としては，人工肺システム，血液透析器，血液フィルタ，血液アフェレーシス機器，血液バッグ及び血液投与用具などがあげられる．

（試験に関する情報）

　通常，ヒト血液を用いて，静置下で医療機器と血液又は血液成分を接触させた後，血液凝固能，血小板活性化，白血球，補体への影響を検出する．試験系の精度や感度，陽性/陰性を判定するためのバリデーションデータを取得して試験を実施する．

8.3.2.3　循環モデル（体内で血液と接触する医療機器）

　医療機器と血液又は血液成分をin vitro循環系で接触させて，血液凝固，血小板活性化，白血球の吸着・活性化，補体活性化の指標を基に，医療機器の血栓性を予測し，血栓症のリスクを評価する．対象となる医療機器としては，抗凝固薬の併用下で循環血液と短期接触する医療機器があげられる．

Supplementary: Some extracorporeal circulation devices, such as cardiopulmonary bypass systems and hemodialysis systems are controlled so that the risk of thrombosis occurring inside the device or accessory is reduced. For example, the devices are instructed to be used under rigorous anticoagulant management, and equipped with an alarm function to detect it. Accordingly, testing is not always required when a minor change is made for a well-established specification. For a novel device, the risk should be evaluated.

Moreover, these devices have a possibility of having some impacts on blood cells and components to cause systemic adverse events, because their blood contact surface area is much larger than others. When they make blood coagulate, they might cause formation of thrombus in the microvasculature. The static condition models described in Section 8.3.2.2 can also be useful for this purpose.

Information related to testing

A closed loop with blood circulation should be designed to simulate the clinical use of device.

Anticoagulant should be used within a range of the clinical dosage. The activated clotting time (ACT) should be measured to conduct the testing, using blood with an ACT similar to that of clinical use. The average or minimum flow rate is recommended as blood circulation condition. The generation of emboli inside the device or circuit system can be detected by raised pressure inside the loop and gross examination after circulation. Risk for induction of disseminated intravascular thromboembolism can be assessed by collecting data for blood coagulation, platelet activation, hematological parameters and/or complement activation simultaneously.

8.3.2.2 Static condition models

The models are intended to evaluate the risk for induction of disseminated intravascular thromboembolism associated with systemic hypercoagulation or platelet activation by the analysis of blood coagulability, platelet activation, effects on leukocytes and/or complement activation under *in vitro* static device/blood contact. Medical devices to be tested with these models include cardiopulmonary bypass systems, hemodialysis systems, blood filters, apheresis and cell separation systems, blood bags and circulatory support devices.

Information related to testing

Human blood or its components is usually used. The parameters of blood coagulability, platelet activation, effects on leukocytes and complement activation should be examined after *in vitro* device/blood contact under static conditions. The information on the validation for testing is necessary to demonstrate the precision and sensitivity of test system and detection method, and the ability to discern between positive and negative responses before testing.

8.3.2.3 Circulation models (medical devices that come into contact with blood *in vivo*)

The models are intended to evaluate the risk of (*in vivo*) thrombosis by predicting the thrombogenicity of the device based on the data from *in vitro* circulation system, such as, blood coagulability, platelet activation, leukocyte attachment and activation and complement activation. Medical devices to be tested with these models include those that temporarily come into contact with circulating blood with the concomitant use of anticoagulant.

　　補足：製造方法の変更など，軽微な変更による血栓症リスクへの影響については，変
　　　　更前の既に実績のある医療機器の結果と比較して評価する.

（試験に関する情報）
　　血栓形成には，材料表面の化学的特性の他，医療機器全体における幾何学的性状も大
きな影響を与える. このため，血液又は血液成分の流れがある循環系に試験試料を留置
する.
　　この際，血液に添加する抗凝固薬や流量，接触時間，回路材料などの条件設定は重要
である. 臨床使用時と同種の薬剤を使用し，陰性／陽性を識別することができる適切な
量を設定しなければならない. これらの条件の適切性を提示するために in vivo で血栓
性が既知の陽性対照材料を設定するか，事前に背景データにより適切性を示したうえで
試験を行わなければならない.
　　一定時間後，得られた血液又は血液成分の凝固能，血小板及び白血球の活性化などの
測定を行う. 同時に試験試料側の影響を肉眼や走査型電子顕微鏡で確認しておくと，血
液と医療機器の相互作用をより詳細に評価できる.
　　補体活性のように医療機器の形状による物理的影響ではなく，材料表面の化学的性質
によって活性化することが知られている試験項目については，8.3.2.2 項の静置モデルを
用いた試験を実施することもできる.

8.4　補体
　　現在，医療機器の補体活性化試験については，標準的な試験方法の規格はない. 以下
に示す情報を基に，試験方法のバリデーションや測定精度を確認して試験方法を設定す
ることが重要である.

8.4.1　評価方法
　　補体活性化の経路として，3 種類（古典経路，第二経路，レクチン経路）が知られて
おり，いずれの経路も C3 が C3a と C3b に分解される. さらに，C3b が C5 を C5a と
C5b に分解し，最終的に膜貫通型タンパク（C5b6789（C5b-9））が生成される. この時，
一定の割合で S プロテインが取り込まれて可溶型になった SC5b-9 が生成するため，こ
の量を測定して補体活性化程度を評価するのが一般的である. C3a を追加して，補体活
性化経路の途中の変化を調べてもよい.

8.4.2　試験系
　　種差がないことや市販の測定キットが適用可能であることから，ヒト血液が使用され
る. 精度の高い測定が可能であれば，全血，血漿，血清のいずれも選択可能である.
　　補体活性化の過程において，カルシウムやマグネシウムイオンが関与することが知ら
れている. またヘパリンは補体の活性化を抑制する可能性も知られている. このため，
ヒト全血や血漿を選択する場合には，使用する抗凝固薬を明確化し，医療機器に起因し
て生じる補体活性化を検出できることを確認して使用する. ヒト血清を使用する場合に

Supplementary: When assessing the impact on thrombosis risk after making minor changes, e.g., changes in the manufacturing method, a comparison should be made with the test results of the marketed unaltered device with a history of safe clinical use.

Information related to testing

In addition to the chemical characteristics of the material surface, the geometric properties of entire device have a significant impact on thrombus formation. For this reason, a test sample should be placed in the circulation system where blood or blood components are flowing.

The conditions such as the anticoagulant used, flow rate, duration of contact and material composing the circulation system are important to conduct testing appropriately. Appropriate dosage of the anticoagulant should be determined to discern between negative and positive response, using the same type of the drug as used during the clinical application. The suitability should be justified to conduct testing by using some relevant background data or a positive control material whose *in vivo* thrombotic properties has been clarified.

After a certain period of device/blood contact, the parameters, such as blood coagulation, platelet activation and leukocyte activation, should be examined. Simultaneous gross examination and SEM of the sample can provide more detailed information on the device/blood interactions.

The static model described in Clause 8.3.2.2 is also available for test categories such as complement activation, which is known to activate in association with the chemical nature on the material surface rather than the shape or the physical properties of material.

8.4   Complement system

There are no established standards which contain a test method for complement activation associated with medical devices. It is important, therefore, to determine a test method following validation of the procedures and confirmation of measurement precision based on the following information.

8.4.1   Tests

Three pathways activate complement system: classical pathway, alternative pathway and lectin pathway. These activation pathways all generate C3a and C3b by breaking C3, and the C3b degrades C5 to produce C5a and C5b, which eventually leads to the production of transmembrane protein (C5b6789 [C5b–9]). During this process, a certain percentage of S protein is taken up to generate SC5b–9, which changes to a soluble form. The amount of the SC5b–9 is commonly measured to evaluate the level of complement activation for medical devices. It is also acceptable to add the measurement of C3a, to trace the changes during the complement activation pathway process.

8.4.2   Test systems

Human blood shall be used for testing, because there are no species differences and commercial test kits are available. Any of the whole blood, plasma and serum can be used if precision measurement is ensured.

It is known that calcium and magnesium ions are involved in the complement activation process. The other anticoagulants, heparin may also suppress complement activation. Accordingly, the anticoagulant used shall be clarified. In addition, the ability to detect device-induced complement activation shall be validated. The factors other than the test material might enhance complement activity when human serum is used. The test results should

も，試験試料以外の要因で補体活性が上昇することもある．いずれの試験系を用いる場合も，陰性対照や陽性対照，使用実績のある医療機器及び背景情報も踏まえたうえで試験結果を考察するのが望ましい．

8.4.3 接触形態

医療機器の形状による物理的影響ではなく，材料表面の化学的性質によって補体活性化が引き起こされると考えられている．したがって，必ずしも血流は必須でない．*In vitro* 静置下で，血液と医療機器を接触させて試験を実施することができる．

8.4.4 接触面積

補体を活性化させる材料においては，接触面積が大きくなるほど補体活性化産物が増加する．試験系との接触比率は，臨床を模擬することが望ましいが，困難な場合は可能な限り接触比率を高くするよう配慮する．ISO 10993-12 の接触条件を基に設定してもよい．

8.4.5 接触時間

補体の活性化は，医療機器と血液の接触初期で生じる．また時間とともに，補体をはじめとした血液成分の変性や活性化が進行することにより，バックグラウンドが高くなり医療機器に起因した補体活性化が高精度に検出できなくなる可能性がある．このため，接触時間を臨床にあわせて長くする必要はない．通常，30～90 分の間で設定される．

8.4.6 対照材料

試験には，必ず陰性対照及び陽性対照を設定して試験系の感度を明確にする．また無処置対照を設けてバックグラウンドを明確にする．

陰性対照材料にはポリプロピレンなど，陽性対照材料には Latex やアセチルセルロースなど，陽性対照物質としてはコブラ毒素が使用されている．

8.4.7 評価

試験試料における補体活性化の程度が無処置対照や陰性対照材料と同等又はそれ以下の場合，補体活性はないと判断される．一方で，無処置対照や陰性対照材料を上回る場合でも，生物学的には影響を与えないことがある．その影響を考察するため，同じ用途で臨床実績のある医療機器を同時に試験して結果を比較してもよい．

8.5 その他の情報

平成 26-28 年度医療研究開発推進事業費補助金 / 創薬基盤推進研究事業「医薬品・医療機器の実用化促進のための評価技術手法の戦略的開発」の分担課題「プラスチック製医療機器の化学物質影響評価法 2 種の開発」において，国内溶血性試験の代替法として開発された簡易溶血性試験法[9]は ASTM 及び NIH 法と同等以上の感度を有しており，

be interpreted in light of the negative and positive control results, history of marketed devices and background information in any test systems.

8.4.3　Form of contact

It is considered that complement activation is induced by the chemical nature of material surface, rather than by the shape or the physical properties of the device. Therefore, blood circulation is not requirement for testing, and this test can be designed to expose a device to contact blood under *in vitro* static conditions.

8.4.4　Blood-contacting surface area

For complement activating material, the amount of complement activation products increase with the area of the materials. The device surface area-to-test system, blood, serum or plasma, volume ratio should be specified according to that of the clinical situation. In case of any difficulty, the ratio should be made as high as possible. It is acceptable to use the conditions of contact described in ISO 10993-12 as the basis.

8.4.5　Duration of contact

Complement activation occurs in the early stage shortly after blood contacts the device. In addition, the degeneration and activation of complements and other blood components are progressive. These might interfere with highly precise detection of device-induced complement activation such as due to increased background noise. For this reason, it is not necessary to extend the duration of contact to that of the clinical use. It is usually from 30 to 90 minutes.

8.4.6　Control materials

A negative and positive controls shall be employed to clarify the sensitivity of test system. An untreated control shall be also used to demonstrate the background. An example of materials and substances used for the controls is following:

　　Negative control material: polypropylene, etc.
　　Positive control materials: latex, acetyl cellulose, etc.
　　Positive control substances: cobra venom, etc.

8.4.7　Evaluation

For general data interpretation, the test sample is not considered to have activated complement system in blood when the level of complement activation (products) is equivalent to or lower than that of the untreated control or negative material control. Even if the complement activation level exceeds that of the untreated control or negative control material, it might have little biological impact in some cases. In order to assess the impact, it is useful to make a comparison by simultaneously testing a clinically well-established device used for the same purpose.

8.5　Other information

The simple hemolysis testing method[9] was invented as an alternative to the previous domestic hemolysis testing method when the task "Development of new methods for evaluating the safety of plastic medical devices" was assigned in relation to the 2014-2016 Medical R&D Promotion Grant/Research on Development of New Drugs "Strategic development of evaluation methods for accelerating novel pharmaceuticals and medical de-

国内 9 機関が参画したラウンドロビンテストにより再現性・頑健性が検証されている. 家兎の飼育, Drabkin's 試薬の使用が不要であり, 小スケールで試験を実施できるため, 材料開発などにおける一次スクリーニング法として利用できる.

　平成 27 - 29 年度医療研究開発推進事業費補助金 / 医薬品等規制調査・評価研究事業「革新的医療機器で用いられる医療材料の生体への安全性等の評価方法等に関する研究」の分担課題「材料表面吸着蛋白質を指標とした血栓性評価法の開発に関する研究」では, ビトロネクチン（VTNC）を 1 次マーカー, C3a 及び C1s を 2 次マーカーとして材料表面への吸着挙動を総合的に評価することにより, 高分子材料の血液適合性を判断する方法が検討されている[10]. 各マーカーの再現性・頑健性は国内ラウンドロビンテストにより検証されているが, 本項で示す医療機器の血液適合性のリスク評価としての有用性は検証されていない.

8.6　その他の留意事項

　本項に掲載されている各種試験は, 生物学的安全性評価のみでなく, その他の目的にも実施できる. 生物学的安全性評価を目的とした試験は GLP に準拠した実施が求められる. ただし,「医療機器の生物学的安全性評価の基本的考え方」の 8 項に記載されているとおり, 性能確認試験など, その他の目的で実施する場合は, 必ずしも GLP 準拠が求められるものではないことに留意する必要がある.

9．薬食機発 0301 第 20 号からの変更点

　ISO 10993-4 が改訂され新たな内容が加わったこと及び実用的にすることを目的に, 全内容について見直した. 主な変更点を以下の 3 項に分けて記載する.

9.1　血液適合性試験法に関する情報の追加や整理

　循環血液と直接接触する医療機器では, 直接的に血液と接触させて相互作用を評価することが原則であり, 試験法は使用環境を考慮して選択されなければならない. 使用環境や接触形態は医療機器により様々であるため, 抽出液を用いた試験とは異なり, 一つの試験デザインで全ての医療機器の血液適合性評価を網羅できる試験はほとんどない. 一方で, 医療機器又は研究機関ごとに適切な試験法が工夫して開発されてきた経緯があり, 医療機器又は血液適合性の評価内容ごとに適切と考えられる試験法は数多く存在する.

　本項では全ての試験法を提示することができないため, 血液適合性の定義（1 項）, 試験目的を明確化又は試験方法の特徴を参考情報などで提示し, 適切な試験方法を設計・選択できるよう配慮している. また注記や補足事項を追加して試験方法に関して参考となる情報を提供している.

vices". The simple method has an equivalent or increased sensitivity compared to the ASTM or NIH methods, and its reproducibility and robustness have been verified by the Round Robin Study participated in by nine domestic institutions. It does not require rabbit housing or Drabkin's reagent, and small-scale testing is possible. For these reasons, the simple method might be useful for primary screening in material development and the like. The 2015-2017 Medical R&D Promotion Grant/Research on Regulatory Science of Pharmaceuticals and Medical Devices, "Study on the safety evaluation methods of medical materials for medical devices with innovative technology" had a task assignment called "Development of the hemocompatibility evaluation method based on behavior of protein adsorption on the surface of medical materials". A method that uses vitronectin (VTNC) as the primary marker and C3a and C1s as the secondary markers is introduced in the task, in which hemocompatibility of polymer materials is determined by comprehensive evaluation of attachment behavior over the material surface[10]. Although reproducibility and robustness of each marker have been verified by the Japanese Round Robin Study, usefulness for hemocompatibility risk assessment has not been verified for the devices mentioned in this Section.

8.6   Other points to note

Biocompatibility testing shall be conducted in compliance with GLP. On the other hand, some of the tests described in this Section are also performed for the purposes other than biological safety evaluation in this guidance. The users should keep in mind that when testing, such as *in vivo* performance study, is conducted with the objective beside biological evaluation, GLP compliance is not always required for it, as described in Clause 8 of "Basic Principles for Evaluating Biological Safety of Medical Device".

9.   Points changed from MHLW Notification, YAKUSHOKUKI-HATSU 0301 No. 20

The overall contents in the previous document were reviewed and revised in this section to make this document more practical and to reflect the information from the revised ISO 10993-4. The main changes are described separately in the following three sections.

9.1   Addition and reconstruction of information related to hemocompatibility tests

In principle, testing is conducted in a way to expose a device to contact with blood to evaluate device/blood interactions, for devices that contact circulating blood directly. A test method should be determined considering the clinical use environment. However, there is a variety of applications for medical devices, and there are various types of blood contact. Therefore, there are few comprehensive test methods that can be applied to most of all medical devices for the evaluation of hemocompatibility, unlike the extracts contact method. On the other side, some tests have been explored and developed historically in each research and development institute to evaluate the hemocompatibility, in association with the cultivation and exploitation of medical device. As a result, there is a variety of appropriate tests for each medical device and purpose. Since it is not possible to present all the test methods, this Section provides the definition of hemocompatibility at Clause 1 and, then the information on the purpose and characteristics of each test as possible as clearly to design and determine an appropriate test. Other useful information on test methods is also presented in the form of note and supplementary.

9.2　ISO 10993-4 の改訂に伴う変更

　試験項目を適切に選択できるように 8.1 項に ISO 10993-4 Table 1 を抜粋して収載した．同表では，機械的因子起因の溶血の試験項目が明記されたことから，8.2.2 項に必要な情報を記載した．

　また ISO 10993-4 では，一般的な評価方法が記載された．これと一致させるため，4 項の評価項目を変更した．

9.3　溶血性試験法の記載変更

（1）　ASTM 法の採用について

　本項では，ASTM 法を採用した．これは，多施設で試験法を検証した結果，ASTM 法の抽出液法で強い溶血性が認められたニトリルグローブについて，従来の国内試験法では，溶血率が低く，施設によっては陰性となる場合があったためである．なお，その他検討された試験試料の溶血率は，ASTM 法の抽出液法と同程度の結果であった．本項では，従来の国内試験法を標準的な評価方法から削除したが，これまで医療機器のリスク評価に使用されてきた実績もあり，一概にリスク評価に使用できないことを示すものではない．

（2）　抽出液法と直接接触法について

　材料起因の溶血については，循環血液と直接接触する医療機器においては，直接接触法と抽出液法の双方を実施することを記載した．ISO 10993-4 では，直接接触法と抽出液法の実施についてまで言及されていないが，材料の溶血特性は抽出液のみでなく，材料表面との直接接触の両面から評価されるのが一般的となっている．

引用規格

1）　ASTM F756-17, Standard Practice for Assessment of Hemolytic Properties of Materials

参考文献又は国際規格

2）　NIH. Evaluation of hemodialyzers and dialysis membranes. Report of a study group for the Artificial Kidney-Chronic Uremia Program NIAMDD-1977. Chapter two. *In vitro* characterization of hemodialyzers. Artifi. Organs. 1977, 1（2）pp.59-77.

3）　N.M.M. Moharram, R.EI Aouad, S. AI Busaidy, A. Fabricius, S. Heller, W.G. Wood, H.U. Wolf and C.C. Heuck. International collaborative assessment study of the AHD_{575} method for the measurement of blood haemoglobin. Eastern Mediterranean Health Journal, Vol. 12, No. 6, 2006.

4）　ISO 7199, Cardiovascular implants and artificial organs-Blood-gas exchangers（oxygenators）

5）　ISO 5840-2, Cardiovascular implants-Cardiac valve prostheses-Part 2; Surgically implanted heart valve substitutes

6）　ISO 7198, Cardiovascular implants and extracorporeal systems-Vascular prostheses-Tubular vascular grafts and vascular patches.

7）　ISO 25539-1, Cardiovascular implants-Part 1: Endovascular devices-Endovascular prostheses

9.2　Changes associated with the revised ISO 10993-4

Table 1 of ISO 10993-4 is presented in Section 8.1 to help determine the appropriate test categories. In the table, the test category of mechanically-induced hemolysis have been clarified. Accordingly, the information is described in Clause 8.2.2. In addition, "Tests" in Clause 4 have been modified to make them harmonize with "the common tests to assess interaction with blood" in ISO 10993-4.

9.3　Changes in the descriptions of material-induced hemolysis testing

(1)　Change to ASTM standards

ASTM standards have been adopted in this Section as material-induced hemolysis testing based on the results in the international multi-center verification test (round robin test). In the test, nitrile gloves showed strong hemolytic in extracts contact method of ASTM standard, but non-hemolytic or mild in the previous domestic method (MHLW method) of some laboratories, though there was no significant difference in the percent hemolysis of other test materials between the MHLW and ASTM extracts contact methods. The MHLW method has not been presented on the list of common tests in this Section. However, it has long been used for the risk assessment of medical devices, and the omission does not mean that it is unusable for any risk assessments.

(2)　Extraction and direct contact methods

This Section demonstrates that both direct contact and extraction methods should be performed to evaluate the material-induced hemolysis risk for the devices that come into direct contact with circulating blood. ISO 10993-4 does not mention it clearly. However, it is common to assess the hemolytic properties of materials in view of not only extracts contact but also direct contact with the material surface.

Normative reference

1)　ASTM F756-17, Standard Practice for Assessment of Hemolytic Properties of Materials

References or international standards

2)　NIH. Evaluation of hemodialyzers and dialysis membranes. Report of a study group for the Artificial Kidney-Chronic Uremia Program NIAMDD-1977. Chapter two. *In vitro* characterization of hemodialyzers. Artifi. Organs. 1977, 1 (2) pp.59-77.

3)　N.M.M. Moharram, R.EI Aouad, S. Al Busaidy, A. Fabricius, S. Heller, W.G. Wood, H.U. Wolf and C.C. Heuck. International collaborative assessment study of the AHD_{575} method for the measurement of blood haemoglobin. Eastern Mediterranean Health Journal, Vol. 12, No. 6, 2006.

4)　ISO 7199, Cardiovascular implants and artificial organs-Blood-gas exchangers (oxygenators)

5)　ISO 5840-2, Cardiovascular implants-Cardiac valve prostheses-Part 2; Surgically implanted heart valve substitutes

6)　ISO 7198, Cardiovascular implants and extracorporeal systems-Vascular prostheses-Tubular vascular grafts and vascular patches.

7)　ISO 25539-1, Cardiovascular implants-Part 1: Endovascular devices-Endovascular prostheses

8)　ISO 25539-2, Cardiovascular implants-Part 2: Endovascular devices-Vascular stents

9)　Haishima Y, Hasegawa C, Nomura Y, Kawakami T, Yuba T, Shindo T, Sakaguchi K, Tanigawa T, Inukai K, Takenouchi M, Isama K, Matsuoka A, Niimi S. Development and per-

8)　ISO 25539-2, Cardiovascular implants-Part 2: Endovascular devices-Vascular stents

9)　Haishima Y, Hasegawa C, Nomura Y, Kawakami T, Yuba T, Shindo T, Sakaguchi K, Tanigawa T, Inukai K, Takenouchi M, Isama K, Matsuoka A, Niimi S. Development and performance evaluation of a positive reference material for hemolysis testing. J. Biomed. Mater. Res. Part B. 102: 1809-1816 (2014).

10)　植松美幸，宮島敦子，野村祐介，蓜島由二，伊佐間和郎，岩﨑清隆，梅津光生. 血液適合性評価法の開発.「医療用バイオマテリアルの研究開発」，シーエムシー出版, 東京，2017，p.26-40.

formance evaluation of a positive reference material for hemolysis testing. J. Biomed. Mater. Res. Part B. 102: 1809–1816 (2014).

10)　Uematsu M, Miyajima A, Nomura Y, Haishima Y, Isama K, Iwasaki K, Umezu M.: Development of hemocompatibility assay. Research and development of biomaterials for medical applications. CMC Publishing CO., LTD., 26–40, Tokyo (2017)

付録

医療機器又は原材料からの抽出液の調製における
試験試料／抽出溶媒比及び抽出温度・時間

1．試験試料／抽出溶媒比

試験試料の形状又は厚さにより，以下に示した試料／溶媒比を用いる．

厚さ（mm）	抽出溶媒 1 mL に対する試験試料の量（許容範囲±10 %）	試験試料の形状の例
＜0.5	6 cm^2	フィルム，シート，チューブ
0.5～1.0	3 cm^2	チューブ，平板，小型の成型物
＞1.0	3 cm^2	大型の成型物
＞1.0	1.25 cm^2	ゴム栓などの弾性材料
不規則な形状の硬質材料*	0.2 g	粉末，ペレット，フォーム状，非吸収性成型物
不規則な形状の多孔性材料*（低密度材料）	0.1 g	メンブランフィルター，繊維製品

*表面積の算出が困難な材料を用いる場合
備考：吸収性材料やハイドロコロイドに適用可能な手順を参考として以下に示す．0.1 g あるいは 1 cm^2 当たりの材料が吸収する抽出溶媒量を求める．抽出を行う際，0.1 g あるいは 1 cm^2 当たりの抽出溶媒量に，先に求めた溶媒量を加える．

2．抽出温度・時間

(1)　121±2℃　　1±0.1 時間
(2)　70±2℃　　24±2 時間
(3)　50±2℃　　72±2 時間
(4)　37±1℃　　72±2 時間

上記条件のうち，試験試料が耐えられる条件を選択する．試験試料が耐えられる条件とは，以下を満たすものである．

1)　抽出温度は材料の融点より低い．
2)　抽出条件で材料が著しく変形しない．
3)　溶出物質が揮発あるいは分解しない．

(1)以外の条件で抽出液を調製する際には，原則，撹拌・循環抽出を行うものとし，抽出完了後，遠心分離，フィルター濾過など，得られた抽出液に影響を与え得る追加処理は行わない．ただし，抽出温度が高い場合には，抽出液を試験に使用できる温度にすることが必要になるため，抽出液中に析出物などが生じないことが確認できる条件下に限り，冷却処理を認めるものとする．また必要に応じて，抽出液の色調変化などを確認・記載すること．なお，各々の試験法において，抽出条件が定められている場合にはその

Appendix

Proportion of test sample and extraction vehicles, and extraction conditions in the preparation of extract solutions from a medical device or their materials

1. Proportion of the test sample and extraction vehicles

The following proportions of the test sample and vehicles should be used depending on the shape or thickness of the test sample.

Thickness (mm)	Surface area or amount of the test sample to each mL of the extraction vehicle (acceptable range ± 10 %)	Example of the shape of the test sample
<0.5	6 cm^2	Film, sheet, tube
0.5~1.0	3 cm^2	Tube, plate, small molding
>1.0	3 cm^2	Large molding
>1.0	1.25 cm^2	Elastic material such as rubber stopper
Hard material in irregular shape*	0.2 g	Powder, pellet, foam, non-absorbable molding
Porous material in irregular shape* (low density material)	0.1 g	Membrane filter, fiber product

*In the case where a surface area of the material is difficult to calculate
Note: The extracting procedure applicable to absorbable materials and hydrocolloids is shown below as a reference. After determine a volume of extraction solvent that 0.1 g or 1 cm^2 of material absorbs, add this volume of solvent to the designated volume of extraction solvent as shown in the above table.

2. Extraction condition (temperature and time)

(1) 121 ± 2 ℃   1 ± 0.1 hours
(2) 70 ± 2 ℃   24 ± 2 hours
(3) 50 ± 2 ℃   72 ± 2 hours
(4) 37 ± 1 ℃   72 ± 2 hours

From the above conditions, an appropriate condition that does not cause significant deterioration of the test sample should be selected. The condition that does not cause significant deterioration of the test sample should satisfy the followings.

1) The extraction temperature is lower than the melting point of the test sample.
2) Under the extracting condition, test samples are not remarkably deformed.
3) The extracted substances from the test sample are not volatilized or degraded.

In principle, extraction should be performed with agitation or circulation of vehicles unless an extract is prepared by the above condition (1). Once extraction is complete, further processing that may cause effects on the extract, e.g., centrifugation, filtration, and so on, should not be performed. When choosing high temperature for the extraction condition, however, it is necessary to adjust the temperature of the extract to enable necessary tests. Therefore, cooling procedures are permitted only if it doesn't cause any changes, e.g., generating precipitates, etc., in the extract. If necessary, visible changes of the extract such as a change of its color should be checked and documented. If extraction conditions are de-

方法に従って抽出液を調製すること.

3．保存温度・時間

　過度な冷却及び冷却保存においても析出物などが生じる可能性があるため，通常，抽出液は 25℃前後で保存し，24 時間以内に使用する．なお，個別の試験方法において，具体的な保存条件が記載されている場合は，その条件に従うこと．

4．有機溶媒抽出の基本的考え方

　ISO 10993-12: 2012 の Annex D には，リスクアセスメントの一環としてのハザード特定を目的に，高分子材料を対象にした過酷な条件下での抽出方法が例示されている．高分子材料においてハザードとなりうる各種低分子物質の分析を目的とした抽出には有機溶媒が用いられていることを考慮して，Annex D では様々な極性，あるいは非極性有機溶媒の使用が推奨されている．またこれらにより得られた抽出物を用いることが適切と考えられる試験として，遺伝毒性試験，感作性試験が挙げられていることなどに鑑み，本ガイダンスでは，これらの試験において，原則，有機溶媒抽出による試験試料調製を求めている．

fined for each test method described in the main contents, the extract should be prepared according to the conditions.

3. Storage temperature and time

Extracts should generally be stored at around 25 ℃ and be used in a test within 24 hours from extraction, as their excessive cooling and/or storage in a cool temperature may generate precipitates. If specific storage conditions are defined for individual test methods, the conditions should be used.

4. Basic concepts of extraction with organic solvents

In Annex D of ISO 10993-12: 2012, exhaustive extraction method of polymeric materials is described to identify hazards as part of risk assessment. In Annex D, it is recommended to select an appropriate solvent from various polar or nonpolar organic solvents for the exhaustive extraction, since organic solvents are usually utilized with reasonable consideration to extract various substances with low-molecular weight that could be hazardous in polymeric material, followed by their chemical characterization. Additionally, this guidance requires preparation of test samples for genotoxicity and sensitization tests by extraction utilizing organic solvents in principle, since it is suggested that the use of extract obtained by the exhaustive extraction may be appropriate.

和英対訳　医療機器の製造販売承認申請等に必要な生物学的安全性
評価の基本的考え方について　第 2 版

2021 年 4 月 25 日　　第 1 刷発行

翻訳：　ISO/TC 194 国内委員会（編集責任者：委員長　蓜島由二）

発行：　株式会社薬事日報社
　　　　〒101-8648　東京都千代田区神田和泉町 1 番地
　　　　電話 03-3862-2141　https://www.yakuji.co.jp/

印刷：　昭和情報プロセス株式会社

表紙デザイン：Atelier Z　たかはし文雄